Length					Weight			
in	cm	cm	in		lb	kg	kg	lb
1	2.54	1	0.4		1	0.5	1	2.2
2	5.08	2	0.8		2	0.9	2	4.4
4	10.16	3	1.2		4	1.8	3	6.6
6	15.24	4	1.6		6	2.7	4	8.8
8	20.32	5	2.0		8	3.6	5	11.0
10	25.40	6	2.4		10	4.5	6	13.2
20	50.80	8	3.1		20	9.1	8	17.6
30	76.20	10	3.9		30	13.6	10	22
40	101.60	20	7.9		40	18.2	20	44
50	127.00	30	11.8		50	22.7	30	66
60	152.40	40	15.7		60	27.3	40	88
70	177.80	50	19.7		70	31.8	50	110
80	203.20	60	23.6		80	36.4	60	132
90	228.60	70	27.6		90	40.9	70	154
100	254.00	80	31.5		100	45.4	80	176
150	381.00	90	35.4		150	66.2	90	198
200	508.00	100	39.4		200	90.8	100	220

1 in = 2.54 cm
1 cm = 0.3937 in

1 lb = 0.454 kg
1 kg = 2.204 lb

From Seidel HM et al: *Mosby's guide to physical examination*, ed 4, St. Louis, 1998, Mosby.

Temperature Equivalents			
Celsius*	Fahrenheit†	Celsius*	Fahrenheit†
34.0	93.2	38.6	101.4
34.2	93.6	38.8	101.8
34.4	93.9	39.0	102.2
34.6	94.3	39.2	102.5
34.8	94.6	39.4	102.9
35.0	95.0	39.6	103.2
35.2	95.4	39.8	103.6
35.4	95.7	40.0	104.0
35.6	96.1	40.2	104.3
35.8	96.4	40.4	104.7
36.0	96.8	40.6	105.1
36.2	97.1	40.8	105.4
36.4	97.5	41.0	105.8
36.6	97.8	41.2	106.1
36.8	98.2	41.4	106.5
37.0	98.6	41.6	106.8
37.2	98.9	41.8	107.2
37.4	99.3	42.0	107.6
37.6	99.6	42.2	108.0
37.8	100.0	42.4	108.3
38.0	100.4	42.6	108.7
38.2	100.7	42.8	109.0
38.4	101.1	43.0	109.4

*To convert Celsius to Fahrenheit: $(9/5 \times \text{Temperature}) + 32$.
†To convert Fahrenheit to Celsius: $5/9 \times (\text{Temperature} - 32)$.

From Hoekelman RA et al: *Primary pediatric care* ed 3, St. Louis, 1997, Mosby.

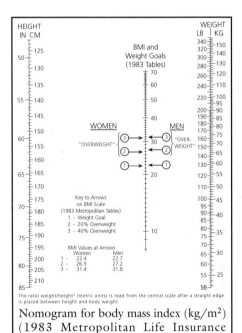

Nomogram for body mass index (kg/m²) (1983 Metropolitan Life Insurance Company tables.) Weights and heights are without clothing. With clothes, add 5 lb (2.3 kg) for men or 3 lb for women and 1 in. (2.5 cm) in height for shoes.

From Burton BT, Foster WR: *Health implications of obesity: an NIH concensus development conference*, J Am Diet Assoc 85(9):1117-1121, 1985.

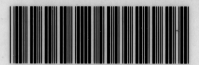

Advanced Health Assessment and Clinical Diagnosis in

Joyce E. Dains, DrPH, JD, RN, CS, FNP
Assistant Professor
Department of Family and Community Medicine
Baylor College of Medicine
Houston, Texas

Linda Ciofu Baumann, PhD, RN, CS-ANP, FAAN
Associate Professor and Nurse Practitioner
School of Nursing
University of Wisconsin—Madison
Madison, Wisconsin

Pamela Scheibel, MSN, RN, CPNP
Clinical Associate Professor
School of Nursing
University of Wisconsin—Madison
Madison, Wisconsin

Mosby

St. Louis Baltimore Boston Carlsbad
Chicago Minneapolis New Yo
London Milan Sydney Tokyo

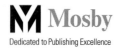

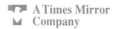

Publisher: Sally Schrefer
Developmental Editor: Rae L. Robertson
Project Manager: John Rogers
Project Editor: Helen Hudlin
Manufacturing Manager: Don Carlisle
Designer: Yael Kats
Cover Design: Liz Young

ACCESSION NO: KH01253
SHELFMARK: 616.075/DAI
1 1364 7453

A NOTE TO THE READER:
The author and publisher have made every attempt to check dosages and content for accuracy. Because the science of pharmacology is continually advancing, our knowledge base continues to expand. Therefore we recommend that the reader always check product information for changes in dosage or administration before administering any medication. This is particularly important with new or rarely used drugs.

Copyright © 1998 by Mosby, Inc.

Printed in the United States of America
Composition by the Clarinda Company
Illustration by the Clarinda Company
Printing/binding by R.R. Donnelley & Sons Company

Mosby, Inc.
11830 Westline Industrial Drive
St. Louis, Missouri 63146

Library of Congress Cataloging-in-Publication Data
Dains, Joyce E.
    Advanced health assessment and clinical diagnosis in primary care
    Joyce E. Dains, Linda Ciofu Baumann, Pamela Scheibel.
        p.   cm.
    Includes bibliographical references and index.
    ISBN 0-8151-3627-7
    1. Diagnosis, Differential.   2. Medical logic.   3. Medical history
taking.   4. Physical diagnosis.   I. Baumann, Linda Ciofu.
II. Scheibel, Pamela.   III. Title.
    [DNLM: 1. Diagnosis, Differential.   2. Diagnostic Techniques and
Procedures.   3. Primary Health Care.   WB 141.5 D133a 1998]
    RC71.5.D35   1998
    616.07′5—dc21
    DNLM/DLC
    for Library of Congress   98-14984
                                                        CIP

98 99 00 01 02 / 9 8 7 6 5 4 3 2 1

Chapter 3

Katharine E. Hohol, MS, RN, APNP-C
Adult Nurse Practitioner
Department of Dermatology
Dean Medical Center
Madison, Wisconsin

Gail A. Viergutz, MS, RN, ANP-C
Clinical Instructor
School of Nursing
University of Wisconsin—Madison
Madison, Wisconsin

Primary Care Nurse Practitioner
Emergency Department/Urgent Care
St. Michael's Hospital
Stevens Point, Wisconsin

Chapter 4

Sandra K. Roof, MSN, RN, CS-ANP
Clinical Associate Professor
School of Nursing
University of Wisconsin—Madison
Madison, Wisconsin

Adult Nurse Practitioner
Physician Plus
Waterloo, Wisconsin

Chapter 6 (Genitourinary Problems in Males; Penile Discharge)

Robert W. Vogler, DSN, RN, CS, FNP
Associate Professor
School of Nursing
University of Texas—Houston
Houston, Texas

Chapters 6 (Urinary Problems in Females and Children), 7, 8

Pam Willson, MSN, RN, CS, FNP
Family Nurse Practitioner Program
College of Nursing
Texas Women's University
Houston, Texas

Patricia Alpert, MSN, MPH, RN-C, PNP
Instructor
Department of Nursing
University of Nevada—Las Vegas
Las Vegas, Nevada

Patricia M. Campbell, MSN, RN, CCRN, ANP, CS
Adult Nurse Practitioner
Emergency Professional Services, Inc.
Good Samaritan Regional Medical Center/Emergency Center
Phoenix, Arizona

Christy L. Crowther, RN, MS, CRNP, CCRN
Nurse Practitioner
Chesapeake Orthopaedic & Sports Medicine Center
Glen Burnie, Maryland

Patricia M. Dieter, PA-C, MPA
Associate Program Director
Physician Assistant Program
Assistant Clinical Professor
Department of Community and Family Medicine
Duke University Medical Center
Durham, North Carolina

Theresa N. Grabo, PhD, CRNP
Associate Professor and Family Nurse Practitioner
Decker School of Nursing
Binghamton University
Binghamton, New York

Brenda Walters Holloway, MSN, RNC, FNP
Clinical Assistant Professor
University of South Alabama
Mobile, Alabama

Ruth M. Kleinpell, PhD, RN, CCRN
Associate Professor
Rush University College of Nursing
Chicago, Illinois

This text is designed for beginning advanced practice clinicians and/or students who will be using history and physical examination skills in the clinical setting. Its purpose is to take the student to the "next step" of health assessment, i.e., beyond basic history and physical examination to using a diagnostic reasoning process. The book is intended to fill the gap between basic physical examination texts and the medical texts that are aimed primarily at disease and disorder management. It is not intended as a substitute for a clinical medicine management text nor does it address management of disorders or diseases. Rather, it is designed specifically to focus on the clinical evaluation of common problems that present in primary care settings, using the tools of history and physical examination to engage in the process of clinical diagnosis.

Each chapter is structured in the context of commonly occurring chief complaints rather than being based on a specific diagnosis or disease entity. These presenting problems are clustered by body system or area for convenience. Patients generally seek care for relief of symptoms and undiagnosed conditions. The initial challenge for primary care providers is to begin the process of differential diagnosis to determine the cause of a disorder, based on history and physical examination and laboratory and other diagnostic tests. However, the steps of the diagnostic reasoning process are seldom articulated in a sequence that reflects the clinician's thought process. Novice clinicians are often left to their own devices, to figure out, for example, which history questions are the most important, which should be asked first and which can be left for later, or to figure out which parts of the physical examination *must* be done as opposed to which will yield little information for a given complaint. This text tries to articulate the reasoning process, order the history questions in a meaningful way, and focus the physical examination for a specific chief complaint.

The diagnostic or clinical reasoning process is woven into each presenting problem. Each symptom begins with a brief introduction, providing the practitioner an overview of causative mechanisms and processes.

The clinical problem-solving process begins with **Diagnostic Reasoning: Focused History,** which walks the practitioner through the thinking process involved in getting a pertinent, relevant, problem-specific history that will assist with differential diagnosis. The section is designed around questions experienced clinicians ask themselves to order and organize the questions to be asked of the patient. These "self-questions" are structured according to what information the clinician needs first or most immediately about the presenting complaint, followed by self-questions that help sort through the possible differential diagnoses. The content and order of the self-questions vary, depending on the presenting problem. Sometimes the self-questions are based on what the condition is most likely to be; sometimes they are based on what is too important to miss.

For each of the self-questions there is a list of **Key Questions** to ask the patient or about the patient if a family member is giving the history. The key questions are followed by an interpretation or explanation of what the patient responses might signify. For ease of format, the key questions are written as though the clinician were addressing the patient. Certainly with young children and sometimes with adults, the clinician will be asking questions of another person about the patient. The intent is to convey *what* questions to ask, rather than to provide every possible format for each question.

Following these two sections is the **Diagnostic Reasoning: Focused Physical Examination** section. It instructs the practitioner in what focused physical examination to perform to assist in the diagnostic process. The section is *not* intended to teach basic physical examination; it assumes the practitioner knows how, using the techniques of inspection, auscultation, percussion, and palpation. This section, rather, provides focus for the examination, explains how to do additional or more advanced maneuvers, and offers an interpretation of the findings.

Following is the section entitled **Laboratory and Diagnostic Studies.** This section provides a brief outline of what kinds of laboratory or diagnostic studies would be appropriate for the chief complaint or suspected diagnosis. Because the goal of the text is clinical diagnosis, the laboratory and diagnostic studies included are those that would be a logical starting point, although perhaps not an ending point.

The final section of each presenting complaint is the **Differential Diagnosis.** It contains the most common differential diagnoses for the chief complaint and summarizes, in a narrative format, the history and physical examination findings, along with the laboratory and diagnostic studies indicated. The section finishes with table(s) of **Differential Diagnosis,** mirroring the narrative summary, which can be used as a quick reference.

The patient focus of *Advanced Health Assessment* is primary care patients. Both adults and children are included, with divergence in questions, examination, or interpretation of findings noted where pertinent. Management of health care problems is intentionally *not* included. Also, no attempt is made to address all possible patient complaints but rather to seek to focus on the most common chief complaints as exemplars of the diagnostic reasoning process.

Joyce E. Dains
Linda C. Baumann
Pamela Scheibel

Contents

Chapter 1

Clinical Reasoning and Differential Diagnosis

Basic health assessment involves the application of the practitioner's knowledge and skills to identify and distinguish normal from abnormal findings. Basic assessment often moves from a general survey of a body system to specific observations or tests of function. Such an approach to assessment and clinical decision making uses a deductive process of reasoning. For example, a specialist, when examining a patient with known hyperthyroidism, would conduct a physical examination to test for deep tendon reflexes. Brisk or hyperreflexic findings would lead the practitioner to conclude that a hyperthyroid state is a likely cause for these findings. This would greatly narrow the choices of diagnostic tests to perform and alternations in treatment to make.

Advanced assessment builds on basic health assessment yet is performed more often using an inductive or inferential process, that is, moving from a specific physical finding or patient complaint to a more general diagnosis or possible diagnoses based on history, physical findings, and laboratory and diagnostic tests. The practitioner gathers further evidence and analyzes this evidence to arrive at a hypothesis that will lead to a further narrowing of possibilities. This is known as the process of diagnostic reasoning.

DIAGNOSTIC REASONING

Diagnostic reasoning is a scientific process in which the practitioner suspects the cause of a patient's symptoms and signs based on previous knowledge, gathers relevant information, selects necessary tests, and recommends therapy. The difference between an average and an excellent practitioner is the speed and focus used to arrive at the correct conclusion and initiate the best course of treatment with minimum cost, risk, inconvenience, and delay (Eddy, 1996).

In using diagnostic reasoning, the practitioner:
- Determines and focuses on what needs to be asked and what needs to be examined
- Performs examinations and diagnostic tests accurately
- Clusters abnormal findings
- Analyzes and interprets the findings
- Develops a list of likely or differential diagnoses

THE DIAGNOSTIC PROCESS

The Primary Care Context

The process of assessment in the primary care setting begins with the patient stating a reason for the visit or a chief complaint. Most visits to primary care providers involve symptoms presented by the patient, such as earache, vomiting, or fatigue. The initial evidence is collected through a patient history. Demographic information, such as gender, age, occupation, and place of residence, is obtained to place the patient in a risk category that can generally rule out certain diagnoses immediately. In most primary care settings, routine vital signs are obtained, which may include height and weight, temperature, pulse, respiratory rate, blood pressure, last menstrual period, and smoking status. As the practitioner is obtaining the history he or she is also making observations of the patient's appearance, interactions with family members, orientation, physical condition, and will note any unusual findings that may help focus the assessment process.

Presenting symptoms need to be explored with further questions about the (1) timing or onset, duration, and frequency; (2) anatomical location; (3) character or quality; (4) setting in which they occur; (5) severity or intensity; (6) aggravating and alleviating factors; (7) associated symptoms; and (8) the patient's perception of the meaning of the symptom. The practitioner then clusters the findings into logical groups based on prior knowledge of symptom clusters associated with specific diagnoses or anatomical locations, which suggests the involvement of a specific body system.

Formulating and Testing a Hypothesis

The practitioner then formulates a hypothesis based on expertise and knowledge of probable processes—e.g., pathological, physiological, psychological. Further interpretation of evidence refines the hypothesis to a working or probable diagnosis. Hypothesis generation, in fact, probably already began based on the patient's age, gender, race, appearance, and presenting problem. Age is the most significant variable in narrowing the probabilities of a problem.

Hypothesis generation forms the context in which further data are collected. This context includes the setting in which care is delivered, such as a hospital, an outpatient setting, or another community-based setting where more than a single individual may be affected. Clinical decision making can be filled with uncertainty and ambiguity. Because available evidence is almost never complete, hypothesis formation involves some element of subjective judgment.

The hypothesis must then be tested and assessed for (1) coherence—are the physiological linkages, predisposing factors, and complications for this disease present in the patient? (2) adequacy—does the suspected disease encompass all of the patient's normal and abnormal findings? (3) parsimony—is it the simplest explanation of the patient's findings? The surest way to make this determination is to ask the patient or the parents why they are seeking care and ask what their perception of the problem is. This is a crucial step since patients must find any treatment recommendation acceptable. And, finally, (4) can a competing hypothesis be eliminated? Are there other disease possibilities that could explain the patient's symptoms?

To confirm the hypothesis, the practitioner establishes a working definition of the problem as a basis for a treatment plan and evaluates the outcome. The goal of a clinical decision is to choose an action that is most likely to result in the health outcomes the patient desires. This step of the decision-making process involves personal preference as to whether benefits are worth the risks involved, the cost is reasonable, or whether the most desired outcomes are short or long term.

Clinicians make extensive use of heuristics, or rules of thumb, to guide the inductive or inferential process of diagnostic reasoning. Heuristics are generally accurate and useful rules to make the task of information gathering more manageable and efficient—rules such as familiarity, salience, resemblance to a patient who has a known disease. However, heuristics can, on occasion, be faulty (if the presentation is atypical or the condition is rare). The clinician must always be open to a low probability or a very serious diagnosis. Heuristics can have negative effects on judgment when stereotypes or biases influence judgment. For example, assuming that a patient is heterosexual can lead to errors in clinical reasoning and differential diagnosis when evaluating the symptom of rectal pain.

EXPERT VERSUS NOVICE CLINICIANS

Students of advanced assessment have a wide variety of backgrounds, with many coming from specialized areas of clinical practice. Such students may have difficulty broadening the scope of their observations and clinical possibilities. In any case, whether specialists or not, non-experts tend to be non-selective in data gathering and clinical reasoning strategies used. Experts, on the other hand, are able to focus on a problem, recognize patterns, and gather only relevant data, with a high probability of a correct diagnosis. The goal for a novice practitioner is to aim for competence and expertise.

The competent practitioner will:

1. *Identify most important cues.* These cues are obtained largely by a thorough symptom analysis, functional assessment, and a history that assesses the patient's beliefs and understanding about the problem or representation of the illness. People's beliefs about an illness or symptom often include a cause, an opinion about the timeline (acute or chronic), consequences of the condition (minor or life threatening), and some type of verbal label used to identify the cluster of symptoms or sensations (e.g., "the flu," "the blues") (Baumann and Leventhal, 1985; Kleinman, Eisenberg, and Good,

1978). Clinicians need to distinguish between the presence of disease, which has a biological basis, and illness, which is the human experience of being sick that may have little correlation with the objective evidence available.

2. *Understand and perform advanced examination techniques.* These techniques may include special maneuvers and closer observation of fine detail during the physical examination, more in-depth interviews using valid and reliable instruments to assess the patient's risk for a specific diagnosis, and "gold standard" diagnostic tests for the identification of a specific disorder.

3. *Test differential or competing diagnoses.* A differential diagnosis results from a synthesis of subjective and objective findings, including laboratory and diagnostic tests, with knowledge of known and recognized patterns of signs and symptoms. When using the "rule-out" strategy, the clinician looks for the absence of findings that are frequently seen with a specific condition; the absence of a sensitive finding is strong evidence against the condition being present. When using the "rule-in" strategy, the clinician looks for the presence of a finding with high specificity (low false positive and high true negative) rate; presence of this finding is strong evidence the condition is present.

4. *See a pattern in the information gathered.* A pattern or cluster of findings may emerge from the subjective and objective data. This pattern may be evident during one patient encounter or it may depend on a pattern of signs and symptoms that develops over time. Often the expert clinician can eliminate competing diagnoses only after the initial treatment pre-

scribed is ineffective, or the symptoms either disappear sooner than expected or persist longer than expected.

DEVELOPING CLINICAL JUDGMENT

Brykcyzynski (1989) conducted a qualitative study on advanced practice nurses to explore how they developed clinical reasoning skills. In her analysis, Brykcyzynski observed that theoretical knowledge about disease and illness was acquired in a decontextual fashion. That is, didactic content in a lecture or in a reference book, which often discusses the classic presentation of a patient with a specific disorder, is unable to bring into the management and assessment plan variables that are present in the actual clinical situation. Thus theoretical knowledge has limitations for the exercising of expert clinical judgment. Even the use of case studies has limitations since the data is presented to the reader, but in actual clinical practice the practitioner has to be ready to begin the clinical reasoning process by knowing what to ask a patient (Ryan-Wenger and Lee, 1997).

Practical knowledge requires actual experience in a situation that is contextual and transactional. Brykcyzynski identified the following themes as emerging only from practice experience: (1) discretionary judgment as a central aspect of "know how" as a practitioner; (2) background knowledge as extremely important in skill development; and (3) practice skills as experience based, acquired only through spending time with patients, practicing focused listening, and gaining experience in recognizing subtle cues.

NEGOTIATING GOALS AND EXPECTATIONS OF A PATIENT ENCOUNTER

Especially in an ambulatory care setting, it is important to identify the patient's goals, expectations, and resources to determine what needs to be achieved during an encounter. A patient who seeks care because of a bothersome symptom may be more interested in having the symptom relieved by a particular date rather than in knowing the cause or diagnostic explanation for the symptom. Other patients may want reassurance that a symptom or sign is not a serious condition and yet do not expect treatment to alleviate the sensations they are experiencing. An explicit discussion between the clinician and patient is necessary to establish what the goals and focus of an encounter will be. Goals can be mutually negotiated to assure clinicians that serious conditions can be 'ruled-out' and to assure patients that their needs and desires are acknowledged.

SUMMARY

In the context of primary care practice, the orientation to the patient should be holistic and general and toward the most prevalent or common conditions in a particular population group. This orientation requires that the expert practitioner develop skills in inductive reasoning to arrive at a diagnosis and treatment plan that is acceptable to a patient. Knowledge of the patient as a person over time greatly enhances the database the clinician works from to arrive at better clinical judgments. Treatment plans in primary care settings rely on low-level technology, stress prevention, and encourage self-care behaviors as well as an open and effective patient-provider communication. Practitioners need to weigh the cost/benefit analysis of clinical decision making and subsequent treatment plans to evaluate diagnostic efficiency. A practitioner can move from novice to expert and become more efficient in exercising clinical judgment but must always be vigilant of the element of uncertainty in clinical situations.

Chapter 2

Common Problems of the Head, Eyes, Ears, Nose, and Throat

Earache

Otalgia, or ear pain, is generally caused by an inflammatory process. In children, inflammation most commonly occurs in the middle ear. Adults more often have an earache from external ear conditions or from referred pain from other head and neck structures. Acute otitis media (AOM) refers to any inflammation of the middle ear and encompasses a variety of clinical conditions. Otitis media with effusion is a collection of fluid in the middle ear. This condition is also known as serous otitis media, secretory otitis, or nonsuppurative otitis. External or middle ear disorders can often be distinguished after a brief history and physical examination. If the physical findings are normal, referred pain is a likely cause. About 50% of referred pain is caused by dental problems, although other causes may include temporomandibular joint (TMJ) disorder, parotitis, pharyngitis, or cervical, mouth, or facial disorders. The most serious, although least common, cause of referred pain is nasopharyngeal cancer. This condition is more common in Asians. Figure 2-1 illustrates the structures of the ear.

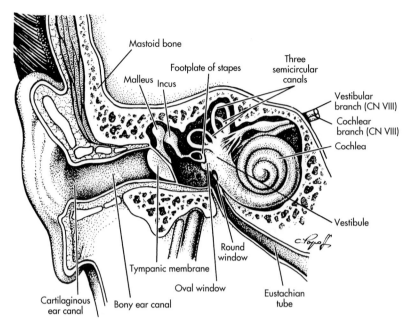

Figure 2-1 External auditory canal, middle ear, and inner ear. (From Barkauskas VH et al: *Health and physical assessment,* ed 2, St. Louis, 1998, Mosby.)

DIAGNOSTIC REASONING: FOCUSED HISTORY

Is this an acute infection?

Key Questions
- How old are you?
- Have you had a fever?
- Have you had an upper respiratory infection?
- Have you had ear infections before?
- Is there a family history of ear infections?

Age. Age is an important clue for the cause of ear pain. The occurrence of AOM declines significantly after age 6. Increased age increases the likelihood of secondary otalgia caused by disorders of the head, face and neck, sinuses, periodontal disease, and malignancy.

Fever. Fever is present in 60% of all children with AOM. In infants younger than 2 months, fever with AOM is uncom-

mon. A high fever accompanying otitis is more likely to occur as part of a systemic illness such as pneumonia or meningitis.

Upper respiratory infection. When the mucous membranes of the nasopharynx and/or sinuses become infected, organisms are forced up the lumen of the eustachian tube. Inflammation of the mucosa or enlarged adenoids obstructs the eustachian opening so that the air in the middle ear is absorbed and replaced by mucus. This mucus creates a mechanical obstruction and can serve as a medium for bacterial growth.

Previous infections. Infants under 3 months who have a first AOM run a high risk of recurrence. Seventy-one percent of children under 3 years old have had at least one episode, and a third have had an average of three episodes. Chronic otitis media can result in anatomical changes to the tympanic membrane and middle ear ossicles, which may predispose the patient to further ear infections.

Family history. Having a sibling or parent with chronic otitis media makes a child twice as likely to develop the illness. The presence of chronic otitis media may also be related to child care practices, such as bottle propping, or environmental exposures, such as secondary cigarette smoke.

What environmental conditions might suggest increased risk?

Key Questions
- Does anyone around you smoke? Do you smoke?
- Does the child attend day care?
- Does the infant take a bottle lying down?
- Do you swim frequently?
- Have you been in an airplane or been diving lately?

Smoke exposure. Second-hand cigarette smoke exposure has been associated with a two- to three-fold increased risk of otitis media. Cigarette smoking leads to functional eustachian tube obstruction and decreases the protective ciliary action in the tube.

Attending day care. Attending a day care setting with other children is associated with increased incidence of otitis media because of exposure to organisms.

Bottle propping. In very young children, lying supine while drinking from a bottle has been associated with acute otitis media. It is postulated that swallowing while lying down allows nasopharyngeal fluid to enter the middle ear, with subsequent infection.

Swimming. Repeated or prolonged immersion in water results in loss of protective cerumen and chronic irritation with maceration from excessive moisture in the canal. This leads to an increased oc-currence of otitis externa, also called swimmer's ear.

Airplane travelers, divers. Barotrauma is a cause of acute serous otitis related to pressure changes from diving or flying. This is often aggravated by recent upper respiratory infection or nasal congestion. Failure of the eustachian tube to open and equilibrate during descent results in collection of serosanguinous fluid in the middle ear. This may be felt as ear pressure that can lead to pain, tinnitus, and temporary deafness. Swallowing, chewing, or blowing out the nose with the mouth and nose occluded can relieve symptoms.

Could this be related to a systemic disease?

Key Questions
- Do you have diabetes?
- Have you ever had dermatitis, eczema, or psoriasis?
- Does the child have an unrepaired cleft palate?

Diabetes mellitus. Diabetes mellitus predisposes adults to otitis externa and can lead to malignant otitis externa, which is a cellulitis involving the ear and surrounding tissue. Persons with diabetes are also at increased risk for otitis media and mastoiditis.

History of seborrheic dermatitis or psoriasis. Chronic inflammatory dermatitis from over-production of sebum can occur in the external canal and cause otitis externa.

Cleft palate. Unrepaired anomalies anatomically predispose a child to otitis media because of functional obstruction of the eustachian tubes.

What does the presence of pain tell me?

Key Questions
- Where specifically is the pain felt? Is it in one ear or both?
- How severe is the pain? Does it inter-

fere with sleeping, eating, or other activities?

- How long have you had this pain?
- Is the pain constant or intermittent? If intermittent, how long does it last?
- Does the pain travel (radiate) to other areas?

Location of the pain. Pain of otitis externa is described as tenderness around the outer ear or opening to the ear canal, which worsens with manipulation of the pinna. Mastoiditis is often associated with severe pain or tenderness over the mastoid bone. If the pain is bilateral, suspect otitis externa. Referred pain or pain of AOM is usually unilateral. Infants cannot assist in location of the ear pain. Instead, they exhibit behavioral changes that may indicate pain, such as irritability, lethargy, poor appetite, vomiting, and diarrhea. Young children may pull or tug at their ears.

Quality of the pain. The pain of AOM is often described as a deep pain or a blockage of the ear. Serous otitis is often painless or may be described as a bubbling, popping, or stuffy sensation in the ear. Otitis externa is a tenderness of the outer ear or ear canal that can be accompanied by itching. A cerumen impaction creates a milder pain or vague discomfort of stuffed ears.

Quantity/severity of the pain. The pain of AOM is severe enough to interfere with sleep and may be suddenly relieved if the eardrum perforates. Chronic ear pain that is unresponsive to treatment may indicate a tumor.

Onset, timing, and duration of the pain. TMJ pain is often described as severe pain lasting a few minutes and recurring three to four times per day, sometimes associated with headache. It is worse in the morning because nighttime teeth grinding is associated with this condition. The pain is intermittent but can be acute, related to trauma or over-extension of the mouth. Chronic pain may be related to dental malocclusion or rheumatoid arthritis. Infants may exhibit crying when sucking to indicate pain with compression and increased pressure in the ears. Nocturnal onset of otalgia from a developing infection is caused by increased vascular pressure in the reclined position, causing the drum to bulge and stimulate pain sensation.

What does the presence of discharge or itching tell me?

Key Questions
- Do you have any discharge from the ear?
- Do you have any itching in the ear?

Itching or drainage. Itching or drainage from the ear usually indicates an infection or inflammation of the external canal. Itching can also be a precursor to herpes zoster of CN V (trigeminal). Drainage may also be present after the tympanic membrane (TM) ruptures from increased middle ear pressure, or it may be from exudate secondary to mastoiditis. Cholesteatoma is an epidermal inclusion cyst of the middle ear or mastoid. It occurs with a perforation of the tympanic membrane and is associated with a foul-smelling discharge.

What does a history of trauma or injury tell me?

Key Questions
- Have you had any recent trauma to the ear?
- Have you had any head trauma?
- How do you clean your ears? Do you use cotton-tipped swabs?
- Do you have a history of excessive ear wax?
- If a child: does the child have a history of putting objects into ears?
- Have you had any recent insect bites around the ear?
- Have you been exposed to any loud noise?

History of ear trauma. Perforation of the eardrum can be caused by blunt or penetrating trauma. Blunt trauma might include a slap to the ear or barotrauma. Penetrating trauma to the canal or tympanic membrane may be self-induced with cotton-tipped swabs or other sharp objects used to remove ear wax or to scratch the canal.

Head trauma. Direct injury to the inner ear by fracture of the petrous temporal bone located at the base of the skull also destroys the inner ear.

History of cerumen impaction. Cerumen is a naturally wet, sticky, honey-colored wax that serves as a lubricant to protect the external ear canal. In some individuals it occurs in a dark scaly form and accumulates in the ear canal. This accumulation may cause hearing loss, tinnitus, pressure sensation, vertigo, and infection. Self-cleaning practices can produce trauma to the canal, or cerumen-softening solutions can cause chemical irritation to the canal tissue.

History of introduction of foreign bodies. Foreign bodies, such as feathers, beads, and insects, especially cockroaches, can produce ear pain and inflammation. Children will often self-insert objects.

Insect bites. Insect bites can lead to acute pain and tenderness of the external canal and may develop into a secondary infection.

Loud noise. Exposure to high-pitched and loud noises for a prolonged period of time destroys the cochlear hair cells. Exposure to noisy work environments, to the operating of heavy machinery, and to loud music increases the risk of injury and eventual hearing loss.

Is hearing loss a clue?

Key Questions

- Do you have any difficulty in hearing?
- Do you have any dizziness?
- Do you have any ringing in the ear?
- Do you think the child can hear normally?
- Does the child turn his or her head to listen?

Difficulty in hearing. Complaints of hearing loss or "difficulty hearing" can indicate blockage of the ear canal by cerumen or a foreign body, inflammation of the middle or inner ear, or a neoplasm. The most frequent cause is a conductive loss, caused by blockage of the external canal, usually by cerumen. Chronic otitis media is usually a condition of adults who have a chronic infection that may destroy the ossicles and spread to the mastoid, labyrinth, and intracranial structures, causing hearing loss. Chronic ear pain is often associated with hearing loss and ear discharge secondary to a perforated non-healing TM.

Hearing loss in children. Chronic otitis media with effusion causes a conductive hearing loss in children. This loss may be caused by negative middle ear pressure, the presence of an effusion in the middle ear, or structural damage to the TM or ossicles.

Dizziness, ringing in ear. Hearing loss associated with dizziness, vertigo, or tinnitus may indicate a serious inner ear condition. Abnormal middle ear ventilation and middle ear effusion are the most common causes of balance disturbance in children. Patients describe tinnitus as snapping, clicking, and popping sounds. These symptoms are caused by re-establishment of aeration in the middle ear cavity as effusion clears.

DIAGNOSTIC REASONING: FOCUSED PHYSICAL EXAMINATION

A correct diagnosis of ear pain requires a good view of the TM and external ear canal. Cerumen obstructions should be removed through lavage or by separating an impaction with an ear curette so that irrigation fluid can penetrate behind the impaction. The curette must be manipulated cautiously because trauma to or inflammation of the sensitive perichondrium that lies just below a thin layer of epithelium in the ear canal elicits excruciating pain and can bleed easily.

Lavage should not be performed if

medical history suggests perforation of the TM. Without visualization of the TM, however, otitis media cannot be ruled out. Lavage solution helps to soften cerumen and can be purchased commercially in kits or a solution can be made of 1 : 1 hydrogen peroxide and water.

Note Behaviors in Children

Otitis media is the most common childhood disorder. Young infants may exhibit nonspecific signs of irritability, poor feeding, congestion, and fever. Older infants and young toddlers are irritable, pull on the painful ear, or bang their head on the affected side. Older children will complain of an earache.

Inspect External Ears

General inspection should begin with the pinna and condition of the skin around the ear, face, and scalp. Hemorrhage over the mastoid bone (Battle's sign) may occur with a basal skull fracture. Eczematous seborrhea or psoriasis is a redness and scaling of the skin that can extend into the external ear canal. Pain in the opening of the ear canal and inflamed skin may suggest a bacterial infection. Fungal and yeast infections appear as white or dark patches. Furuncles or lesions secondary to trauma or irritation appear as localized areas of tenderness or swelling. A hot, swollen, and erythematous ear and surrounding skin indicates cellulitis. Redness and painful swelling over the mastoid process is a sign of infection in the mastoid air cells.

Palpate External Ears

Palpate the pinna and tragus for tenderness. In mastoiditis, the pinna is displaced forward and swelling may be present behind the ear. Palpation of the mastoid process elicits severe tenderness. Otitis externa is associated with pain on manipulation of the pinna. With referred pain, the structures will appear normal although palpation over the TMJ may elicit tenderness,

and movement of the jaw may create a clicking sound.

Palpate the pre- and post-auricular area on the right and left simultaneously to elicit pain. Palpate anterior and posterior cervical lymph nodes and over the mastoid process. Pre-auricular nodes may be enlarged in AOM and otitis externa. Post-auricular swelling may indicate extension of infection into the mastoid cavity.

Inspect Ear Canals

With the otoscope, observe for patency of the canal, condition of the skin of the ear canal, and the presence of cerumen. With cerumen impaction, the ear canal will appear normal but no structures can be visualized. A foreign body is easily visualized. Vesicles on the external ear canal and auricle may indicate herpes zoster (Ramsay Hunt syndrome).

Visualize any discharge, noting color, consistency, and odor. Discharge is usually indicative of an active infection. However, cranial trauma with cerebral spinal fluid leakage must be kept in mind. Cheesy, green-blue, or gray discharge can be seen with otitis externa.

Inspect Tympanic Membranes

Visualize the TM, noting light reflex and anatomical structures. The appearance of a normal TM is translucent and pearly gray in color. Mild diffuse redness can occur from crying or coughing. Mild vascularity is sometimes seen in the normal eardrum, especially on the handle of the malleus. Localized redness is a sign of inflammation. Scarring and effusion can cause whitening and opacification of the TM.

The contour of the normal TM is somewhat concave. Fullness or bulging indicates either increased air pressure or, more commonly, increased hydrostatic pressure within the middle ear. Fullness of the eardrum is seen first around the periphery of the TM. As pressure increases, central fullness becomes visible. Concavity or retraction of the eardrum is associated

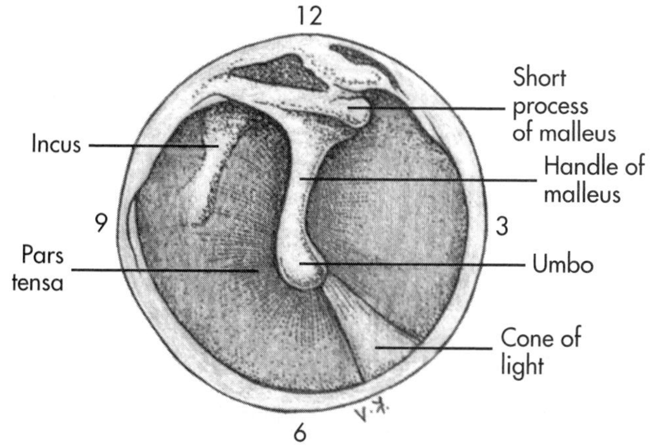

Figure 2-2   Usual landmarks of the right tympanic membrane with a "clock" superimposed. (From Wong DL, Perry S: *Maternal child health,* St. Louis, 1998, Mosby.)

with negative middle ear pressure or post-inflammatory adhesions. As the eardrum retracts, the handle of the malleus short process becomes more visible.

Myringitis is a red inflamed eardrum without effusion. Bullous myringitis describes an extremely painful condition of small blisters on the tympanic membrane caused by a bacterial otitis media. Figure 2-2 illustrates the usual landmarks of a normal right tympanic membrane. Chronic otitis media can lead to cholesteatoma, or a cyst-like mass behind the eardrum, caused by proliferation of squamous epithelium. The mass can grow to cause necrosis of the ossicles. Examination will reveal a collection of white granulation tissue with perforation of the TM.

Perform Pneumatic Otosocopy (Insufflation)

The normal eardrum is suspended from its margins and responds to slight pressure changes. Insufflation tests the mobility of the TM. It can be an insensitive test for otitis media if poor technique fails to create a seal. Properly performed, however, it is more reliable than visualization alone.

To perform insufflation, a large speculum is needed to create a seal. A normal finding elicits a slight motion of the TM when air is insufflated. This movement is compared to the opposite ear. A TM that has been retracted as a result of negative middle ear pressure or adhesions does not move with inflation, but rebound mobility is seen when the bulb is released. Any accumulation of liquid in the middle ear (e.g., effusion) or scarring of the TM inhibits movement when air is insufflated.

Test Hearing Acuity

Test hearing acuity using the whisper test and the tuning fork for the Rinne and Weber tests. The sensory function of the acoustic nerve (CN VIII) should be tested to determine whether air or bone conduction loss is present with ear pain.

The Weber test is done with a 512-Hz or higher frequency tuning fork. To perform the test, firmly place the vibrating tuning fork on a midline point of the skull. If there is unilateral conductive hearing loss, sound will lateralize to the ear with loss because the better ear is being distracted by ambient noise. Alternately, if the client has unilateral sensorineural loss, the sound will lateralize to the better ear because the neural pathway is interrupted on the affected side. Equal perception of vibration can indicate normal hearing or bilateral hearing loss. The Rinne test compares air conduction (AC) to bone conduction (BC); AC:BC should be 2:1. A 20- to 30-decibel conductive loss would result in better sound transmission through bone than through air. Conductive hearing loss results when sound transmission is impaired through the external or middle ear. Sensorineural hearing loss results from a defect in the inner ear.

Examine Related Body Systems

Examine other regional body systems of the head and neck, including inspection of the conjunctiva, mucosa and patency of the nose, percussion and palpation of frontal and maxillary sinuses for tenderness, and inspection of the posterior pharynx for lymphedema, color, and presence of exudate. Inspecting the condition of the oral mucosa—teeth and gums—will provide information about possible causes of referred pain. A focused physical examination for head and neck symptoms should include palpation of cervicofacial lymph nodes, especially the pre- and post-auricular nodes.

Perform an Intraotic Manipulation

If referred pain is suspected, do a more extensive neurological examination and assess for TMJ disorder. TMJ pain can be replicated by instructing the patient to open the mouth wide. Face the patient and insert a single fingertip in each ear and pull toward you as the patient is instructed to open and close the mouth. Pain will be elicited in 90% of patients with TMJ disorder.

Evaluate Cranial Nerves V, VII, and IX

Observe jaw and facial muscle movement for symmetry and strength by palpating over the masseter muscles and asking the client to bite and clench the teeth (CN V). Assess intactness of sensation to pain and light touch using a sharp-dull stimulus over the three branches of CN V. Both

cranial nerves VII (anterior two thirds) and IX (posterior third) innervate taste sensation to the tongue as well as sensation to the external ear. Test taste sensation by having the client protrude the tongue and apply sweet and salty substances separately to each half of the tongue to test CN VII and bitter and sour substances to test CN IX.

LABORATORY AND DIAGNOSTIC STUDIES

Tympanometry

Tympanometry involves inserting a probe into the external ear canal while pressure against the eardrum is continually changed to assess the mobility of the TM. The tympanogram provides an indirect measure of pressure in the middle ear. Under normal middle ear pressure, the TM absorbs the sound energy waves and produces a bell-shaped pattern that peaks when sound pressure is introduced. With positive or negative middle ear pressure, the tympanogram results in a flat pattern or an early peak pressure. Figure 2-3 illustrates examples of various tympanogram results.

Audiometry

Audiometry assesses both the frequency and intensity of sound that can be perceived. An air conduction audiometer transmits via earphones a pure tone that has variable frequency and intensity settings to test each ear separately. The goal of audiometry is to test the lowest decibel intensity that can be heard for each frequency tested. An individual trained in the proper technique will produce reliable, reproducible, and valid test results. A threshold of up to 20 decibels (dB) is considered normal for adults. Above that dB, hearing loss is graded as mild, moderate, moderately severe, severe, and profound.

Mastoid Process X-Ray

X-rays of the mastoid bone show clouding of the air cells when otitis media is present.

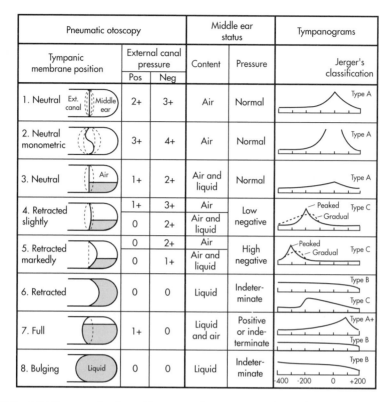

| Pneumatic otoscopy | | | Middle ear status | | Tympanograms |
| Tympanic membrane position | External canal pressure | | Content | Pressure | Jerger's classification |
	Pos	Neg			
1. Neutral Ext. canal / Middle ear	2+	3+	Air	Normal	Type A
2. Neutral monometric	3+	4+	Air	Normal	Type A
3. Neutral Air	1+	2+	Air and liquid	Normal	Type A
4. Retracted slightly	1+	3+	Air	Low negative	Peaked Type C / Gradual
	0	2+	Air and liquid		
5. Retracted markedly	0	2+	Air	High negative	Peaked / Gradual Type C
	0	1+	Air and liquid		
6. Retracted	0	0	Liquid	Indeterminate	Type B / Type C
7. Full	1+	0	Liquid and air	Positive or indeterminate	Type A+ / Type B
8. Bulging Liquid	0	0	Liquid	Indeterminate	Type B
					-400 -200 0 +200

Figure 2-3   Middle ear evaluation with pneumatic otoscopy and impedance tympanograms. (From Daeschner CW Jr: *Pediatrics: an approach to independent learning,* New York, 1983, John Wiley & Sons.)

Chronic mastoiditis may reveal decalcification of the bony wall between the mastoid air cells.

Computed Tomography (CT) Scan

A CT scan of the temporal bone is helpful in diagnosing cholesteatoma, congenital syndromes, and acoustic neuroma.

DIFFERENTIAL DIAGNOSIS

External Otitis

External otitis is more common in adults than children and often presents as bilateral pain that worsens with manipulation of the pinna. The patient complains of a stuffed ear, and occasionally conductive hearing loss may occur. Discharge and itching that occurs 1 to 2 days after swimming may be associated with otitis externa. The affected canal may be swollen shut. Palpation will often reveal enlarged pre- or post-auricular nodes.

Acute Otitis Media

Acute otitis media most often occurs in children under 6 years of age and is associated with an upper respiratory infection. It is an acute infection associated with ear pain and a bulging, red eardrum. The pain of otitis media is severe enough to interfere with sleep and may be suddenly relieved if the eardrum perforates. Swelling of the pre-auricular node is sometimes seen in children with AOM.

Serous Otitis

Serous otitis commonly occurs in children, often without pain. It is caused by a mechanical process or eustachian tube blockage that leads to inadequate ventilation of the middle ear and a collection of fluid that resembles mucus. In serous otitis, the TM may be injected and immobile, either bulging or retracted, as noted by the shape of the cone of light reflex and pneumatic otoscopy. In adults, serous otitis is associated with recent upper respiratory infection.

Cholesteatoma

Cholesteatoma is an epidermal inclusion cyst formation in the middle ear and mastoid cavity. It is often the sequel of chronic otitis media. The formation occurs with the migration of skin cells from the external ear canal through a perforation in the tympanic membrane. Once established in the middle ear, the cells desquamate and form the cholesteatoma. This condition is life threatening if left untreated because it will continue to erode away medially to impinge on intracranial structures. A cholesteatoma appears as a cyst or collection of granulation tissue on the TM, commonly located in the pars flaccida area in the superior anterior quadrant of the TM.

Mastoiditis

Mastoiditis is an infection of the soft tissue surrounding the air spaces in the mastoid bone and is connected to the middle ear space. Mastoiditis usually occurs with bacterial otitis media and is associated with fever. More advanced mastoiditis is manifested by swelling, erythema, and tenderness over the mastoid bone. Swelling can displace the position of the auricle. The swelling can extend to the facial nerve causing paralysis, or to the labyrinth or cerebrospinal fluid, causing meningitis or brain abscess. Advanced mastoiditis requires immediate referral and surgical management.

Foreign Bodies

Foreign bodies are easily visualized on examination of the ear canal and can produce a foul-smelling ear drainage secondary to infection or abscess.

Cerumen Impaction

Impaction of cerumen is likely if the patient complains of a stuffed-up ear or decreased hearing acuity. An impaction may also produce pain if cerumen is pressed against the TM. Examination reveals cerumen occluding the external canal.

Barotrauma

Barotrauma produces an acute serous otitis that is caused by pressure changes (e.g., in divers or airplane travelers) and is often aggravated by a recent URI or nasal congestion. Serosanguinous fluid collects in the middle ear and during descent this may be felt as ear pressure, pain, tinnitus, or temporary deafness. Swallowing, chewing, or blowing out the nose with the mouth and nose occluded can relieve symptoms.

Trauma

Blunt or penetrating trauma can perforate the TM. A hole in the TM is visible on examination or the examiner may notice an absence of normal landmarks. A perforated eardrum does not significantly impair hearing or result in vertigo and usually heals within 4 to 6 weeks without sequelae. Assess the extent of other damage to the ear when perforation is identified.

Cervical Lymphadenitis

Anterior cervical lymphadenitis is a common cause of referred ear pain in children. This may be seen with strep throat, as well as in cases of mononucleosis with extensive cervical node swelling in adolescents or young adults.

Referred Pain From Cervical Nerves

Cervical nerves 2 to 3 innervate the skin and muscles of the neck and include the great auricular nerve, which supplies the external canals and posterior auricular area. Pain is perceived in these areas. The ear examination will be normal.

Referred Pain From Cranial Nerves

Cranial nerves (CN) associated with referred ear pain include the trigeminal nerve (V), which supplies the anterior portion of the auricle and tragus, the anterior and superior auditory canal, and the anterior TM, and the facial (VII), the vagus (X), and the glossopharnyngeal nerves (IX), which innervate the posterior portion of the TM and the external auditory canal. Inflammation of CN X is associated with lesions of the larynx, esophagus, trachea, and thyroid. With referred pain, the structures of the ear will appear normal.

TMJ Disorder

TMJ disorder is a common secondary cause of ear pain. Diagnosis of the disorder is likely if palpation over the TMJ elicits tenderness, and movement of the joint creates a clicking sound. Examination of the ear is normal. Pain also increases with intraotic manipulation. TMJ pain is often worse in the morning. The pain can be acute, related to trauma or over-extension of the mouth, or chronic, related to dental malocclusion or rheumatoid arthritis.

Table 2-1

Differential Diagnosis of Common Causes of Ear Pain

Condition	History	Physical Findings	Diagnostic Studies
External otitis	More common in adults, especially those with diabetes, ear pickers, or swimmers; bilateral itching; pain	Discharge; inflamed, swollen external canal; pain with movement of the pinna; TM normal or not visible	None
Acute otitis media	More common in children <6 years; those with smoke exposure, recent URI; severe or deep pain; unilateral; sensation of fullness	Red, bulging TM; fever; decreased light reflex; opaque TM; decreased TM mobility	None initially

Continued

Table 2-1

Differential Diagnosis of Common Causes of Ear Pain—cont'd

Condition	History	Physical Findings	Diagnostic Studies
Serous otitis	More common in children but occurs in adults with recent URI; unilateral pain; sensation of crackling or decreased hearing	Fluid line or air observed behind TM; conductive hearing loss; decreased TM mobility	Tympanogram
Cholesteatoma	Hearing loss; recent perfo-rated TM	Pearly white lesion on or behind the TM	Immediate referral
Mastoiditis	History of recent otitis media; chronic otitis pain behind ear	Swelling over mastoid process; fever, palpable tenderness, and erythema over mastoid process	X-ray of mastoid sinuses reveals cloudiness; re-ferral
Foreign body or cerumen impac-tion	Both children and adults have pain or vague sensa-tion of discom-fort; decreased hearing	Visualize foreign body or ceru-men; may detect foul odor; con-ductive hearing loss	None
Barotrauma	History of flying, diving; severe pain; hearing loss; sensation of fullness; his-tory of recent nasal congestion	Retraction or bulging of TM; perforation of TM, fluid in canal	Tympanogram
Trauma	History of blunt trauma, pen-etrating trauma	Perforation of TM	X-rays/CT scan as directed by injury
Cervical lymphadenitis	History of cervical node swelling; pain in ear common in children	Enlarged, tender, cervical lymph nodes; may see early onset of AOM in children	Throat culture if indicated; in adolescents mono spot if indicated
Cervical nerves 2, 3 (referred pain)	Pain in skin and muscles of the neck and in ear canal	Dermatome evalu-ation for cervical nerve	None

Table 2-1

Differential Diagnosis of Common Causes of Ear Pain—cont'd

Condition	History	Physical Findings	Diagnostic Studies
Cranial nerves (referred pain)	History, depending on CN involved	Test function of CN V, VII, IX, X; ear exam normal	X-rays/CT scan, directed by cranial nerve involvement
TMJ disorder	More common in adults; 50% related to dental problems; discomfort to severe pain; unilateral; pain worse in morning	Malocclusion; bruxism; normal external and middle ear structures and function; jaw click; abnormal cranial nerve function; ear exam normal	None

Sore Throat

Sore throat is most often the result of an inflammation of the mucosa of the oropharynx, secondary to an infectious cause (e.g., viral, bacterial, fungal, spirochetal). Less commonly sore throat may be a symptom of systemic illness, such as mononucleosis. The posterior pharnyx is also vulnerable to irritants from the environment and drainage from the nose and sinuses. Thus pharyngitis begins as an inflammation of the mucous membranes with secondary involvement of the lymph node drainage system, rarely progressing to deep neck and mediastinal involvement. Throat pain can also be referred from other structures, most commonly the ears and thyroid gland.

Sore throats can be classified as those with pharyngeal ulcers and those without. The classification serves as a device to sort out those relatively few sore throats caused by specific viral or fungal infections that produce pharyngeal ulcers and those caused by agents and processes characterized by an absence of pharyngeal ulcers.

The goals of assessment and diagnosis are to identify those patients with group A beta-hemolytic streptococcal (GABHS) infection (because they are at risk for rheumatic fever and glomerulonephritis), to reduce the possibility of sequelae of peritonsillar and retropharyngeal abscess, and to identify epiglottitis.

DIAGNOSTIC REASONING: FOCUSED HISTORY

Is this an emergency?

Key Questions
- Have you been drooling?
- Have you been unable to swallow?
- Have you been unable to lie down?
- Have you been restless, unable to stay still?
- Have you been unable to carry on a conversation?

The previous complaints signal acute epiglottitis. The history is usually elicited from another individual as the ill person is either a child or is too ill to talk. Acute epiglottitis is rare, with an incidence of $10:100,000$ in pediatric patients <15 years and $1\text{-}8:100,000$ in adult patients. The morbidity and mortality because of airway obstruction, however, are significant.

Symptoms of epiglottitis are sore throat, difficulty swallowing, and respiratory distress, characterized by drooling, dyspnea, and inspiratory stridor. *Hemophilus influenzae* type b is the most common pathogen. Streptococci are rarely responsible. The incidence of *H. influenzae* type b epiglottitis is highest in children ages 2 to 5 years. It is uncommon in children less than 2 years of age but can occur at any age.

Epiglottitis is a rapidly progressive illness with a potentially fatal outcome and must be recognized and referred immediately.

Is the sore throat related to an infectious cause?

Key Questions

- Is anyone else at home sick?
- Are any of your friends or co-workers sick?
- When did the pain start?
- How severe is the pain?

Exposure. Exposure to other ill individuals increases the likelihood of viral or bacterial infection. Respiratory illness caused by GABHS is spread within families, with approximately 20% of family members becoming infected. Epstein-Barr virus is not highly contagious and requires intimate contact between susceptible individuals and symptomatic shedders of the virus. Transmission is primarily through saliva.

Onset. Sudden onset of sore throat is often caused by GABHS. The organisms invade the pharyngeal epithelium where they multiply and cause an intense immune response. Gradual onset is more common in infectious mononucleosis. The Epstein-Barr virus infects B lymphocytes of the pharynx with resultant dissemination throughout the lymphoreticular system, resulting in an immune response that is more gradual in onset.

In viral pharyngitis, a sore throat begins a day or so after the onset of other illness symptoms, reaching its peak by the second or third day.

Non-infectious causes of sore throat typically have an insidious onset. The patient often is not able to pinpoint when the sore throat started but notes that it has been persistent.

Severity. Throat pain associated with streptococcal infection is usually intense. Throat pain associated with influenza and adenovirus is severe, with prominent edema of the throat. Severe throat pain with trismus (spasm of the jaw muscles) and refusal to speak indicates severe peritonsillitis, which may lead to peritonsillar abscess formation (quinsy). The throat pain produced by non-infectious causes tends to be less severe and may be described as "scratchy" or "annoying."

Young children may not be able to express the sensation of a sore throat or the severity of it. Instead, they may refuse to eat or drink. Pain in the younger child, if present, more commonly indicates the presence of epiglottitis or laryngitis, abscess, diphtheria, or scarlatina.

What does the presence of fever tell me?

Key Questions

- Have you had a fever?
- When did it start?
- How high has it been?

Fever is almost always present with GABHS and is the most commonly occurring symptom in children. The fever is of sudden onset and rises above 38.5° C (101.5° F), with malaise, headache, and painful swallowing.

Influenza is characterized by abrupt onset of fever, ranging from 37.8° to 40° C (100° to 104° F). Adenoviral infection in children typically presents with a temperature of more than 40° C (104° F). Patients with Epstein-Barr virus have a low-grade fever.

Fever, followed by an interval of several days without fever, then recurrent fever, or a continuing fever for several days may indicate peritonsillar abscess.

The absence of fever suggests a non-infectious cause. Patients with candidiasis and aphthous stomatitis may also present without a fever.

What does the presence of upper respiratory symptoms tell me?

Key Questions

- Do you have a cough?
- Have you had a runny nose? What color is the drainage?
- Do you have mucus dripping from the back of your nose down your throat?
- Do you have any eye redness or discomfort?
- Have your eyes been itchy or watery?
- Have you had any hoarseness?
- Have you been sneezing?

Cough and rhinorrhea. Cough, rhinitis, conjunctivitis, and hoarseness rarely occur with streptococcal pharyngitis, and the presence of two or more of these signs or symptoms suggests a viral infection.

Influenza is often associated with several days of fever, cough, and rhinorrhea. Pharyngitis associated with common cold viruses is characterized by a sore, scratchy throat, nasal symptoms such as stuffiness and rhinorrhea, and a cough.

Clear nasal discharge is common in allergic pharyngitis and may produce post-nasal drip that causes a sore throat.

Conjunctivitis. Conjunctivitis rarely occurs with streptococcal pharyngitis. Mild conjunctivitis is common with viral infection. Watery or itchy eyes are associated with exposure to allergens.

Sneezing. Sneezing is common both with viral infection and with allergen exposure. The sneezing associated with allergic pharyngitis is more persistent and enduring and is often seasonal.

Hoarseness. Hoarseness is not uncommon in allergy-associated sore throat and may be present with viral infection as well. Inflammation produces laryngeal edema that results in hoarseness. Hoarseness is not typically associated with GABHS infection.

What do associated symptoms tell me?

Key Questions

- Do you have muscle aches?
- Have you had any nausea, vomiting, or diarrhea?

Systemic complaints. Systemic complaints such as myalgia are common in influenza and GABHS infection. Streptococcal pharyngitis or influenza in children over 2 years of age is associated with complaints of headache, abdominal pain, and vomiting.

Influenza is often associated with several days of fever and systemic symptoms such as myalgias, cough, and rhinorrhea. Pharyngitis associated with common cold viruses is also often associated with systemic symptoms such as myalgia.

Does the presence of risk factors help me to narrow the cause?

Key Questions

- How old are you?
- What is your smoking history?
- What kind of work do you do?
- Do you engage in oral sex?
- Are you taking any medications?
- Do you have any chronic health problems?
- Are your immunizations up to date?

Age. Group A streptococcal infection is primarily a disease in children 5 to 15 years of age. GABHS is rare in children below 3 years. Influenza affects all ages, whereas parainfluenza and respiratory syncytial viruses primarily affect children.

Adenoviruses, the major viral agents isolated in exudative pharyngitis in younger children, are endemic. In military populations, adenovirus type 4, and, to a lesser extent, types 3, 7, and 21 are the most common causes of pharyngitis.

Adolescents and young adults are more likely to have a sore throat associated with mononucleosis caused by the Epstein-Barr virus. Mononucleosis occurs in older adults but often without pharyngitis, adenopathy, or splenomegaly.

Irritant exposures. Agents, such as tobacco smoke, smog, dust, and allergens, can irritate the throat. These agents cause mucosal irritation and set up the inflammatory process. People who work outdoors may have greater exposure to environmental allergens. Housekeepers may have an increased risk of exposure to dust mites or chemical irritants.

Sexual behavior. Pharyngitis from *Chlamydia trachomatis* and *Neisseria gonorrhea* is more prevalent in persons with a history of oral-genital sexual activity. Gonococci pharyngitis is present in about 10% of patients with anogenital gonorrhea.

Medications/chronic health problems. Immunosuppression increases susceptibility to viral agents that produce pharyngeal ulcers (e.g., herpangina, herpes simplex). Persons with diabetes and those taking broad-spectrum antibiotics are more susceptible to candidiasis. Persons with a history of gastroesophageal reflux disease (GERD) may have a sore throat secondary to reflux of gastric contents.

Immunizations. Lack of immunization to diphtheria can place a person at risk for diphtheria.

DIAGNOSTIC REASONING: FOCUSED PHYSICAL EXAMINATION

Assess Degree of Illness

Assessment of the patient begins with general observation about the severity of illness. Severe illness, with signs of upper airway obstruction, such as restlessness, stridor, difficulty breathing, drooling, inability to swallow, and very high fever, signal epiglottitis and require immediate referral. Further examination could trigger laryngospasms and lead to airway obstruction.

Inspect the Mouth

Examine the buccal mucosa, tongue, and sublingual area for presence of ulcers. Note the location, number, size, and appearance of any lesions.

The lesions produced by the group A coxsackie virus (herpangina) first appear as small, grayish, papulovesicular lesions on the soft palate and pharynx. These progress to shallow ulcers, usually less than 5 mm in diameter.

Vincent's angina (necrotizing ulcerative gingivostomatitis) is a fusospirochetal infection of the gingiva. The gingiva appear inflamed and ulcerated, often covered with a gray slough. As the infection spreads, ulcers may appear on the oral mucosa and posterior pharnyx.

Aphthous stomatitis lesions affect about 20% of the general population and are associated with immunological mechanisms. They occur most often on the buccal mucosa, tongue, and soft palate. The lesions first appear as indurated papules and then progress to shallow ulcers. The ulcers have a yellow membrane and red halo.

Herpes simplex lesions involve the anterior oral mucosa and the gums. Herpetic pharyngitis is manifested by vesicles, ulcers, or exudate of the oral and pharyngeal mucosa. Specifically, the lesions involve the tonsils, pharynx, uvula, and edges of the soft palate. Vesicular lesions may or may not be intact.

Inspect the Posterior Pharynx and Observe Swallowing

Look for edema, color, exudate, presence, size (Table 2-2), and condition of the palatine tonsils. Good visualization is critical for accurate diagnosis. Use a good light source and ask the patient to open wide and say "ah" but not to protrude the tongue. If you cannot view the pharynx, depress the tongue firmly with a tongue blade, far enough back to get a good view but not enough to cause the patient to gag. Use two tongue depressors to retract tissues medially and laterally when examining areas such as the retromolar region and floor of the mouth and the orifices of Wharton and Stensen's ducts (Figure 2-4). The best visualization is achieved with a headlight.

Drooling may indicate peritonsillar abscess or epiglottitis partially occluding the pharynx and esophagus. Only occasionally can the red, swollen epiglottis be visualized above the base of the tongue. If you suspect epiglottitis, do not examine the pharynx because manipulation may precipitate laryngospasm and airway obstruction. Refer the patient immediately for specialist evaluation and further diagnosis that may involve soft tissue x-rays of the head and neck and laryngoscopy.

Table 2-2	
Grading Tonsillar Size	
GRADE	**TONSIL LOCATION**
1	Behind pillars
2	Between pillars and uvula
3	Touching the uvula
4	Extending beyond midline of the oropharynx

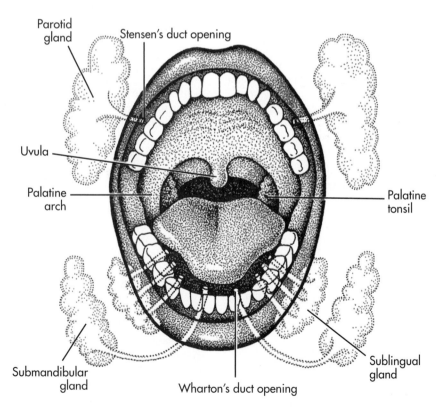

Figure 2-4 Anatomical structures of the mouth. (From Barkauskas VH et al: *Health and physical assessment,* ed 2, St. Louis, 1998, Mosby.)

Edema of the affected tonsil, with movement of the tonsil toward midline indicates peritonsillar abscess. Diphtheria may appear as a thick, gray tonsillar exudate or pseudomembrane, spreading to the tonsillar pillars, uvula, soft palate, posterior pharyngeal wall, and larynx. The exudate is not easily removable and bleeds easily.

Pharyngeal or tonsillar exudate can be present with either a bacterial or viral infection. A yellowish exudate of GABHS pharyngitis is often present. Generally the exudate of viral agents tends to be whiter than that from GABHS.

A bright red uvula and the presence of petechiae on the posterior pharnyx and palate indicates group A streptococcal pharyngitis. "Doughnut lesions" or red, raised hemorrhagic lesions with a yellow center are highly diagnostic of streptococcal pharyngitis.

Post-nasal drainage can irritate the posterior pharynx and should be observed for color. Purulent drainage that is yellow or greenish in color is associated with infectious sinusitis. White curdy patches that bleed on scraping are characteristic of oral candidiasis.

When examination reveals normal findings, suspect a systemic referred cause for the sore throat, particularly acute otitis media, sinusitis, or thyroiditis.

Palpate the Cervicofacial Lymph Nodes

In streptococcal pharyngitis, the anterior cervical lymph nodes are often enlarged and tender. In viral infections, posterior cervical nodes are more often enlarged. Lymphadenopathy is a cardinal sign of infectious mononucleosis, with over 90% of patients having enlarged posterior cervical nodes.

Inspect the Nasal Mucosa

Red swollen turbinates indicate an infectious process, while pale boggy turbinates indicate an allergic process. Presence of mucoid discharge occurs in allergic rhinitis. Purulent discharge suggests infectious sinusitis.

Inspect the Conjunctiva

Injected conjunctiva associated with a sore throat may indicate pharyngoconjunctival fever. It is caused by an adenovirus and is often associated with nonpurulent discharge, fever, and pharyngitis. It frequently occurs in epidemics. Mild conjunctivitis in the presence of itching eyes and with a clear watery discharge is associated with an allergic process.

Inspect the Tympanic Membrane

Evidence of otitis media with effusion may indicate nontypical *H. influenzae* acute otitis media (conjunctivitis-otitis syndrome). Earache can be caused by referred pain, especially from the tonsils.

Palpate the Thyroid

Acute thyroiditis is associated with a sore throat in the presence of a normal throat examination but with an enlarged and tender thyroid gland.

Inspect the Skin

Evidence of a fine maculopapular erythema that has a generalized distribution with accentuation in the skinfolds, circumoral pallor, and sparing of the palms and soles indicates scarlet fever. The rash characteristically is followed by a fine desquamation, starting at the hands.

Auscultate the Lungs

Mycoplasma pneumoniae is frequently associated with sore throat in adolescents and young adults. If pneumonia is present, palpation, percussion, and auscultation of the lungs will reveal an area of consolidation and adventitious breath sounds (see

Chapter 4 for further discussion of the lung examination).

Palpate the Abdomen

Splenomegaly is found in about half the cases of mononucleosis, although hepatomegaly is rare. GERD may be associated with palpable upper epigastric tenderness.

LABORATORY AND DIAGNOSTIC STUDIES

The laboratory evaluation of sore throat is generally limited to the identification of GABHS. Other infectious causes, such as gonorrhea or diphtheria, are rare and testing is done only if the history indicates exposure. The importance of diagnosing streptococcal pharyngitis is to treat it promptly with antibiotics, avoiding serious sequelae such as peritonsillar abscesses or rheumatic fever.

Rapid Screening Tests

A throat swab is a rapid screen for streptococcal antigens and should be done if GABHS is suspected. If it is positive, the patient is treated without follow-up cultures. If the swab is negative, a throat culture is obtained. The test has a sensitivity of 75% to 85% and a specificity of 95% to 98%.

The monospot is a rapid slide test that detects heterophil antibody agglutination; it is not specific for Epstein-Barr virus (EBV). It is most sensitive 1 to 2 weeks after symptoms appear and remains positive for up to 1 year. If chronic fatigue syndrome is being considered as a differential diagnosis, specific EBV antibody tests should be considered.

Culture

A throat culture to detect group A beta-hemolytic streptococcus is the "gold standard" of diagnosis, with a 10% or lower false negative rate. When obtaining a culture, first remove crusts from lesions, taking care to touch only the throat or tonsils with the sterile swab. Avoid touching the tongue. Roll the throat swab over one tonsil, proceed across the posterior pharynx, and then swab the other tonsil. A culture for gonorrhea can confirm a diagnosis of gonococcal pharnygitis.

ASO Titer

Group A beta-hemolytic streptococci produce enzymes that include streptolysin. An ASO titer is a serological test that detects the presence of a previous streptococci infection. This titer does not increase until 1 to 6 months post-infection so it is of no diagnostic value. It is used to aid in the diagnosis of streptococcal-associated infections, such as rheumatic fever, glomerulonephritis, and pericarditis. A caution, however, is that in as many as 50% of positive streptococcus cultures, an elevated ASO titer post-infection will not be found.

CBC with Differential

Test results that show 50% lymphocytes and at least 10% atypical lymphocytes confirm the diagnosis of mononucleosis.

CT Scan

Suspicion of an obstruction or swelling of the throat should be referred for further radiographic evaluation with a CT scan.

Nasal Smear

Nasal cytology can be performed on nasal secretions obtained by having the patient blow the nose into a paper or by using a cotton-tipped swab to obtain secretions from the nose. The presence of esosinophils on a nasal smear stained with Wright's stain viewed under a high-power microscope suggests an allergic, inflammatory process.

DIFFERENTIAL DIAGNOSIS

PHARYNGITIS WITHOUT ULCERS

Epiglottitis

Epiglottitis is caused by infection with *H. influenzae* type b that produces inflammation and edema of the epiglottis and the surrounding areas, obstructing the flow of air. The edematous epiglottis may be pulled into the larynx during inspiration and can completely occlude the airway. Symptoms are respiratory distress, sore throat, difficulty with secretions, drooling, pain on swallowing (seen in pediatric patients >2 years), and a toxic appearance. The infection occurs in both children and adults.

Peritonsillar/Retropharyngeal Abscess

A peritonsillar abscess, also called quinsy, is a collection of pus between the tonsil and the capsule of the tonsillar pillar. This condition occurs in children but is more common in adults, especially in persons with a history of recurrent tonsillitis. The patient usually presents with a history of respiratory symptoms, difficulty swallowing, otalgia, malaise, fever, and cervical lymphadenopathy. On examination there may be trismus, asymmetrical swelling of the uvula, tonsils, posterior pharynx, or a visible abscess.

Viral Pharyngitis

Most sore throats are caused by viral infections. Patients usually display systemic symptoms of malaise, fever, headache, cough, and fatigue. The pharynx is usually erythematous or it may be pale, boggy, and swollen. There is usually no tonsillar or pharyngeal exudate or tonsillar enlargement present, although infection with an adenovirus may produce pharyngeal exudate. The presence of concomitant upper respiratory symptoms such as cough and congestion makes the diagnosis of viral pharyngitis more likely than that of streptococcal. Common cold viruses cause sore throats most frequently during the colder months of the year.

Streptococcal Pharyngitis

The major differential diagnoses for sore throat will be viral or bacterial infection. Fewer than 10% of adults and 30% of children who seek care for sore throat symptoms have streptococcal tonsillopharyngitis. However, reliance on clinical impression to arrive at a specific diagnosis is problematic. The symptoms most likely to occur with streptococcal pharyngitis include a fever of 38.5° C (101.5° F) or higher, tonsillar exudate, anterior cervical adenopathy, and a history of recent exposure. Streptococcal pharyngitis increases from 10% in the summer and fall to 40% during the winter and early spring. GABHS cannot be reliably diagnosed on the basis of signs and symptoms, and, even when cultures are obtained, a causative agent may not be identified in 50% of patients. Table 2-3 shows the groups at risk for GABHS.

Mononucleosis

Mononucleosis causes about 5% of sore throats. It is most often a disease of young adults, and the causative agent is the Epstein-Barr virus in over 90% of cases. History reveals a gradual onset, low-grade temperature, mild sore throat, posterior cervical lymphadenopathy, and pronounced malaise and fatigue. Diagnosis can be confirmed with a positive monospot test and a CBC that reveals greater than 50% lymphocytosis. Splenomegaly occurs in about 50% of cases, while palatine petechiae are less common symptoms. GABHS occurs concomitantly in 10% to 20% of cases.

Gonococcal Pharyngitis

This is a fairly rare form of pharyngitis that can occur in patients who are at risk (i.e., those with a history of orogenital sexual activity). The patient may have

---

Table 2-3

Groups at Risk for Group A Beta-Hemolytic Streptococcus (GABHS) Pharyngitis

RISK FACTORS	DIAGNOSTIC TESTS
High Risk Tonsillar exudate Fever >38.5° C (101.5° F) Cervical lymphadenopathy Existing valvular rheumatic heart disease	None; treat on basis of risk factors
Presumed Strep Scarlet fever Strep epidemic Antibiotics already started	None; treat

Medium Risk
Exudate or nodes or fever
Prior rheumatic fever
"Low risk" by PE but:
   Young <25; with no URI
   Diabetic
   Recent "strep" exposure
	Rapid strep screen; if positive, treat; if negative, do culture; treat if culture positive; do not treat if culture negative

Low Risk No exudate or nodes or fever	Rapid strep screen; if positive, treat; if negative, do not culture; do not treat if culture negative

---

no symptoms. Examination shows an exudative pharyngitis with bilateral cervical lymphadenopathy. Diagnosis is confirmed through Gram staining or culture.

Inflammation

Inflammatory sore throat occurs in the presence of sinusitis or exposure to local irritants. The patient often complains of a post-nasal drip and allergic symptoms (itchy, watery eyes; runny nose). On examination, the patient may have sinus tenderness. The pharynx may be swollen or pale, and posterior drainage may be apparent. The patient has no fever or lymphadenopathy. Patients with allergies report symptoms that regularly follow seasonal patterns.

PHARYNGITIS WITH ULCERS

Herpangina

Herpangina is an infection caused by the coxsackie virus. The patient complains of a painful sore throat, fever, and malaise. Headache, anorexia, neck pain, abdomen and extremity pain may occur. Within 2 days of onset, small, grayish, papulovesicular lesions appear on the soft palate and pharynx. These progress to shallow ulcers, usually less than 5 mm in diameter. Outbreaks occur during summer months. Coxsackie virus peaks in August, September, and October, although some cases occur during the winter months. It is more common in children and in immunosuppressed patients. Diagnosis is based on symptoms and characteristic oral lesions. An antibody titer can confirm diagnosis.

Vincent's Angina

Vincent's angina is caused by a fusospirochetal infection that results in necrotizing ulcerative gingivostomatitis. Patients present with complaints of painful ulcers, foul breath, and bleeding gums. Without secondary infection, there is usually no fever. On examination, gray, necrotic ulcers without vesicles are apparent on the gingivae and interdental papillae. Gram staining shows spirochetes and confirms the diagnosis.

Aphthous Stomatitis

Aphthous stomatitis or "canker sores" appear as discrete ulcers without preceding vesicles. The ulcers are located on the inner lip, tongue, and buccal mucosa. Lesions last about 1 to 2 weeks. Etiology of the lesions is unknown, but immunological mechanisms play a major role.

Herpes Simplex

Herpes simplex virus (HSV) type 1 (can also include HSV type 2) is an infection manifested by fever, headache, sore throat, and lymphadenitis. Characteristic clusters of yellow vesicles appear on the palate, pharynx, and gingiva. Lesions last 2 to 3 weeks. Recurrent lesions are characterized by prodromal symptoms of burning, tingling, or itching. Active lesions are usually painful. Recent studies indicate that infections afflict about 20% to 45% of the U.S. population.

Candidiasis

Candidiasis is a yeast infection that produces white plaques over the tongue and oral mucosa with erythema; the plaques bleed when scraped. *Candida* infection occurs commonly in otherwise normal infants in the first weeks of life, in immunocompromised persons, including those with diabetes, and in persons taking antibiotics or using inhaled steroids.

Table 2-4

Differential Diagnosis of Common Causes of Sore Throat

Condition	History	Physical Findings	Diagnostic Studies
Pharyngitis Without Ulcers			
Epiglottitis	Sore throat, difficulty with secretions, odynophagia (seen in pediatric patients >2 years), unable to lie flat, can't talk	Respiratory distress, drooling, toxic appearance; DO NOT EXAMINE PHARYNX	Refer immediately
Peritonsillar/ retropharyngeal abscess	History of recurrent tonsillitis; sore throat, difficulty swallowing, respiratory symptoms, fever, malaise	Orthopnea, dyspnea, asymmetrical swelling, abscess, trismus	Refer immediately: CT scan; head and neck x-rays; laryngoscopy

Table 2-4

Differential Diagnosis of Common Causes of Sore Throat—cont'd

Condition	History	Physical Findings	Diagnostic Studies
Viral pharyngitis	Scratchy, sore throat, malaise, myalgias, head-ache, chills, cough, rhinitis	Erythema, edema of throat, tender posterior cervical nodes	None
Group A beta-hemolytic strep-tococcal pharyngitis	Most common in persons 5-15 years; known exposure; fall/winter season; sudden onset of fever, severe sore throat, and malaise; absence of cough and upper respiratory symptoms	Fever >38.5° C (101.5° F); exudate; anterior cervical lymph-adenopathy	Positive rapid strep antibody screen; strep culture
Mononucleosis (Epstein-Barr virus)	Young adults; slow onset of malaise, low-grade tem-perature, mild sore throat	±Pharyngeal exudate, pala-tine petechiae, posterior cervical lymphadenop-athy, spleno-megaly	Positive monospot; CBC with differ-ential; >50% leukocytes
Gonococcal pharyn-gitis	History of orogeni-tal sexual activ-ity; may be asymptomatic	Pharyngeal exu-date; bilateral cervical lymph-adenopathy	Gram stain; gonor-rhea culture
Inflammation	Exposure to irri-tants; post-nasal drip; allergic symptoms	Sinus tenderness, pale or swollen pharynx, post-nasal drainage visible, no fever or lymphade-nopathy	Esosinophils in nasal secretions with allergies

Continued

Table 2-4

Differential Diagnosis of Common Causes of Sore Throat—cont'd

Condition	History	Physical Findings	Diagnostic Studies
Pharyngitis With Ulcers			
Herpangina (coxsackie virus)	More common in children; immunosuppressed; painful throat; fever, malaise	Lymphadenopathy; small grayish papulovesicular lesions on the soft palate and pharynx, progressing to shallow ulcers, usually less than 5 mm in diameter	Serology
Fusospirochetal infection (Vincent's angina)	Poor oral hygiene; painful ulcers, foul breath, bleeding gums	Gray necrotic ulcers without vesicles on the gingival margins and interdental papillae	Gram stain reveals spirochetes
Aphthous stomatitis	Oral trauma, ill-fitting dentures; painful ulcers vary in size; absence of other symptoms	Shallow ulcers, no vesicles; indurated papules that progress to 1 cm ulcers; ulcer has yellow membrane and red halo; no fever or nodes	None
Herpes simplex infection	History of trauma to the mucosa; pain, fever, headache	Perioral lesions; lymphadenitis; vesicles on palate, pharynx, gingiva	Viral culture
Candidiasis	Immunosuppressed; persons on antibiotics or with diabetes; sore mouth/throat	Curdy white plaques that bleed when scraped off	KOH smear shows hyphae; culture

Nasal Symptoms and Sinus Congestion

Concern about symptoms of the "common cold" account for a significant proportion of primary care visits by both children and adults, especially in the winter months. Symptoms include nasal congestion, rhinorrhea, post-nasal drip, sneezing, itchy nose, watery and itchy eyes, and frontal headache. Severe symptoms are associated with aguesia (loss of taste) and anosmia (loss of smell).

The nose humidifies, warms, and filters inspired air. The nasal turbinates promote turbulent air flow that causes particulate matter to fall on the mucosa where it is swept away by ciliated psuedostratified columnar cells to the nasopharynx. Rhinitis, or inflammation of the mucous membranes, is a frequent nasal symptom and is caused by bacterial or viral infection, a response to allergens, or a response to medication or extremes in environmental temperature.

Nasal obstruction can be caused by nasal polyps, septal deviation, or congenital anomaly. In children, nasal obstruction is very frequently unilateral and may be secondary to a foreign body inserted into the nose.

Respiratory epithelium lines the paranasal sinuses and creates drainage into the nasal cavity via the superior meatus and middle meatus. The maxillary sinus is the most frequently involved paranasal sinus because its ciliated cells carry maxillary sinus drainage against gravity. When drainage systems become impaired as a result of mucosal edema, mechanical obstruction, or impaired ciliary activity, viruses and bacteria proliferate.

The paranasal sinuses include the frontal, ethmoid, maxillary, and sphenoid. Most sinus infections are caused by bacteria common to the nasopharynx that proliferate when local or systemic defenses are impaired. The most common causative organisms producing bacterial sinusitis in both adults and children are *Streptococcus pneumoniae* and *Hemophilus influenzae*. Sinusitis may also be associated with allergies and asthmatic exacerbations or with contiguous infection of the mouth or face.

DIAGNOSTIC REASONING: FOCUSED HISTORY

What are the primary symptoms that will help me narrow the possibilities?

Key Questions
- How long have these symptoms been present?
- Do you have a history of nasal or sinus problems?
- Do the symptoms occur at any particular time of the year or season?
- Is there a family history of allergies or asthma?
- Do you have other symptoms?

Acute symptoms. Acute symptoms of rhinitis or sinus congestion, usually lasting 48 to 72 hours, are caused by edematous mucosa obstructing the sinus ostia. If a person has no previous history of similar symptoms but has systemic symptoms such as fever, myalgias, and chills, acute infectious rhinitis caused by rhinoviruses or parainfluenza virus is likely.

Chronic symptoms. Chronic rhinitis lasting weeks to years is rarely infectious. Rather it is often associated with anatomical abnormalities that impair the sinus drainage system, although the mucociliary clearance mechanisms are normal.

Allergic symptoms. Suspect allergic rhinitis if a person describes nasal symptoms, associated with sneezing, wheezing, and itchy or burning eyes, that are a seasonal occurrence. A distinguishing feature of the allergic individual is the propensity to develop sustained IgE response following antigenic stimulation. IgE is an antibody capable of interacting with target cells that release mediators on contact with specific antigens. This reaction is the manifestation of an allergy.

Persons wth perennial allergies have the allergen present in the environment year round from sources such as animal dander, house dust, mold, feathers, and cockroaches. Seasonal allergies have three distinct seasons, early spring (tree pollens), early summer (grass pollens), and early fall (weed pollens). A family history of asthma or allergies is frequently associated with allergic rhinitis. Other symptoms may include a sensation of head stuffiness, ear discomfort, fatigue, and a scratchy or mild sore throat.

If I suspect sinus problems, what do I need to know?

Key Questions

- Do you have a history of sinus problems?
- Do you have pain? Please point to the areas.
- Do your symptoms change with position changes?
- How long have you had these symptoms?

Acute symptoms. Acute sinusitis is an abrupt onset of infection of one or more of the paranasal sinuses and occurs when the sinus ostia become obstructed usually after an upper respiratory infection. Sinusitis is frequently associated with a sore throat often irritated by post-nasal discharge, facial or tooth pain, headache over the affected sinus, as well as morning periorbital swelling, fever, and malaise. Other less common causes include anatomical abnormality, adenoid hypertrophy, or contiguous infection, such as a dental abscess or periorbital cellulitis.

Location of pain. An adult patient with sinusitis most often complains of a prolonged cold with symptoms of nasal congestion and facial pain. Children rarely complain of headache or facial pain. The location of pain may indicate which sinus is involved. Pain of maxillary sinusitis occurs over the sinuses and is sometimes perceived as a maxillary toothache. Frontal sinusitis produces a frontal headache that is worse on morning wakening. Ethmoid sinusitis causes pain that refers to the vertex, forehead, occipital or temporal region, while the pain of sphenoid sinusitis is perceived on the top of the head.

Position change. Maxillary sinusitis produces pain that worsens with bending or leaning forward. The post-nasal discharge associated with sinusitis produces a cough that worsens while lying down.

Chronic symptoms. In children chronic sinusitis is defined as the presence of symptoms for more than 30 days. The cause can be prolonged obstruction of the osteomeatal complex, which leads to dysfunction of ciliary motility and movement of mucus within the sinuses. Local factors causing mechanical obstruction include adenoid hypertrophy, conchas bullosa, nasal polyps, foreign bodies, and nasal deviations.

Do associated symptoms provide any clues?

Key Questions

- Do you have other acute symptoms such as cough, fever, muscle aches?
- Do you have other chronic symptoms, such as eye pain, bad breath, fatigue?

Other acute symptoms. Acute bacterial infection of the nasal and sinus mucosa is characterized by the presence of purulent nasal discharge. Acute rhinitis caused by a bacterial or viral infection produces systemic symptoms such as fever, myalgia, and chills.

Allergic rhinitis is associated with sneezing, nasal congestion, clear and profuse rhinorrhea, and pruritis of the nose, palate, pharynx, and middle ear. Eye complaints include conjunctival irritation, itching, erythema, and tearing. Ear complaints involve a feeling of fullness in the ears with popping. Sinus complaints are pressure and/or pain of the cheeks, forehead, or behind the eyes.

Acute sinusitis in children involves the presence of symptoms for less than 30 days, a persistent cough, fever >39° C (102.2° F) for longer than 3 days, and malodorous breath. The maxillary and ethmoid sinuses are most commonly affected, with occasionally the frontal sinus and rarely the sphenoid sinus.

Chronic symptoms. Chronic sinusitis involves long episodes of inflammation or repeated infections that lead to anatomical destruction. The recurrent symptoms interfere with daily activities and are not relieved with nonpharmacological measures or over-the-counter medications. Patients often complain about a cold that doesn't go away, eye pain, halitosis, chronic cough, fatigue, anorexia, malaise, and low-grade fever.

Is it viral or bacterial?

Key Questions
- What color is your nasal drainage?
- How long have you had these symptoms?

Acute rhinitis caused by a bacterial or viral infection produces yellow or green purulent nasal discharge. Watery or clear discharge occurs with allergic reactions. Symptoms of viral upper respiratory infections in children persist 5 to 10 days, then gradually subside. Many children may have up to eight colds per year.

Are symptoms unilateral or bilateral?

Key Question
- Is the symptom on one side or both sides?

Infectious and allergic rhinitis are usually bilateral. Unilateral symptoms are more indicative of an anatomical cause, such as nasal polyps, septal deviation, or a foreign body, in a child.

Are there risk factors that will narrow the diagnosis?

Key Questions
- Do you smoke?
- Are you exposed to others who smoke?
- Do you have any other health problems?
- Have you had a recent history of head or facial trauma?
- Have you been diving or swimming?
- Have you been exposed to infections in day care, school, or work settings?
- Are you pregnant?

Smoking history. Smokers have an increased risk of sinusitis. Smoking can lead to production of more tenacious mucus and lead to temporary paralysis of the nasal cilia. Exposure to passive smoke causes an increased risk of upper and lower respiratory tract infections.

Trauma history. Nasal trauma or fracture will lead to nasal congestion. A rare but serious post-trauma cerebrospinal fluid rhinorrhea can be present. Up to 80% of head injuries involve the paranasal sinuses.

Diving, swimming. Sinusitis from diving or swimming is secondary to barotrauma, infection from contaminated water, or an allergic response to chlorine.

Exposure. Exposure to viral infections increases when children are exposed to other children. The spread of a virus is by direct secretion of droplets or by contaminated wet objects.

Pregnancy. The hormonal changes of pregnancy can cause nasal congestion.

Is the patient using any drugs that would cause nasal congestion?

Key Questions
- Are you using nasal sprays or drops?
- Do you use cocaine or other drugs?
- What other medications are you taking?

Nasal spray. Use of topical sympathomimetic sprays or drops for more than a week can lead to rebound nasal congestion or vasodilation after short periods of vasoconstriction. Use of decongestants and antihistamines with low ambient humidity leads to excessive dryness and impaired ciliary function.

Drug use. Chronic or acute cocaine use can also cause rebound nasal congestion. Nasal congestion associated with conjunctivitis and irritation of the eyes may be seen in persons who abuse drugs by inhalation.

Medications. Oral contraceptives, phenothiazines, angiotensin-converting enzyme (ACE) inhibitors, and beta-blockers may cause nasal congestion.

Is there systemic disease present?

Key Questions
- Have you noticed any other general body symptoms?
- Do you have any chronic health problems?

Systemic disorders. Systemic causes of decreased mucociliary clearance include cystic fibrosis, ciliary dyskinesia syndrome, or immunoglobulin deficiency. Persons with congenital or acquired immune deficiencies, such as diabetes mellitus, leukemia, AIDS, and cystic fibrosis, have an increased risk of developing acute and chronic sinusitis. Hypothyroidism, acromegaly, Horner's syndrome, neoplasm, and granulomatous disorder can also cause nasal symptoms.

DIAGNOSTIC REASONING: FOCUSED PHYSICAL EXAMINATION

Perform a General Inspection

Note general appearance. Observe for signs of impaired mental status. A severe unremitting or new-onset headache, vomiting, or alteration in consciousness requires consideration for immediate referral.

Take Vital Signs

Persons with acute viral rhinitis or acute sinusitis may be afebrile or have low-grade fever. Persons with allergic rhinitis are afebrile. The presence of mouth breathing suggests chronic nasal obstruction caused by hypertrophied pharyngeal lymphoid tissues.

Inspect the Face

Children with chronic allergic conditions have an allergic "salute." This is a crease on the nose from continued wiping up of nasal drainage. Allergic "shiners" are dark circles under the eyes suggestive of venous congestion and stasis. Observe for facial symmetry and signs of periorbital edema. Periorbital cellulitis is the most common serious complication of severe bacterial sinusitis.

Perform a Regional Examination of the Head and Neck

Examine the eyes (including visual acuity), ears, and cervicofacial lymph nodes. Complications of severe fulminate sinusitis are rare and are caused by direct spread of infection, secondary to destruction of the wall between the sinuses and the orbit. Symptoms can include a sudden increase in pain, acute edema of the eyelids, periorbital edema and erythema, decreased visual acuity, diplopia, and displacement of the eye laterally. The patient may experience pain on testing of extraocular muscles (EOMs). These symptoms mandate immediate referral.

Observe for symptoms of coryza as well as ear and eye drainage. Erythematous tympanic membranes are seen in acute viral rhinitis.

Examine the Mouth and Teeth

Examine the teeth for the presence of abscesses, especially the first and secondary maxillary molars and the alveolar margin of the teeth. Tenderness elicited by tapping on the maxillary teeth with a tongue blade may indicate dental root infection or maxillary sinusitis. Mouth breathing is associated with hypertrophied gingival mucosa and halitosis.

Children with acute viral rhinitis have mild erythema of the tonsils and posterior pharynx. If there is vasomotor rhinitis, mucus is present in the posterior pharynx.

Inspect Condition of Nasal Mucosa and Turbinates

Test for smell. Severe nasal congestion or ethmoid sinusitis causes anosmia. Use a nasal speculum and head mirror to optimally visualize the condition of the nasal mucosa and turbinates. A topical vasoconstrictive agent may be needed to shrink the swollen mucosa to visualize the middle meatus.

In infants and young children, the nares tend to open forward, and simply tilting the tip of the nose up with the thumb and directing the light into the nares will allow inspection of the nasal cavities.

Pale, boggy turbinates are seen with allergic rhinitis. Inflamed mucous membranes are seen with acute coryza or hay fever. Allergic rhinitis may also produce a violet-colored mucous membrane. Ulceration of the nasal mucosa may be

found in persons who abuse drugs by inhalation.

Inspect for Masses

Observe for presence of nasal polyps, which look like skinned grapes and are usually bilateral and hang from the middle turbinate into the lumen of the nose. Septal deviation or anatomical anomalies may predispose to infection. Nasal septum deviation can also lead to nasal obstruction. A squamous cell carcinoma usually occurs unilaterally. Masses that increase in size and pulsate on Valsalva may indicate an encephalocele or meningocele.

Note for Presence and Color of Any Discharge

Pus in the ostium of the middle turbinate suggests a bacterial sinusitis. Cerebrospinal fluid drainage will increase in a forward position. Identify cerebrospinal fluid (CSF) by testing nasal drainage for glucose and protein levels comparable to CSF. Foul-smelling nasal discharge is a characteristic feature of sinusitis of dental origin.

Transilluminate the Sinuses

Light will pass through air-filled sinuses. Transillumination is used to assess presence of fluid in the frontal and maxillary sinuses and cannot be used to examine the ethmoid or sphenoid sinuses. Normal transillumination of the frontal sinus rules out frontal sinusitis in 90% of cases. Complete opacity of sinuses suggests infection. However, results of transillumination are often nonspecific, such as reduced illumination, and do not lead to a diagnosis.

Transillumination of maxillary sinuses can be done two ways. Place a transilluminator over the infraorbital rim, blocking light from the examiner's vision with the free hand, and judge the amount of light transmission (opaque, dull, normal) through the hard palate. This should be performed in a completely darkened room. Dentures must be removed. A second method is to place the transilluminator in the patient's mouth, sealing the lips, and observe the amount of light transmitted through the maxillary sinuses. Frontal sinuses can be transilluminated by placing the instrument below the supraorbital rim.

Palpate and Percuss Frontal and Maxillary Sinuses for Tenderness

Percuss and palpate the cheeks for tenderness and swelling, indicating maxillary sinusitis of dental origin. Gentle pressure on the floor of the sinuses beside the nose may cause severe pain in frontal sinusitis. Direct percussion may elicit tenderness over the affected sinus.

Test for Facial Fullness and Pressure

Bending forward from the waist (with head dropping downward) or performing a Valsalva maneuver will worsen the symptoms if a partial or complete sinus obstruction is present.

Examine the Lungs

Auscultate the lungs for signs of wheezing, rales, and loudness of breath sounds. Peak flow volume or pO_2 saturation using a pulse oximeter will detect the presence of reactive upper airway disease.

Perform Neurological Testing If Indicated

Assess neurological and cranial nerve function if the patient appears severely ill to detect any complications from sinusitis. Severe complications of sinusitis are cavernous sinus thrombosis and brain abscesses.

LABORATORY AND DIAGNOSTIC STUDIES

Nasal Smear

A nasal smear done to detect for eosinophils confirms the diagnosis of allergic rhinitis. Nasal scraping of the surface epithelium along with a sample of secretions is more reliable in detecting the presence of eosinophils than is sampling secretions alone. Either method can be used to detect the presence of neutrophils. Specimens are graded using a semiquantitative scale of 0 to 4+, based on the concentration of cells. Table 2-5 illustrates the diagnostic classifications found with varying nasal smears.

Sinus X-Rays

X-rays are not routinely indicated but may be done in patients who have severe symptoms, fail to respond to treatment, or have chronic and recurrent sinusitis. Severe symptoms may indicate complications of sinusitis, such as orbital cellulitis, brain abscess, osteomyelitis, or cavernous sinus thrombosis.

A sinus radiographic series consists of four views that include an anteroposterior (Caldwell) view of the ethmoid sinus, a view (Chamberlain) of the frontal sinus, a lateral view of the sphenoid and frontal sinuses, and an occipitomental (Waters) view of the maxillary sinuses. The series is up to 96% as accurate as aspiration and culture for diagnosing maxillary sinusitis. A single Waters view is the most commonly ordered view. Figure 2-5 (see p. 36) illustrates the three radiographic views of the maxillary, ethmoid, and frontal sinuses.

Abnormal mucosal thickening will show up on radiographs when chronic sinusitis is present. Findings of partial or complete opacification of a sinus, air-fluid levels, or mucosal thickening greater than 5 mm suggests sinusitis. False-negative x-rays are more likely in the early stages of a sinus infection. Sinus x-rays will also reveal osteomyelitis or

Table 2-5

Diagnostic Classifications of Nasal Smear Specimens

NASAL SMEAR	DIAGNOSTIC CLASSIFICATION
Increased eosinophils	Allergic or nonallergic eosinophilia; aspirin intolerance
Increased basophils	Same as above; nonallergic basophilia
Increased neutrophils	
With intracellular bacteria	Nasopharyngitis; sinusitis
With ciliary tophthoria	Viral upper respiratory infection (URI)
With fungi	Fungal URI
With no bacteria	Irritant reaction
Bacteria (2-4+)—intracellular	Nasopharyngitis or sinusitis
No eosinophils or basophils, 2+ or fewer neutrophils, few bacteria	Normal finding

From Mygind N, Naderio R: *Allergic and non-allergic rhinitis*, Copenhagen, Denmark, 1993, Munksgaard International Publishers.

squamous cell carcinoma of the maxillary sinus.

Computed Tomography (CT) Scan

CT scan shows air, bone, and soft tissue and optimally facilitates definition of regional anatomy and the extent of disease. CT scan is done when sinusitis becomes chronic and does not respond to symptomatic or antibiotic treatment.

Sinus Aspiration

Sinus aspiration is the only way to confirm the diagnosis of bacterial sinusitis and is performed by an otolaryngologist. A trochar is introduced into the maxillary sinus through the upper gingival recess.

Allergy Skin Testing

Results of skin testing can confirm immunological disease and identify specific antigens responsible for allergic rhinitis, which may come from exposure to irritants in the patient's environment. Presence of serum IgE antibody suggests an allergic response.

DIFFERENTIAL DIAGNOSIS

Infectious Rhinitis

Infectious rhinitis is an acute condition frequently associated with a history of recent URI. A definitive sign of this condition is the presence of yellow or green purulent discharge and red nasal mucosa.

Allergic Rhinitis

Allergic rhinitis is distinguished by a recurrent rhinorrhea with clear watery mucus, sneezing, and pruritis. Nasal turbinates are pale and swollen. Family history of allergies is often positive. About 25% of the population has some type of allergy. IgE-mediated reactions to aeroallergens are based on a combination of history, physical examination, and skin tests. Nasal smears can be tested for the presence of eosinophils to confirm an allergenic response.

Seasonal allergies are associated with short bursts of intense exposure to an allergen that creates symptoms consistent with a histamine-mediated response, such as pruritis, swelling, sneezing, and rhinorrhea. A common seasonal allergy is polli-

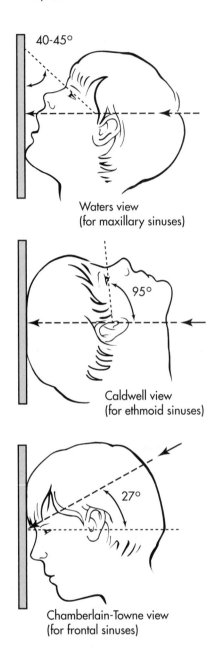

Waters view
(for maxillary sinuses)

Caldwell view
(for ethmoid sinuses)

Chamberlain-Towne view
(for frontal sinuses)

Figure 2-5   Radiographic views of the maxillary, ethmoid, and frontal sinuses. (Modified from Reilly BM: *Practical strategies in outpatient medicine,* ed 2, Philadelphia, 1991, WB Saunders.)

nosis or hay fever. A history or pattern of symptoms and exposure is critical in diagnosis.

Perennial allergies are caused by continuous exposure to allergens associated with chronic congestion. Common indoor allergens are animal dander, dust mites, and cockroaches. Outdoor allergens often include grasses, trees, pollens, and weeds.

Non-Allergic Rhinitis

Non-allergic rhinitis can be associated with or without eosinophilia on nasal smear. Non-allergic rhinitis with eosinophilia syndrome (NARES) is a diagnosis based on nasal cytology and involves symptoms similar to allergic rhinitis without an identifiable allergen cause. A history will reveal aspirin or NSAID intolerance and rhinorrhea. Non-eosinophilia is associated with any other non-allergic cause of rhinitis.

Rhinitis Medicamentosus

A drug-induced rebound congestion can follow long-term use of topical nasal decongestants. Rhinitis medicamentosus is also used to describe nasal symptoms secondary to other medications, such as nasal congestion associated with hormone changes of pregnancy. Other drugs that have vasodilatory effects include antihypertensives that interfere with adrenergic neuronal function and hormones in oral contraceptives. Nasal vasoconstriction response is completely abolished after administration of reserpine.

Acute Sinusitis

Acute sinusitis is characterized by purulent nasal discharge, post-nasal drip, and localized facial pain over the sinus involved. It often follows a viral URI. However, symptoms such as halitosis, reduced sense of smell, or morning cough have been reported in children in the absence of facial pain. Physical examination will elicit localized tenderness to palpation or percussion over the affected sinus. Pressure and pain will increase in a forward-bending position. Purulent discharge may be visible in the posterior pharynx or may be seen coming from the ostia of the middle turbinate. Transillumination will indicate unilateral or bilateral obstruction. Ciliary function is impaired with infection and may not be completely restored for 2 to 6 weeks. Diagnosis of sinusitis in children requires two major criteria (cough, purulent nasal discharge, or purulent pharyngeal drainage), or one major and two minor criteria (sore throat, wheezing, foul breath, facial pain, periorbital edema, headache, earache, fever, and toothache).

Chronic Sinusitis

An incompletely treated acute sinusitis can lead to a chronic condition. The patient presents with persistent symptoms of low-grade infection and intermittent acute exacerbations typical of acute sinusitis. Symptoms are recurrent and not controlled with over-the-counter or nonpharmacological remedies. Multiple pathogens may be causative organisms, with the most common being *M. catarrhalis*, *H. influenzae*, and *S. pneumoniae*. Sinus x-rays or CT scan will reveal mucosal thickening of 5 mm or greater. Allergy testing may reveal a perennial allergy that creates chronic inflammation.

Nasal or Sinus Obstruction

A history of aspirin intolerance or asthma with polyps is associated with obstruction. Acute obstruction suggests edema secondary to infection, allergic response, exposure to irritants, or foreign body in children. Chronic obstruction may be secondary to congenital deformity, nasal polyps, or septal deviation. In infants, congenital choanal atresia can cause obstruction.

Nasal Polyposis

This syndrome has multiple causative factors, including a history of asthma and aspirin intolerance. The polyps are translucent grapelike growths that are mobile, rarely bleed, and prolapse into the nasal cavity. The resulting obstruction can be associated with chronic sinusitis. Any suspicious polyps should be biopsied.

Osetomyelitis of the Frontal Bone

Osteomyelitis can occur as a complication of sinusitis. Osteomyelitis occurs in children and young adults and may follow head trauma or scuba diving. *Staphylococcus pyogenes* or anaerobic streptococcus are causative organisms. Patients appear severely ill and may have edema of the upper eyelid and puffy swelling over the frontal bone. Diagnosis is by x-ray and blood culture.

Table 2-6

Differential Diagnoses of Common Causes of Nasal Symptoms and Sinus Congestion

Condition	History	Physical Findings	Diagnostic Studies
Infectious rhinitis	Perennial but more common in winter months; recent URI	Red, swollen mucosa; purulent discharge	Nasal smear for neutrophils, intracellular bacteria

Continued

Table 2-6

Differential Diagnoses of Common Causes of Nasal Symptoms and Sinus Congestion—cont'd

Condition	History	Physical Findings	Diagnostic Studies
Allergic rhinitis	Family history of allergies; sneezing; recurrent pattern; more common in children and young adults	Pale, boggy mucosa; rhinorrhea with clear, watery mucus	Nasal smear for eosinophils; allergy testing
Non-allergic rhinitis	No allergenic cause identified	Similar to allergic rhinitis	Absence of eosinophilia on nasal cytology
Rhinitis medicamentosus	History of medication use: oral contraceptives, nasal sprays, antihypertensives; nasal congestion	Swollen mucosa; clear mucus or dry mucosa	None
Acute sinusitis	Smoker; recent URI; winter months; frontal headaches made worse with forward bending; sensation of fullness or pressure	Purulent discharge; maxillary toothache on percussion; postnasal drainage; decreased transillumination	Sinus x-rays (Waters view)
Chronic sinusitis	History of previous sinus infections; dull ache or no pain; persistent symptoms	Same as above; decreased or no transillumination; obstruction such as deviated septum, polyps	Sinus x-rays; sinus aspiration and culture
Obstruction	History of asthma, aspirin intolerance; foreign body in children; tumor in adults; infants with choanal atresia: difficulty feeding; cyanosis if bilateral	Increased pain with forward motion or Valsalva; pain with percussion and palpation of sinuses; no transillumination; septal deviation	Sinus x-rays; CT scan
Nasal polyposis	History of asthma, aspirin intolerance	Presence of polyps	May require biopsy
Osteomyelitis of the frontal bone	History of head trauma, diving	Appear severely ill; periorbital and frontal edema	Sinus and skull x-ray; blood culture

Hoarseness

Hoarseness is a disturbance of the normal voice pitch by processes that affect the structure or function of the vocal cords. It is a term used to describe an unnaturally rough, harsh, or deep voice. Voice is the sound produced when the vocal folds are approximated, and expired airflow between the cords causes them to vibrate. The sound produced by the larynx is amplified by the pharynx, oral cavity, sinuses, and nasal cavity and is modified by movements of the tongue, uvula, and soft palate. Hoarseness may be an early sign of local disease or a manifestation of a systemic illness. Hoarseness is a cardinal symptom for laryngeal disease.

The larynx includes the glottis, or true vocal cords, the supraglottic area that includes the vestibular folds (false vocal cords), arytenoids, aryepiglottic folds, and the laryngeal surface of the epiglottis. It separates the upper from the lower respiratory tract and, therefore, may be affected by disease from above or from below. Many benign conditions cause hoarseness, such as functional disorders from voice overuse. Functional causes are unrelated to organic disease and may have a psychosocial component, such as restraint in expressing anger, or crying, or a history of psychological trauma.

However, persistent hoarseness for more than 3 weeks in an adult and 1 week in a child may indicate secondary changes to the vocal cords. These changes may be caused by structural changes resulting from palsies, polyps, cysts; laryngeal neoplasm; or congenital disorders of the larynx. Hoarseness may also be a symptom of systemic disease, such as hypothyroidism or a symptom of inflammation caused by a variety of processes. Many forms of laryngitis that appear alike on physical examination may have very different causes. Critical clues to the specific etiology for laryngitis depend on a careful history.

DIAGNOSTIC REASONING: FOCUSED HISTORY

Is the hoarseness acute or chronic?

Key Questions
- How long has the symptom been present?
- Has this happened before? Is it recurrent?
- Is it getting worse?

Duration. Symptoms of less than 3 weeks' duration are considered to be acute; the most likely etiology is a viral upper respiratory infection. Inflammation secondary to acute viral infection or voice overuse are the most common causes of acute laryngitis. Chronic symptoms suggest structural change in the larynx or hoarseness secondary to disorders such as gastroesophageal reflux disease (GERD) or systemic disease. If the duration of hoarseness is longer than 3 weeks, referral to an ENT specialist is indicated to evaluate for neoplasm, most often squamous cell carcinoma, since chronic laryngitis is rarely of infectious etiology.

Recurrence. Recurrent episodes of hoarseness may indicate allergies or sinusitis with post-nasal drip.

Progression. Progressive hoarseness usually indicates a lesion such as laryngeal or hypopharyngeal cyst.

What does the onset of hoarseness tell me?

Key Questions
- How did the hoarseness develop?
- Did it come on suddenly or gradually?
- Is there any history of trauma to the throat?
- Have you had any recent surgery around the throat or neck?

Onset. In children, hoarseness of acute onset is usually the result of infection or trauma. The trauma can be from direct injury (foreign body, accidents) or overuse from screaming. The overuse can be gradual, resulting in progressive hoarseness and vocal cord changes. This hoarseness is worse in the afternoon or evening. Hoarseness from birth may indicate a congenital problem, such as laryngeal web, cyst, palsy, or angioma. Newborns with aphonia or a hoarse cry that does not resolve may have a congenital anomaly, papilloma, or vocal cord paralysis.

Trauma. External trauma to the throat is a rare cause of hoarseness but can result in hematoma formation in the laryngeal soft tissues. There can also be mucosal lacerations, arytenoid cartilage dislocation, or fracture of the laryngeal cartilage. Internal trauma can occur with intubation associated with surgery, when a tracheostomy tube catches on laryngeal structures and is pushed against resistance.

Surgical history. Tonsillectomy, thyroidectomy, or rhinoplasty can alter the quality of the voice secondary to structural change and scarring. Cardiac surgery has also been cited as a cause of injury when the vagus nerve (CN X) is damaged in its course around the aorta.

Does the presence of risk factors help narrow the diagnosis?

Key Questions
- Have you had a recent cold or upper respiratory infection (URI)?
- Do you have allergies or asthma?
- Do you smoke? For how long?
- How much alcohol do you drink?
- Describe your voice habits, such as singing, talking, shouting.
- Are you frequently exposed to dust, fumes, or loud noise?
- Are your immunizations up to date?

Upper respiratory infection (URI). Acute laryngitis, epiglottitis, and acute laryngotracheobronchitis (croup) are sequelae from a viral URI that can result in vocal cord inflammation. Post-nasal discharge that is thick and purulent may pool around the larynx and cause chronic secondary edema. Nasal congestion that leads to mouth breathing produces laryngeal dryness, with resultant hoarseness on arising in the morning.

Children who have epiglottitis are not hoarse, but, as the epiglottis swells, the voice becomes muffled and drooling is observed.

Allergies and asthma. Poorly controlled or undiagnosed asthma can result in a chronic cough with subsequent hoarseness. Allergies can cause chronic or recurrent irritation and swelling of both the upper and lower airways. Children who have a history of allergies can develop vocal cord edema and inflammation and hoarseness.

Smoking. Cigarette smoking is the most significant risk factor for laryngeal cancer. Smoking is also a risk factor for acute or chronic laryngitis because smoke irritates all mucous membranes and impairs ciliary function, causing pooling of secretions around the larynx.

Alcohol consumption. Chronic consumption of hard liquor is a direct irritant to the throat and is associated with laryngeal cancer.

Voice habits. Voice misuse occurs when the true vocal cords are forced to vibrate under undue stress and tension. Voice abuse is exuberant overuse and can lead to inflammation of the larynx and edema, hemorrhage, or vocal cord polyps. A gradual progression of hoarseness may go unnoticed by the patient. Often a precipitating incident produces acute laryngitis, such as shouting, excessive speaking, or singing. Specific questions may need to be asked to make the patient aware of conditions that lead to voice abuse, such as:
- Have others noticed a change in the quality of your voice?

- Do you talk frequently to persons who are hard of hearing?
- Do you yell at children?
- Do you work in an environment that is noisy or contains dust or fumes?
- Have you attended a recent sporting event?

Exposures. Patients who are chronically exposed to work environments that contain dust, fumes, or a high noise level that leads to chronic voice abuse are at increased risk for laryngeal cancer.

Immunizations. Laryngeal diphtheria should be considered in patients who have failed to update their diphtheria immunization. Updating the tetanus-diphtheria (Td) immunization is recommended every 10 years after the primary immunization series is completed. Laryngeal diphtheria usually develops as a downward progression of the tonsillar-pharyngeal membrane.

What other clues will help narrow the diagnostic possibilities?

Key Questions
- Does the hoarseness change during the day?
- Is it painful?
- What other symptoms are present?
- Do you have a neurological disorder?

Timing. Hoarseness that is altered by a position change suggests a mobile lesion such as a pedunculated polyp. Patients with myasthenia gravis have a normal voice in the morning with progressive hoarseness throughout the day.

Pain. Pain may be associated with an inflammatory process, such as a viral URI or GERD. Pain occurs late in laryngeal cancer. Neurological and hormonal causes do not usually produce pain.

Associated symptoms. The presence of cough, shortness of breath, weight loss, dysphagia, ear pain, or throat pain should raise concerns about neoplasm, systemic disease, or neurological causes. Hormonal disorders, such as hypothyroidism, will also produce signs and symptoms that vary in severity, according to the duration and degree of hormone deficiency. Early symptoms of hypothyroidism include cold intolerance, heavy menses, weight gain, dry skin, fatigue, and constipation. Later signs and symptoms include hoarseness, very dry skin, hair loss of lateral eyebrows, and neurological symptoms such as delayed deep tendon reflex (DTR) recovery, depression, and mental confusion.

Neurological disease. Patients with Parkinson's disease, myasthenia gravis, or amyotrophic lateral sclerosis have progressive dysarthria and dysphagia. As neurological disease progresses, patients will develop a chronic cough and throat clearing caused by microaspiration of pooled secretions.

Gastroesophageal reflux disease (GERD). Reflux of gastric contents causes inflammation of the posterior larynx, especially the arytenoid mucosa. The patient may also report a habit of frequent throat clearing and a sensation of a lump in the throat. Chronic cough or throat clearing further damages already irritated vocal folds. In children, GERD presents with dysphagia, vomiting, and failure to thrive.

DIAGNOSTIC REASONING: FOCUSED PHYSICAL EXAMINATION

Listen to the Quality of Voice

Acoustic evaluation criteria for voice include range (monotonal to extremely variable), loudness (soft to loud), pitch (low-pitched voice requires more effort to produce adequate volume; also sudden changes in pitch), register (temporary loss

Table 2-7		
Criteria Used in Evaluating Voice		
ACOUSTIC QUALITY	**MEASUREMENT**	**DISORDER**
Range	Monotonal to extremely variable	Monotonal: Parkinson's disease, depression
Loudness	Soft to loud	Environmental, psychological, systemic disease
Pitch	Low to high; glottal, raspy to falsetto	Variable: puberty Low: male gender, overuse
Register	Presence of voice	Vocal fatigue, overuse
Quality	Breathy to resonant	Vocal cord mass, paresis, bowing, atrophy

of voice because of abductor spasm), and quality (roughness, breathiness, and hoarseness). Table 2-7 lists common criteria used in evaluating the voice.

Examine the Respiratory System

If the patient is able to cough and laugh but cannot speak, this indicates a functional problem since coughing and laughing require total adduction of the vocal cords. Auscultate the lungs for quality of breath sounds, asthmatic wheezing, and signs of consolidation.

Perform a General Inspection

Note hair distribution, especially signs of hair loss over lateral eyebrows and hair loss on scalp, to assess thyroid function. Look for the placement of the trachea and thyroid gland. Bulges or asymmetry of the neck suggest a tumor. A head and neck hemangioma or lymphangioma increase the possibility of a similar laryngeal lesion as the source of hoarseness.

Examine the Head and Neck

Examine the oral, pharyngeal, and nasal mucosa for signs of excessive dryness, inflammation, or infection. Excessive mucosal dryness, including the conjunctiva, may be secondary to medication use, such as decongestants and antidepressants, or may be a symptom of an autoimmune disorder such as Sjogren's syndrome.

Otoscopy may point out otitis media with effusion, contributing to hearing loss, a factor to be considered in voice abuse. Inspect the nasal mucosa for color, edema, purulent discharge, and the nasal septa for deviation that may cause obstruction. Hypertrophic tonsils and severe dental abnormalities (malocclusion, cleft palate) can contribute to hoarseness.

Any indication of airway obstruction associated with hoarseness is a potentially life-threatening situation. Do not perform a physical examination of the pharynx if you suspect acute epiglottitis. Examination may trigger laryngeal spasm and airway obstruction. Refer immediately for emergency treatment and airway support.

Examine the larynx indirectly using a laryngeal mirror. Patient cooperation is critical. Ask the patient to open the mouth wide and extend the neck while protruding the tongue. The mirror is advanced to contact and lift the uvula while the patient breathes through the mouth. Focus the light on the mirror after the mirror is angled to visualize the larynx. Ask the patient to say "e" or "a" to observe movement. Sometimes the epiglottis obscures visualization. Direct examination of the larynx with a laryngoscope requires the skill and experience of a specialist.

Observe the larynx for presence of secretions, evidence of ulcers, polyps, masses, edema, or redness. Observe for vocal cord motion, especially adduction and abduction of vocal cords, and presence of spasm or tremor.

Assess Cranial Nerve Function

Most of the cranial nerves (CN) play a part in speech and voice production, and any disease process that affects neurological function, especially vocal cord paralysis, may affect the voice. Specifically examine CN V, VII, VIII, IX, X, XI, and XII.

Assess Hearing (CN VIII)

Voice or whisper testing for hearing acuity is the first level of hearing screening. An audible whisper is approximately 20 dB and normal speech is about 50 dB. Patients with neurosensory hearing loss may use abnormally loud speech.

Palpate Lymph Nodes

Palpate cervicofacial lymph nodes. Tender nodes indicate inflammation; non-tender nodes may indicate neoplasm. Enlarged nodes in the deep cervical chain in the absence of other symptoms may indicate laryngeal cancer.

Palpate Thyroid

Palpate the thyroid for size, tenderness, and crepitus by moving the thyroid cartilage across the cervical spine.

LABORATORY AND DIAGNOSTIC STUDIES

Flexible Fiberoptic Laryngoscopy

Laryngoscopy allows direct examination of the hypopharynx and larynx. Local anesthesia is applied to the oral or nasal mucosa, and the instrument is passed through the nose or oral cavity for excellent visualization of laryngeal structures. Laryngoscopy is also performed under general anesthesia.

X-Rays

Lateral view x-rays of soft tissues of the neck are used to evaluate structures for abnormality.

Barium Esophogram With Fluoroscopy

This contrast endoscopic technique can be used to detect gastroesophageal reflux.

DIFFERENTIAL DIAGNOSIS

Acute Laryngitis

Acute laryngitis is a self-limiting condition caused by a viral infection, environmental irritants, or voice overuse. The loudness and quality of voice is affected, and the patient may complain of a sore throat. Hoarseness often progresses throughout the course of the day. Indirect examination of the larynx reveals redness and edema of the vocal cords. Physical pathology may be absent in mild cases.

Acute Epiglottitis

Adults will complain of severe and rapidly progressing symptoms of sore throat, dyspnea, and hoarseness. In children, there is no cough or hoarseness, and drooling with a forward leaning posture is observed. This condition is most commonly associated with *Hempohilus influ-*

enzae infection. Voice quality is froglike. The patient will also have a high fever and be anxious, fearful, and restless with respiratory distress.

Trauma

Any swelling in response to trauma, directly to the larynx or indirectly to the throat, will cause hoarseness. Swelling might be secondary to head and neck surgery such as dental surgery, tonsillectomy, or thyroidectomy. Post-intubation trauma may be acute if secondary to inflammation or chronic if neurological or structural damage is irreversible. Mucosal abrasion or ulcer may be caused by direct trauma to the larynx and is associated with painful phonation and a breathy voice.

Acute Laryngeal Edema

Laryngeal edema may be one symptom in a generalized allergic response that involves the lips, tongue, and other hypopharyngeal structures. Drug reactions and food allergies, especially to seafood and nuts, often precipitate this response. This condition is a medical emergency because of the high risk of airway obstruction.

Laryngotracheobronchitis (Croup)

Subglottic edema is caused by a viral infection, most often parainfluenza 1 virus, that can obstruct the airway. This condition is most common in children 3 months to 3 years of age and is more prevalent in the fall and winter. It is associated with a barking cough, dyspnea, wheezing, low-grade fever, and hoarseness. Inspiratory stridor occurs abruptly because of narrowing of the passage, causing negative pressures generated on inspiration. Physical examination can determine the degree of respiratory distress, such as color, stridor, nasal flaring, and level of consciousness.

Chronic Laryngitis

This condition is associated with a combination of chronic exposure to working conditions with high levels of dust, fumes or noise, hard liquor consumption, cigarette smoking, and a history of frequent and persistent cough. Physical examination reveals edema or nodules of the vocal cords.

Polyps

Vocal cord polyps develop as a result of chronic inflammation from voice abuse, allergies, or GERD. Voice quality is breathy. With dependent polyps, the patient may report that symptoms of hoarseness change with position.

Neoplasm

Laryngeal cancer usually occurs in patients who have a long history of cigarette smoking and drinking alcohol. Hoarseness is characterized by a raspy or harsh voice. Physical examination may reveal leukoplakia, or a white scaly appearance of the vocal cords. Patients do not usually complain of pain until carcinoma is advanced. Pain secondary to ulceration is late and is often perceived as ear pain, especially when swallowing.

Gastroesophageal Reflux Disease (GERD)

Patients with GERD will complain of retrosternal burning (heartburn) that radiates upward. The regurgitation of gastric acid is exacerbated by large meals, a supine position, or bending over. Patients may describe a sour taste, experience salivary hypersecretion, have painful swallowing, or have a chronic cough or habit of throat clearing. Physical examination will be normal or epigastric tenderness may be elicited by abdominal examination. Inflammation or ulceration may be visible on the vocal cords.

Hypothyroidism

One symptom of hypothyroidism is a low, gravelly voice. The degree of hoarseness depends on the severity of thyroid deficiency. Usually the diagnosis of hypothyroidism is suspected when other symptoms are present, such as cold intolerance; rough, scaly skin texture; weight gain; and signs such as bradycardia and prolonged DTR recovery. Risk factors for hypothyroidism include increased age, postpartum in women, and a family history of thyroid disease. The thyroid gland may be nonpalpable or goiterous. Examination of the larynx may reveal edema or polyps. An elevated serum thyroid-stimulating hormone (TSH) level will confirm the diagnosis.

Vocal Cord Paralysis

Paralysis is usually unilateral and produces a weak, breathy voice. A unilateral abductor paralysis on the left side is caused by pressure on the vagus or recurrent laryngeal nerve by a mass of malignant glands in the superior mediastinum or carcinoma of the thyroid or esophagus.

Psychogenic Hoarseness

Patients with psychogenic hoarseness will have a low, breathy voice caused by voluntarily abducting the vocal cords during phonation. Physical examination will be normal. Psychogenic hoarseness may follow a traumatic event.

Laryngeal Papillomas

These are the most common benign laryngeal tumors that occur during childhood. Most patients are between the ages of 2 and 7 and present with hoarseness. Occasionally papillomas, caused by the human papilloma virus, are seen in newborns. On direct laryngoscopy, they appear as white, wartlike proliferations, arising in the glottic region.

Table 2-8			
Differential Diagnosis of Common Causes of Hoarseness			
Condition	History	Physical Findings	Diagnostic Studies
Acute laryngitis	Voice overuse, exposure to environmental irritants, recent URI	Voice quality: aphonia, cervical lymphadenopathy; pharyngitis; edema and redness of vocal cords	None, if duration of hoarseness is less than 3 weeks
Acute epiglottitis	Adults: rapid onset of sore throat, dyspnea, hoarseness; child: drooling, forward leaning posture	Voice quality frog-like; fever, signs of respiratory distress; drooling	Possible airway support; lateral and AP x-ray views of the neck

Continued

Table 2-8

Differential Diagnosis of Common Causes of Hoarseness—cont'd

Condition	History	Physical Findings	Diagnostic Studies
Trauma	Hoarseness after intubation; direct throat trauma or foreign body	Subluxation of the cricoarytenoid joint	Lateral and AP x-ray views of the neck; laryngoscopy
Acute laryngeal edema	History of food or drug allergy	Edema of the lips, tongue, and hypopharynx; observe for respiratory distress; voice quality breathy	Possible airway support
Laryngotracheo-bronchitis (croup)	Children 3 months to 3 years; recent URI	Barking cough, low grade fever, wheezing, hoarseness; edema of vocal cords; observe for signs of respiratory distress	None initially, airway support may be necessary
Chronic laryngitis	Chronic history of smoking and alcohol use; exposure to environmental irritants; chronic cough; duration of hoarseness more than 3 weeks	Edema of vocal cords; nodules may be present	Lateral and AP x-ray views of the neck; laryngoscopy
Polyps	History of allergy; voice abuse, GERD, smoker; duration of symptoms longer than 3 weeks; progressive hoarseness, worse at end of day, but near normal in the morning; hoarseness may change with position	Polyps visible on vocal cords	ENT referral for biopsy

Table 2-8

Differential Diagnosis of Common Causes of Hoarseness—cont'd

Condition	History	Physical Findings	Diagnostic Studies
Neoplasm	Smoking, airborne exposure, chronic alcohol use, history of chronic cough, hoarseness for more than 3 weeks	Tracheal deviation; pain with advanced tumor; hoarseness may be the only sign	ENT referral for biopsy
GERD	History of UGI burning and cough especially at night; chronic use of alcohol, NSAIDS, or aspirin; history of ulcer disease, smoker, below 45 years; frequent throat clearing	May have epigastric tenderness on palpation; vocal cord inflammation or ulcers	Referral for endoscopy if symptoms not relieved with medication or dietary alterations
Hypothyroidism	Presence of systemic symptoms such as cold intolerance, weight gain, fatigue; persons over 65 years; postpartal women; family history of thyroid disease	Normal or enlarged thyroid gland, coarse hair, very dry skin, prolonged DTR recovery	TSH, free T4 index
Vocal cord paralysis	Chronic cough; inspiratory or expiratory stridor with exertion	Breathy, weak, soft voice; abnormal movement (usually unilateral) of vocal cords; examination may suggest specific CN involvement	Refer for ENT evaluation

Continued

Table 2-8

Differential Diagnosis of Common Causes of Hoarseness—cont'd

Condition	History	Physical Findings	Diagnostic Studies
Psychogenic hoarseness	History of psychiatric illness or psychological trauma	Breathy, low voice; larynx will appear normal	As indicated to rule out other causes (i.e., lateral and AP x-ray view of the neck); laryngoscopy
Laryngeal papillomas	Children 2-12 and may occur in infants; history of maternal human papilloma virus; may be recurrent, progressive	Faint cry, severe stridor, voice change, or complete aphonia	Refer for ENT evaluation

Red Eye

The term red eye is used to denote a myriad of different ocular entities. The anatomical location in and around the eye and the probable cause of the eye disorder is an important framework to use in assessment. General anatomical locations are the ocular adnexa, conjunctiva, cornea and anterior segment, and the posterior eye (Figure 2-6).

The eye has two major defense mechanisms. The first is tears, which contain immunoglobulin A and lysozymes that provide an important washing action. The second defense mechanism is a conjunctival immune system of lymphocytes, plasma cells, and neutrophils. Inoculation of the eye with virulent organisms or trauma disrupts these normal defense mechanisms, leading to a red eye.

Although most cases of red eye are caused by viral or bacterial conjunctivitis, other possibilities exist. Some of these are trauma, glaucoma, systemic disease, and congenital anomalies. Determining etiology is an important step in assessment of the condition.

DIAGNOSTIC REASONING: FOCUSED HISTORY

Is this a chemical emergency?

Key Question
- Did you get a chemical into your eye?

Chemical injury. Chemical burns of the conjunctiva and cornea represent one of the true ocular emergencies. Alkali burns usually result in greater damage to the eye than acid burns because alkali compounds penetrate ocular tissues more rapidly.

All chemical burns require immediate and profuse irrigation and immediate referral to an ophthalmologist. Irri-

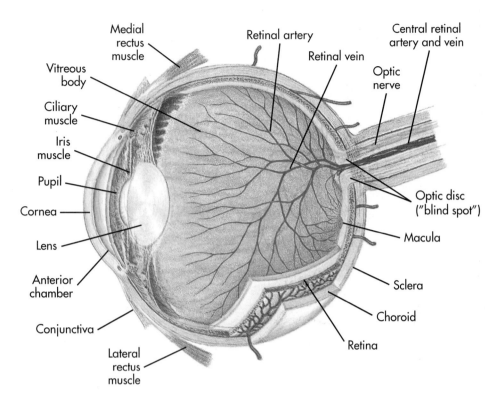

Figure 2-6   Anatomical structures of the eye. (From Seidel HM et al: *Mosby's guide to physical examination,* ed 3, St. Louis, 1995, Mosby.)

gate the eye with water while obtaining history of the incident and possible chemical contact.

Could this be caused by an orbital infection?

Key Questions

- Do you notice any swelling or tightness around the eye(s) or of the eyelid(s)?
- Does it hurt to move your eye around?
- Do you have a fever?
- Have you had a recent sinus infection?

Swelling, redness, fever. Orbital or periorbital cellulitis can present with conjunctivitis and signal a medical emergency. They can occur as a complication of sinusitis. Complaints of swelling, redness, and fever should alert you to these

conditions. Both conditions require immediate referral. Orbital cellulitis is life threatening.

Pain on attempted motion of the eye. Orbital cellulitis causes pain on movement because of the collection of pus between the periosteum and the wall of the orbit. The inflammation continues to all tissues in the orbit, and proptosis and impairment of ocular motility is seen.

Fever. Bacterial conjunctivitis is not associated with a fever. Otitis-conjunctivitis syndrome begins with a low-grade to moderate fever, mucopurulent rhinorrhea, and a cough. Three or four days after onset of fever the child wakes up with eyelashes crusted together. Ear complaints begin the same day as eye symptoms.

Recent sinus infection. Sinusitis is the most common predisposing condition in patients with orbital cellulitis. The ethmoid sinuses are most commonly involved, with the maxillary sinus next.

Can I rule in or rule out trauma?

Key Question

- How has your eye been injured? (e.g., foreign body, chemical, blow, stab, cut)

History of blunt trauma to the ocular adnexa can cause lid swelling and/or discoloration. Rupture of the globe, fractures of the orbital bones, and internal bleeding may also be possible. Sharp trauma to the area can cause lacerations of the lid and underlying lacerations of the globe. Internal bleeding may be subconjunctival (between the conjunctiva and sclera) or intraocular (hyphema). The cornea may have a foreign body and/or abrasions.

History of forceful trauma causing laceration or perforation of the globe is a surgical emergency and should be immediately referred without manipulation of the eye or eyelid.

Is this an acute or chronic condition?

Key Questions

- When did the redness start? How long has it been red?
- Did the redness start abruptly or was it gradual?
- Have you had this redness before? When?

Onset. An abrupt onset of redness typifies trauma, chemical burn, foreign body, ultraviolet (UV) exposure, or contact lens problems. Onset over a few hours may indicate infection from adjacent structures (periorbital, orbital, or sinuses). Onset over a few days is characteristic of conjunctivitis.

Duration. Acute redness can be caused by infection of the conjunctiva and/or eye-lids. Common causative organisms include *Staphylococcus aureus, Streptococcus pneumoniae,* group A streptococcus, *Hemophilus influenzae,* and *Neisseria gonorrhea.* Recurrent redness is often the result of allergic conjunctivitis from hypersensitivity reaction to a specific antigen. Iritis from systemic causes can also produce recurrent redness because of collagen destruction.

Can I narrow the problem by location?

Key Question

- Does one eye or do both eyes bother you?

Unilateral redness is more likely to indicate trauma or infection. Bilateral redness is more likely to indicate allergy and underlying systemic process. Blepharitis, inflammation of the eyelids, causes itching and crusting of the lash line and is usually bilateral. A hordeolum (sty) produces redness at the base of eyelashes and is usually unilateral. A chalazion is a chronic granulomatous inflammation of the meibomian gland. It is found in the mid-eyelid, often on the conjunctival side, and is usually unilateral. Some conditions can present with either unilateral or bilateral symptoms. Conjunctivitis often starts in one eye and then spreads to the other eye. Subconjunctival hemorrhage is often unilateral but may involve both eyes. Herpetic infection may be unilateral or bilateral.

A unilaterally painful, inflamed eye with photophobia and often a foreign body sensation *without* a history of significant trauma may indicate acute glaucoma.

What does the presence or absence of pain tell me?

Key Questions

- Is there any pain in your eye? What does it feel like?
- Does it hurt when you move your eye around?
- Does it feel like there is something in your eye?

Box 2-1			

Differential Diagnosis Based on Symptoms of Pain and Visual Loss

Red Eye No Pain or Visual Loss	Red Eye Painful	
	Vision Normal	*Vision Impaired*
Conjunctivitis	Episcleritis	Iritis
Subconjunctival hemorrhage	Keratitis	Glaucoma
Episcleritis	Cluster headache	Orbital cellulitis
	Corneal abrasion	Scleritis
	Corneal ulcer	Corneal abrasion
		Keratitis
		Corneal ulcer

Location of pain. Decide whether the pain is coming from the eye itself or is referred from surrounding structures. The ophthalmic nerve innervates the lid, conjunctiva, cornea, and uveal tract. The retina, the vitreous, and the optic nerve are less well innervated and seldom are a source of pain. Referred pain can come from contiguous structures or from inflamed structures innervated by the meningeal branches of the ophthalmic nerve.

Severity of pain. Bacterial conjunctivitis causes minimal pain; most patients complain of discomfort from the discharge and matting. There may be an itching/burning pain with allergy, moderate pain with iritis, and severe pain with corneal abrasion/ulcer. Constant, boring, throbbing pain, often severe enough to interfere with sleep, can result from ocular inflammation associated with iritis, acute glaucoma, and scleritis.

Foreign body sensation. Foreign body in an eye is a likely cause of pain. Viral causes of conjunctivitis produce a gritty sensation in the eye. A scratchy sensation often accompanies conditions that lead to dry eye, such as Sjogren syndrome. Patients who over-wear contact lenses frequently complain of pain in the eye,

caused by corneal hypoxia, several hours after removing contacts.

Do I need to worry about vision changes?

Key Questions

- Have you noticed any loss of vision?
- Have you had any blurred vision, double vision, halos, or floaters?

Visual decrease/loss. Distinguish visual loss from blurry vision caused by the discharge associated with conjunctivitis. No decrease in vision is seen in bacterial and allergic conjunctivitis, beyond that reasonably related to blurring from the heavy discharge. Vision is mildly decreased in iritis, but markedly decreased in acute glaucoma and with corneal abrasions/ulcers. Box 2-1 lists differential diagnoses based on symptoms of pain and visual loss.

Sudden diminution or loss of visual acuity is an ocular emergency and may indicate corneal or uveal tract disorders, acute glaucoma, or orbital cellulitis.

Blurring. True blurring is caused by an ocular problem. When the cornea, lens, aqueous humor, or vitreous are hazy, vision blurs and often there is dazzle in bright light. Some patients describe both refractive errors and double vision as blurred vision. Heavy discharge associated with conjunctivitis can also produce perceived blurring of vision.

Double vision. True double vision becomes single when one eye is covered. Sudden onset usually indicates a neurological problem. Chronic diplopia may be caused by muscular problems. Monocular diplopia usually indicates either corneal or lens changes.

Halos. Halos result from prismatic effects. They can be visual signs of corneal edema, caused by an abrupt rise in corneal or intraocular pressure (acute glaucoma). Less serious causes are water drops in the cornea or lens (seen in corneal edema or cataract).

Floaters. Floaters and/or flashing lights occur with vitreoretinal traction. The traction may progress to a retinal tear or detachment. With a tear, patients may complain of spaghetti-like strands floating in their vision. With a detachment, patients will give a history of blurred or blackened vision over several hours that progresses to complete or partial monocular blindness.

What does the presence or characteristics of the discharge tell me?

Key Questions
- Do you have any discharge from your eye?
- What are the color, consistency, and characteristics of this discharge?

A watery, nonpurulent discharge usually indicates allergic conjunctivitis. Discharge that is purulent or mucopurulent may indicate bacterial conjunctivitis and often affects both eyes. Viral conjunctivitis discharge is watery and may affect only one eye. Corneal abrasions and ulcers also produce watery/purulent discharge and are usually unilateral.

In the neonate 24 hours old, mucoid or purulent discharge indicates chemical conjunctivitis from prophylactic instillation of silver nitrate and other medications. Severe, bilateral purulent conjunctivitis 3 to 7 days after birth may indicate gonococcal infection of the eye. Discharge that is seen 5 to 30 days postpartum may indicate chlamydial conjunctivitis.

What does the presence of photophobia tell me?

Key Question
- Does light bother you/hurt your eye(s)?

Photophobia usually indicates ocular inflammation or irritation. Intraocular inflammation (iritis or generalized uveitis) causes pain on pupillary changes and thus leads to avoidance of bright light. This symptom may be mild and is often not reported unless the patient is asked. There is no photophobia with bacterial conjunctivitis. In infants and young children, photophobia signals a serious condition, such as juvenile arthritis, intraocular tumors, congenital glaucoma, or trauma.

What other things do I need to consider?

Key Questions
- Has there been any swelling?
- Do you have excessive tearing?
- Do your eyes itch?
- Does the itching occur at different times of the year?

Swelling. The orbital septum is a continuation of the periosteum of the bones of the orbit. It extends to the margins of both the upper and lower eyelids. Any conditions occurring in these areas can cause swelling. Secondarily, the skin of the eyelids is a very thin subcutaneous tissue that is musculofibrous and contains no fat. Thus the eyelid can allow a considerable amount of fluid to accumulate in a short period of time. Swelling and erythema under, and associated with, the medial canthus of the affected eye may indicate dacryocystitis. Swelling of the lids may be associated with inflammation, local infection, or trauma. Periorbital swelling may indicate cellulitis.

Tears. The lacrimal gland, which is situated in the upper lateral orbit, produces tears that are then carried across the eye to the puncta on the nasal side of the upper and lower lid. Obstruction of the passage of tears via the nasolacrimal duct to the nose causes regurgitation of fluid down the cheek (tearing). Epiphora (excessive production of tears) is common with viral conjunctivitis, corneal abrasions, infantile glaucoma, and nasal lacrimal duct stenosis.

Itching and tearing. The hallmark of an allergic conjunctivitis is itching and tearing disproportionate to findings. Vernal conjunctivitis is seasonal, recurrent, and bilateral. Itching is intense in the spring and fall months.

DIAGNOSTIC REASONING: FOCUSED PHYSICAL EXAMINATION

Test Visual Acuity

In adults and children over the age of 3½, use a Snellen, tumbling E, or Lippman chart. In children, the referral standard is 20/50 or worse in both eyes or a two-line difference between eyes. Retesting before referring children is suggested because they may do better (within normal limits) on the second examination.

For children less than 3½, use an ophthalmoscope. Darken the room. Stay at arm's length from the child and look at the eyes at a distance of 1 meter or more. When the child looks at the light, look at both red reflexes simultaneously and compare them. They should be red and equal in coloration. This indicates that the vision and binocular alignment are good and that no major pathology of the cornea, lens, vitreous, or retina is present. If the reflexes are not equal, a referral is required to an ophthalmologist.

Test Visual Fields

Testing of visual fields assesses the function of the peripheral vision and the central retina, optic pathways, and cortex. The peripheral field is damaged in glaucoma and by tumors or vascular lesions involving the visual fibers from the chiasm to the occipital cortex.

Inspect the Lids and Lid Margins and Periorbital and Orbital Tissues

Note redness or swelling of the lids. Look for lid lesions. Inspect the lid margins. Evert the lids and note appearance.

Unilateral inflammation of the lids and periorbital tissues without proptosis or limitation of eye movement characterizes periorbital cellulitis. If proptosis and/or limitation of eye movement are present, orbital cellulitis is the cause.

Erythematous swelling without systemic signs may be caused by contact dermatitis. All exposed skin should have the same coloring. Magenta discoloration of the eyelid is caused by *H. influenzae*.

A lid that is injected, swollen, and irritated may be so because of an underlying disease process in the conjunctiva, cornea, sclera, or intraocular area.

Examine for the presence of focal or diffuse inflammation. Blockage of the glands along the lash line may produce localized or diffuse redness or flaking of the skin as a result of staphylococcal or seborrheic causes.

Lids that appear to have follicular changes (small aggregates of lymphocytes) in the palpebral conjunctiva are commonly seen with viral conjunctivitis. Lids that have large, flattened, cobblestone-like papillary lesions of the palpebral conjunctivae are characteristic of vernal conjunctivitis.

Inflammation of the lid margins in all four lids and with associated loss of eyelashes is common in children. This condition is known as blepharitis. The lashes are waxy, scaling, red, irritated, and the eyes have slightly swollen lid margins.

Eye pain with no external inflammation suggests referred causes, such as sinusitis, carotid artery aneurysm, temporal arteritis, migraine or cluster headache, or trigeminal neuralgia. Optic neuritis can also cause eye pain without inflammation.

Observe for Entropion and Ectropion

Entropion occurs when the eyelid margin turns inward. The eyelashes contact the corneal and conjunctival surfaces, and the patient complains of discomfort. Scarring can occur.

Ectropion occurs when the eyelid margin turns outward. A pool of stagnant tears results and does not allow proper mechanical protection of the cornea and conjunctiva. The exposed tarsal conjunctiva is also susceptible to repeated trauma.

Evert the Eyelid If Indicated by History

Eversion of the eyelid is necessary to detect a possible foreign body. This is done by first having the patient look down. Hold the upper eyelashes straight forward. Push down on the upper tarsal border with a cotton tip applicator. The lid everts. Hold the eyelid in this position by moving fingers to the brow. To undo, hold the lashes and pull gently forward while asking the patient to look up.

Inspect the Conjunctiva

Note bilateral or unilateral redness. Note where the redness occurs on the conjunctiva. Distinguish between peripheral or circumcorneal injection (ciliary flush). Ciliary flush is the deep conjunctival or episcleral blood vessel injection around the limbus (junction between the cornea and conjunctiva), dilating in response to corneal disease or injury. It is frequently associated with keratopathy, uveitis, and episcleritis/scleritis. Abrasions and ulcers of the cornea cause increased redness of the globe around the corneal limbus, appearing as a reddish ring surrounding the cornea. Note any discharge. Look for visible lesions or foreign bodies on the conjunctiva.

Conjunctival inflammation as a result of infection causes a red eye with peripheral injection that is maximal toward the fornix (the fold between globe and lid). Peripheral injection involves the bulbar conjunctiva without edema or exudate, and the cornea is spared.

Subconjunctival hemorrhage causes a bright red splash of blood that is visible on the conjunctiva and sclera. Without a history of trauma or bleeding diathesis and no presence of retinal hemorrhage, the cause may be intravascular pressure from coughing, sneezing, or straining.

Systemic autoimmune processes such as juvenile rheumatoid arthritis, serum sickness, and Stevens-Johnson syndrome may cause conjunctivitis. Perilimbal conjunctival injection is seen in juvenile rheumatoid arthritis.

A localized degenerative process of the substantia propriae of the conjunctiva, known as pinguecula, may invade the superficial cornea. There are yellow, elevated nodules of fibropathic material that are usually adjacent to the cornea on the nasal side.

Look at the palpebral conjunctiva and the fornices for foreign bodies and pterygia, which are neovascularized structures that can encroach on the cornea and form a pannus interfering with vision.

Inspect the Sclera

Note the color. The sclera gives the eye its white appearance. Inflammation (scleritis) causes a dusky red color.

Examine the Cornea

Test the corneal light (red) reflex. Note if the cornea is hazy or has opacities. Look for visible foreign bodies.

The normal cornea is transparent, with blood vessels only at the limbus (the junction between cornea and conjunctiva). Illumination of the cornea tangentially may show abnormalities, such as abrasions or foreign bodies. These imperfections of the corneal surface will produce an abnormal light reflex or a break in the image as the light reflects off the cornea. The blood vessels around the limbus dilate in response to corneal disease or injury.

Topical application of fluorescein to the cornea that reveals dendrite ulcers should lead you to suspect herpes simplex virus.

When looking for the red reflex, note any corneal opacity as well as the depth of the opacity. Corneal opacities move in the opposite direction of the opthalmoscope, lens opacities stay still, and vitreous opacities move in the same direction as the opthalmoscope. Corneal clouding (edema) is seen with glaucoma.

Examine the Iris, Pupil, and Lens

Note pupil size and equality. Note transparency of lens. Test pupillary reaction (direct and consensual). Note any photophobia.

The anterior chamber should contain only clear aqueous humor. Trauma may cause blood to accumulate in the chamber; this is known as a hyphema. The shock wave produced by the sudden compression and decompression of the cornea is transmitted through the eye and may result in a tear in the ciliary body. Disruption of the anterior arterial circle of this structure produces bleeding that accumulates. The hyphema appears as a bright or dark red fluid level between the cornea and iris or as a diffuse murkiness of the aqueous humor. Pus may also accumulate in this space in association with corneal infection. This is known as hypopyon.

All hyphemas are abnormal and must be referred to an ophthalmologist.

The pupil is the central aperture of the iris. It floats in the aqueous humor and divides the anterior segment into anterior and posterior chambers, which communicate throughout the pupillary aperture. It slides freely on the anterior surface of the lens when dilating and contracting. Conditions that affect this anatomy cause pupil abnormalities. Inflammation of the iris (iritis) causes reduction in the reactive capacity of the iris and inequality of pupils. Acute increased intraocular pressure causes the space in the anterior chamber to become very shallow, resulting in a dilated, fixed, oval pupil.

The lens is normally transparent and not visible on inspection; however, any visible clouding of the lens as seen through the pupil is indicative of cataract formation.

Perform Ophthalmoscopy

Look for a large and deepened cup if you suspect glaucoma. Early in the course of the disease, the funduscopic examination may be normal. Do not use mydriatic agents if you suspect glaucoma.

Test Extraocular Movements (EOMs)

Test eye movement in all six fields of gaze. Note pain or restriction. Inflammation or underlying periostitis and impaired venous drainage as a result of reactive inflammation causes restrictive eye movement and proptosis (exophthalmos). Decreased range of motion can also occur with orbital cellulitis.

Palpate the Lid/Lacrimal Puncta

Observe for edema and note pain or tenderness on palpation. The lacrimal puncta should be turned backward slightly to catch the pool of tears in the inner canthus. Tears should not spill over the cheeks. Note if gentle palpation of each lacrimal sac produces any material that regurgitates into the eye. Unilateral swelling over the lacrimal sac on the lid margin at the side of the nose because of infection or obstruction of the lacrimal drainage system is common. Infection of the meibomian glands of the eyelids (hordeolum or internal sty) and the glands of Zeis or Moll (hordeolum or external sty) produces pain on palpation. Internal sties are generally large, very tender, and may point to the conjunctiva or epidermis part of the lid. External sties are small, superficial, and point only to the epidermis side.

Granulomatous inflammation of a meibomian gland nodule that is firm, not tender, and with no inflammatory signs is a chalazion.

Examine the Tympanic Membranes

Examination of the TM is necessary because of the frequent association with atypical *H. influenzae* acute otitis media (conjunctivitis-otitis syndrome).

Palpate Pre-Auricular Nodes

Pre-auricular nodes are usually palpable with a viral infection of the eyes.

LABORATORY AND DIAGNOSTIC STUDIES

Fluorescein Staining

Dendrite etchings on the anterior part of the cornea are seen in herpes infection. Nodules near the limbus with surrounding hyperemia are seen in keratoconjunctivitis. Hypertrophy of the dorsal conjunctiva with elevated grayish areas near the limbus is consistent with vernal conjunctivitis. Under a blue light, a corneal abrasion and foreign body will stain bright green with fluorescein.

Culture

Moisten a sterile alginate (not cotton) swab with sterile saline and wipe the lid margin or conjunctival cul-de-sac. The culture medium is then inoculated directly with the swab tip. Place on solid media, writing *R* for right eye, *L* for left eye, and *Z* for another culture site. The tip of the applicator may then be broken off and dropped into the tube of liquid culture medium.

Cultures should be taken before instilling topical anesthetics because preservatives will reduce the recovery of some bacteria.

Gram Stain

Gram-positive cocci in pairs may indicate *S. pyogenes*. Gram-negative diplococci indicate *Neisseria gonorrhea*. Large Gram-negative diplobacilli indicate *Moraxella catarrhalis; H. influenzae* stains as a Gram-negative coccobacillus.

Complete Blood Count (CBC)

A complete blood count with differential is done to establish systemic infection. An increase in WBCs and bands is seen with systemic infection.

Blood Cultures

Blood cultures are done on any suspected orbital cellulitis or when there is reason to suspect a clinically significant bacteremia. *Hemophilus influenzae, Streptococcus pneumoniae, Staphylococcus aureus, Streptococcus pyogenes,* or anerobes are possible infecting organisms.

CT Scan

A CT scan is used to determine the presence and extent of an abscess and/or to localize the site of infection in the periorbital region as well as in the sinuses.

Intraocular Pressure

Intraocular pressure is measured with a Schiötz tonometer. The technique is as follows: after instillation of a local anesthesia, the patient is placed in a supine position and asked to look directly upward. The lids are held separated and the instrument is placed gently in a vertical position directly over the cornea, with the plunger placed on the cornea. A reading on the scale is then taken. A pressure elevated greater than 21.5 is seen in acute closed-angle glaucoma.

DIFFERENTIAL DIAGNOSIS

LACRIMAL SAC

Dacryocystitis

Infection of the lacrimal sac occurs secondary to obstruction. In infants it is a complication of congenital dacryostenosis. In adults duct obstruction results from nasal trauma, deviated septum, hypertrophic rhinitis, and mucosal polyps. The patient experiences pain, swelling, and redness around the lacrimal sac with tearing. Conjunctivitis, blepharitis, and leukocytosis are associated with an acute condition; with a chronic condition the only symptom may be slight swelling of the sac. Pus may regurgitate through the punctum.

EYELIDS

Blepharitis

Blepharitis is the most common inflammation of the eyelids. It usually involves the lid margins and frequently is associated with conjunctivitis. It is bilateral, not painful, and has no associated photophobia. The lids are inflamed and scaling of the lid margins is seen. Loss of eyelashes occurs late. Visual acuity is unimpaired.

Hordeolum

Hordeolum is caused by infection of the glands of Zeis or Moll along the lash line. It develops acutely and manifests as a palpable indurated area along the lid margin, with a purulent center and surrounding erythema. It spontaneously drains within 1 to 2 weeks. The patient presents with swelling of the eyelid and local pain. It is limited to the lids.

Chalazion

A chalazion is a granulomatous reaction in the meibomian gland on the tarsal plate of the lid. This is usually a chronic condition. The lesion is usually painless and indurated. When symptoms are present, they include pruritis and redness of the involved eye and eyelid.

Entropion and Ectropion

Malposition of the eyelid causes local irritation and may be a cause of red eye. In entropion the lid is turned inward; in ectropion the lid is turned outward.

CONJUNCTIVA

Bacterial Conjunctivitis

Bacterial conjunctivitis is most commonly caused by *S. aureus, S. pneumoniae,* group A streptococcus, *H. influenzae,* and *N. gonorrhea.* The onset is gradual, begins unilaterally, and often becomes bilateral. The patient usually complains of a scratchy sensation instead of pain. There is generally no photophobia. Examination reveals peripheral injection, purulent discharge, and matted eyelids. Visual acuity is not affected, although the presence of discharge may produce "blurring" of vision.

Viral Conjunctivitis

Occurring most commonly in young adults, viral conjunctivitis is caused by such viruses as adenovirus, picornavirus, rhinovirus, and herpes virus. The onset is gradual and unilateral early in the course and then may become bilateral. The patient complains of a scratchy, rather than painful, sensation. On examination, peripheral injection with watery discharge is apparent. Visual acuity is intact. Lids may have follicular changes (small aggregates of lymphocytes) in the palpebral conjunctiva.

Allergic Conjunctivitis

Allergic conjunctivitis is a chronic, seasonal condition caused by hypersensitivity reaction to a specific allergen. It is bilateral, itchy, and painless. The conjunctival injection is peripheral. There is ropy, mucoid discharge. The palpebral conjunctiva has a cobblestone appearance. Visual acuity is unaffected.

N. gonorrhea Conjunctivitis

The *Neisseria gonorrhea* organism can produce a bacterial conjunctivitis in newborns. It is bilateral, with very purulent discharge 48 to 72 hours after birth. Although rare in adults, it can occur through direct transmission via finger contact or via contact of the eyes in a nonchlorinated swimming pool.

Chemical Conjunctivitis

Chemical conjunctivitis occurs with instillation of chemical prophylaxis in the neonate. A bilateral reaction occurs within the first 24 hours.

Subconjunctival Hemorrhage

Subconjunctival hemorrhage is usually the result of a small blood vessel rupture in the conjunctival tissue and frequently develops after episodes of coughing or straining. It is painless although often frightening to the patient. Visual acuity is not impaired.

Hyphema

Hyphema is caused by blood in the anterior chamber of the eye usually produced by trauma to the eye. The patient has a marked decrease in vision, with red cells present diffusely throughout the anterior chamber. A settled layer of blood present inferiorly or a complete filling of the anterior chamber is possible, obscuring the visual examination of the posterior chamber. The pupil is irregular and poorly reactive.

Episcleritis

Often a benign inflammatory condition of the covering of the sclera, episcleritis is bilateral, with mild stinging. Peripheral injection is present. There is no discharge, but some lacrimation and photophobia may be present. Visual acuity is unimpaired.

Scleritis

Inflammation of the sclera can result in severe destructive disease. It is usually a unilateral inflammatory condition associated with rheumatoid arthritis, systemic immunological disease, or other autoimmune disorders. There is pain and ciliary injection. Lacrimation is present and visual acuity is variable.

CORNEA

Keratitis

Bacterial, fungal, and viral organisms can cause infection of the cornea. Moderate to severe eye pain is present, there is some discharge, and visual acuity is decreased. Pupils are equal and normal, but the cornea appears cloudy. Peripheral injection is present and diffuse. A ciliary flush is also present.

Corneal Abrasion

Corneal abrasion may be superficial, lying on top of the anterior surface of the cornea, or it may be subtarsal and become implanted on the palpebral conjunctiva, causing the cornea to become irritated when the patient blinks. The patient usually has a history of a foreign body on the anterior surface of the eye. The abrasion causes moderate to severe pain with discharge present. Visual acuity may be normal or decreased, photophobia is present, and pupil size and reaction is normal. Fluorescein stain is taken into the ulcer and can be seen under the Wood's lamp.

Herpetic Infection

Caused by the herpes simplex virus, this infection occurs unilaterally or bilaterally. The patient presents with pain, photophobia, and diffuse or ciliary injection. Discharge is variable, and visual acuity is markedly decreased. Dendrites are seen on fluorescein staining.

ORBIT

Periorbital Cellulitis

The patient presents with unilateral swelling of lid, redness, fever, and hotness. The conjunctiva is clear, the eye moves freely, and vision is not impaired.

Orbital Cellulitis

The patient presents with unilateral lid swelling, fever, and pain. Examination reveals proptosis, chemosis, and conjunctivitis. There is limitation of eye motion on testing of EOMs. The patient appears ill. This condition is life threatening and requires immediate intervention.

UVEAL TRACT

Iritis

Characterized by inflammation of the iris and ciliary body, iritis may be idiopathic and develop in response to coexistent conjunctivitis, keratitis, or eye trauma, or it may occur with chronic inflammatory or infectious processes. Eye pain is moderate and aching, visual acuity is decreased, and photophobia is present. There is minimal eye discharge, the affected pupil is smaller, and the cornea appears normal. There is central redness of the eye, with ciliary flush present.

GLAUCOMA

Acute Closed-Angle Glaucoma

The patient presents with unilateral, deep eye pain and photophobia. There may be a complaint of halos around visualized objects. There is ciliary injection with tears and decreased visual acuity. The pupil is mid-dilated and has decreased reactivity to light. The cornea is cloudy. There is diffuse redness of the eye with intraocular pressure (IOP) of greater than 21.5. This condition requires emergency referral.

Table 2-9

Differential Diagnosis of Common Causes of Red Eye Complaints

Condition	History	Physical Findings	Diagnostic Studies
Lacrimal Sac Dacryocystitis	Unilateral, acute onset; pain	Swelling and redness around lacrimal sac; tearing; may have pus through punctum	CBC: leukocytosis

Continued

Table 2-9

Differential Diagnosis of Common Causes of Red Eye Complaints—cont'd

Condition	History	Physical Findings	Diagnostic Studies
Eyelids			
Blepharitis	Bilateral, gradual onset; no pain	Lids inflamed; scaling on margins; visual acuity OK; loss of lashes (late)	None
Hordeolum/sty	Unilateral; pain	Swelling of eyelid; indurated lesion with central pus and surrounding erythema	None initially; if repeated, screen for diabetes
Chalazion	Unilateral; chronic; painless	Indurated lesion on tarsal plate of lid; may have pruritis and redness of the involved eye and eyelid	None
Entropion/ ectropion	Unilateral or bi-lateral	Lid turned inward or outward; local irritation and tearing; peripheral injec-tion	None
Conjunctiva			
Bacterial conjunctivitis	Gradual onset, unilateral early, bilateral late; scratchy (no pain); photo-phobia	Peripheral injec-tion; purulent discharge; matted eyelids; visual acuity OK	None initially; if not better with treatment, ob-tain culture and sensitivities, Gram stain
Viral conjunctivitis	Gradual onset, unilateral early, bilateral late; scratchy (no pain)	Peripheral injec-tion; watery discharge; visual acuity OK; fol-licular changes (small aggre-gates of lympho-cytes) in the palpebral con-junctiva	As for bacterial conjunctivitis

Table 2-9

Differential Diagnosis of Common Causes of Red Eye Complaints—cont'd

Condition	History	Physical Findings	Diagnostic Studies
Allergic conjunctivitis	Chronic; seasonal; bilateral; itchy (no pain)	Peripheral injection; ropy, mucoid discharge; cobblestone mucosa; visual acuity OK	Fluorescein staining: hypertrophy of dorsal conjunctiva with elevated gray areas near limbus with vernal conjunctivitis
N. gonorrhea conjunctivitis	Bilateral; newborn	Purulent discharge 48-72 hours after birth	Culture on Thayer-Martin plate; Gram stain
Chemical conjunctivitis	Bilateral	Neonate: within first 24 hours	None
Subconjunctival hemorrhage	Unilateral; painless; coughing or straining	Splash of blood in conjunctiva and sclera; visual acuity OK	None
Hyphema	Unilateral; trauma to eye	Red cell in anterior chamber; visual acuity decreased; pupil irregular and poorly reactive	Refer to ophthalmologist
Episcleritis	Bilateral; mild stinging	Peripheral injection; no discharge; visual acuity OK	None
Scleritis	Unilateral; deep boring pain	Ciliary injection; teary; visual acuity variable; photophobia	Associated with systemic immunological disease
Cornea			
Keratitis	Bilateral; moderate to severe pain	Discharge; pupils normal; cornea cloudy; visual acuity decreased	Test for bacterial, fungal, viral infection
Corneal abrasion/ foreign body	Unilateral; pain/ photophobia	Diffuse injection; tears; visual acuity variable	Fluorescein stain positive

Continued

Table 2-9

Differential Diagnosis of Common Causes of Red Eye Complaints—cont'd

Condition	History	Physical Findings	Diagnostic Studies
Herpetic keratitis	Unilateral or bilateral; pain; photophobia	Ciliary flush; discharge variable; visual acuity markedly decreased	Fluorescein stain shows dendrites
Orbit			
Periorbital cellulitis	Unilateral	Swelling of lid, fever, redness, conjunctiva clear, eye moves freely, vision not impaired	CBC—leukocytosis, blood cultures
Orbital cellulitis	Unilateral; pain	Proptosis, lid swelling, chemosis, conjunctivitis, limitation of eye motion	CBC, blood cultures; CT scan; life threatening
Uveal Tract			
Iritis	Unilateral; moderate aching pain; photophobia	Tearing; affected pupil smaller; cornea normal; ciliary flush	Refer
Glaucoma			
Acute closed-angle glaucoma	Unilateral; deep pain; photophobia; halos	Ciliary injection; tears; visual acuity decreased	Tonometry; emergency referral

Chapter 3

Common Problems of the Skin

≡ Rashes and Skin Lesions

Dermatological problems result from a number of mechanisms, including inflammatory, infectious, immunological, and environmental (traumatic and exposure induced). At times, the mechanism may be readily identified, such as the infectious bacterial etiology in impetigo. However, some dermatological lesions may be classified in more than one way. Most insect bites, for example, involve both environmental (the bite) and inflammatory (the response) mechanisms. Awareness of the potential mechanism of any skin rash or lesion is most helpful in identifying the risk a person may have for other illnesses. For example, persons with eczema are also frequently at risk for or have other atopic conditions, notably asthma and/or allergies. Thousands of skin disorders have been described, but only a small number account for the vast majority of patient visits.

Evaluation of rashes and skin lesions depends on a carefully focused history and physical examination. For this, the provider needs to be familiar with characteristics of various skin lesions; anatomy, physiology, and pathophysiology of the skin; clinical appearance of the basic lesion; arrangement and distribution of the lesion; and clinicopathological correlations. Common symptoms associated with specific lesions, such as itching or fever, are also important to know. It is necessary to quickly identify life-threatening diseases and those that are highly contagious. Ultimately, competence in dermatological assessment involves recognition through repetition.

DIAGNOSTIC REASONING: INITIAL FOCUSED PHYSICAL EXAMINATION

Initial Inspection

Dermatological assessment is similar to assessment of most other body systems in that it depends on patient history and physical assessment. However, sometimes a brief initial physical assessment preceding the history can assist in the development of the initial differential diagnosis, followed by a focused history and further physical examination.

Morphological Criteria

Examination involves the classification of the lesion based on a number of morphological features. Evaluation should be systematic. Generally, each of the following morphological features should be analyzed (examples are listed in Table 3-1; also consult a physical examination or dermatology text for a complete review of these terms):
- Identify the location of the lesion(s)
- Identify the distribution of the lesions as localized, regional, or generalized
- Identify whether the lesion is primary (appearing initially) or secondary (resulting from change in a primary lesion)
- Identify the shape of the lesion and any arrangement if numerous
- Describe the margins (borders)
- Describe the pigmentation, including variations
- Palpate the texture and consistency
- Measure the size of an individual lesion or estimate if numerous or widespread

Erythema in dark-skinned persons may be difficult to appreciate. It often is seen as post-inflammatory hyperpigmentation.

Gloves are not necessary unless there are open, draining, or exudative lesions.

Examination in a systematic manner and, in part, before obtaining the majority of the history, provides greater relevance to the data.

DIAGNOSTIC REASONING: FOCUSED HISTORY

Is the rash associated with an immediate life-threatening condition?

Key Questions
- Do you have a fever?
- Are you short of breath or do you have difficulty swallowing?
- Is the rash tender with fever and mucosal involvement?

Fever. Fever is common in viral exanthems (rashes), and the accompanying condition is usually not life threatening. However, fever with irritability, hypotension, and sepsis with a macular or petechial rash may indicate meningococcemia. Treatment needs to be immediate to be life saving.

Allergic reaction. Urticarial allergic reactions may be associated with angioedema (swelling) of the extremities, face, lips, tongue, and/or airway; cough; wheezing; shortness of breath; or heart palpitations. The sooner symptoms occur after the exposure to the allergen the more severe the reaction. Treatment needs to be instituted immediately.

Rash with fever and mucosal involvement. Toxic epidermal necrolysis (Stevens-Johnson syndrome) is a tender, morbilliform, erythema multiforme-like rash accompanied by fever, conjunctivitis, oral ulcers, and diarrhea. Immediate hospitalization is required, usually in a burn center, to treat exfoliation of large areas of skin. The condition is usually drug induced.

Table 3-1

Morphological Criteria of Rashes and Skin Lesions

NATURE OF LESION	DESCRIPTION	EXAMPLES
Primary Lesions (develop initially in response to a change in the internal or external environment of the skin)		
Macule	Discrete flat change in color of the skin; usually <1.5 cm diameter	Freckle, lentigo, purpura
Patch	Discrete flat lesion (large macule); usually >1.5 cm diameter	Pityriasis rosea, melasma, lentigo
Papule	Discrete palpable elevation of the skin; <1 cm diameter; origin may be epidermal, dermal, or both	Nevi, seborrheic keratosis, dermatofibroma
Nodule	Discrete palpable elevation of the skin; may evolve from papule; may involve any level of skin from epidermis to subcutis	Nevi, basal cell carcinoma, keratoacanthoma
Plaque	Slightly raised lesion, typically with a flat surface; >1 cm diameter; scaling frequently present	Psoriasis, mycosis fungoides
Wheal	Transient pink/red swelling of the skin; often displaying central clearing; various shapes and sizes; usually pruritic and lasts less than 24 hours	Urticaria
Tumor	Large papule or nodule; usually >1 cm diameter	Basal cell carcinoma, squamous cell carcinoma, malignant melanoma
Pustule	Raised lesion <0.5 cm diameter containing yellow cloudy fluid (usually infected)	Folliculitis, acne (closed comedones)
Vesicle	Raised lesion <0.5 cm diameter containing clear fluid	Herpes simplex, herpes zoster, contact (irritant) dermatitis
Bulla	Vesicle >0.5 cm diameter	Bullous pemphigoid, contact (irritant) dermatitis, blisters of second-degree sunburn
Cyst	Semi-solid lesion; varies in size from several mm to several cm; may become infected	Sebaceous cyst

Continued

Table 3-1

Morphological Criteria of Rashes and Skin Lesions—cont'd

NATURE OF LESION	DESCRIPTION	EXAMPLES
Secondary Lesions (appear as a result of changes in primary lesions)		
Crust	Dried exudate that may have been serous, purulent, or hemorrhagic	Impetigo, herpes zoster (late phase)
Scale	Thin plates of desquamated stratum corneum that flake off rather easily	Xerosis, icthyosis, psoriasis
Excoriation	Shallow hemorrhagic excavation; linear or punctate; results from scratching	Contact (irritant) dermatitis
Lichenification	Thickening of the skin with exaggeration of the skin creases; it is the hallmark of chronic eczematous dermatitis	Chronic eczema
Erosion	Partial break in the epidermis	Herpes simplex or zoster, pemphigus vulgaris
Fissure	Linear crack in the epidermis	Xerosis, angular chelitis, severe eczema
Distribution of Lesions		
Localized	Lesion appears in one small area	Impetigo, herpes simplex (e.g., labialis), tinea corporis ("ringworm")
Regional	Lesions involve a specific region of the body	Acne vulgaris (pilosebaceous gland distribution), herpes zoster (nerve dermatomal distribution), psoriasis (extensor surfaces and skinfolds)
Generalized	Lesions appear widely distributed or in numerous areas simultaneously	Urticaria, disseminated drug eruptions
Shape/Arrangement		
Round/discoid	Coin- or ring-shaped (no central clearing)	Nummular eczema
Oval	Ovoid shape	Pityriasis rosea
Annular	Round, active margins with central clearing	Tinea corporis, sarcoidosis
Zosteriform (dermatomal)	Following a nerve or segment of the body	Herpes zoster

Table 3-1		

Morphological Criteria of Rashes and Skin Lesions—cont'd

NATURE OF LESION	DESCRIPTION	EXAMPLES
Shape/Arrangement—cont'd		
Polycyclic	Interlocking or coalesced circles (formed by enlargement of annular lesions)	Psoriasis, urticaria
Linear	In a line	Contact dermatitis
Iris/target lesion	Pink macules with purple central papules	Erythema multiforme
Stellate	Star-shaped	Meningococcal septicemia
Serpiginous	Snake-like or wavy line track	Cutanea larva migrans
Reticulate	Net-like or lacy	Polyarteritis nodosa, lichen planus lesions of erythema infectiosum
Morbilliform	Confluent and salmon-colored	Rubeola
Border/Margin		
Discrete	Well-demarcated or defined, able to draw a line around it with confidence	Psoriasis
Indistinct	Poorly defined, having borders that merge into normal skin or outlying ill-defined papules	Nummular eczema
Active	Margin of lesion shows greater activity than center	Tinea species eruptions
Irregular	Non-smooth or notched margin	Malignant melanoma
Border raised above center	Center of lesion is depressed compared to the edge	Basal cell carcinoma
Advancing	Expanding at margins	Cellulitis
Associated Changes Within Lesions		
Central clearing	Erythematous border surrounds lighter skin	Tinea eruptions
Desquamation	Peeling or sloughing of skin	Rash of toxic shock syndrome
Keratotic	Hypertrophic stratum corneum	Calluses, warts
Punctation	Central umbilication or dimpling	Basal cell carcinoma
Telangiectasias	Dilated blood vessels within lesion blanch completely; may be markers of systemic disease	Basal cell carcinoma, actinic keratosis

Continued

Table 3-1

Morphological Criteria of Rashes and Skin Lesions—cont'd

NATURE OF LESION	EXAMPLES
Pigmentation	
Flesh	Neurofibroma, some nevi
Pink	Eczema, pityriasis rosea
Erythematous	Tinea eruptions, psoriasis
Salmon	Psoriasis
Tan-brown	Most nevi, pityriasis versicolor
Black	Malignant melanoma
Pearly	Basal cell carcinoma
Purple	Purpura, Kaposi's sarcoma
Violaceous	Erysipelas
Yellow	Lipoma
White	Lichen planus

Is the rash acute or chronic (recurrent)?

Key Questions
- How long have you had this?
- Have you ever had anything like this before?

Onset. Diagnosis of skin lesions is initially aided by categorizing the lesion as acute versus chronic or recurrent. Acute eruptions, such as urticaria or various fungal rashes (tinea), are classified as such because they have a tendency to be self-limiting or to not recur after effective treatment. Chronic rashes, such as psoriasis or eczema, may persist or be recurrent with exacerbations and remissions. Box 3-1 shows common rashes categorized by duration.

Ascertain the duration of the eruption at presentation. A word of caution, however, is in order as the initial occurrence of a chronic rash may present acutely. Conversely, an acute eruption not optimally treated may present as a chronic problem.

Where is the rash in its evolution?

Key Questions
- What did this look like initially?
- Has it changed? If so, how?
- Has it spread? Where?

Initial presentation. Most skin lesions evolve over time, although this varies from minutes in urticaria to weeks or even months with psoriasis or mycosis fungoides.

Change in lesion. Determining whether there has been a change from the initial appearance of a lesion gives diagnostic clues. The eruption of pityriasis rosea classically begins with a "herald patch," a single, scaly, erythematous patch usually on the trunk, followed within days by a regional outbreak of numerous smaller erythematous patches, thus providing a key diagnostic clue. The rash may look like ringworm, but it appears too quickly to be ringworm. Another example of evolutionary change is the eruption of herpes simplex virus,

Box 3-1

Duration of Rash

Acute	**Chronic**
Allergic or contact dermatitis	Acne vulgaris
Candida dermatitis (diaper rash, intertrigo)	Bullous pemphigus
	Eczema
Erythema infectiosum (fifth disease)	Erythema nodosum
Erythema multiforme	Kaposi's sarcoma
Fixed drug eruptions	Mycosis fungoides
Folliculitis	Polyarteritis nodosa
Herpes simplex virus (HSV)*	Psoriasis
Herpes zoster/varicella zoster (HZ)	Rosacea
Impetigo	Seborrheic dermatitis
Infestations (scabies, pediculosis)	Systemic lupus erythematosus
Insect bites	
Kawasaki disease	
Pityriasis rosea	
Septicemia (meningococcal)	
Scarlet fever	
Tinea (corporis, pedis, versicolor)	
Urticaria*	
Viral exanthems (measles)	

*Occasionally recurrent.

which begins with small vesicles that later umbilicate, possibly ooze, and eventually crust before healing. A rash may appear in different ways, depending on the point at which evaluation is sought.

Spread. The way a rash spreads is helpful in diagnosing the specific rash. There are three general ways a rash can spread: centripetal or moving to the center, centrifugal or moving away from the center, or caudal or moving down (see Table 3-2 at the end of this chapter for a description of the characteristic distribution and spread of common rashes).

What does pruritus tell me?

Key Question
• Does it itch?

Itching. All dermatoses can be classified into three groups: a small group that

always itches, those that never itch, and an intermediate group where itching is variable (Box 3-2). Pruritus is often reported to be worse at night. However, during the day, pruritus is less troublesome because the patient is distracted by daily routines. It is only at bedtime, while trying to sleep, that the slightest sensation of pruritus becomes overwhelming because the patient has nothing else on which to concentrate. Once the patient scratches the area, histamine is released from the inflammatory cells (especially mast cells), and this causes more pruritus and an itch-scratch cycle is established.

Swimmer's itch occurs in areas unprotected by a swimsuit. Seabather's itch occurs in areas under the swimsuit. Nocturnal pruritis most typically occurs in scabies infestations. Itching in the absence of rash may be an important clue to internal disease.

Box 3-2		

Itching: Comparison

Always Itch	**May Itch**	**Never Itch**
Atopic dermatitis	Psoriasis	Warts
Urticaria	Impetigo	Neurofibromatosis
Insect bites	Tinea	Vitiligo
Scabies	Pityriasis rosea	Nevi
Pediculosis		
Lichen planus		
Chickenpox		

What does associated pain tell me?

Key Questions
- Is it painful or sore?
- Does it burn?

Pain. Pain is a rare symptom. The classic painful rash is associated with herpes zoster, including post-herpetic neuralgia, although severe psoriasis or eczema, when associated with fissures and bleeding, may be described as painful by some patients. Soreness is a more common symptom and may be associated with numerous rashes. Tender erythema may be associated with toxic epidermal necrolysis.

Burning. Burning is infrequently reported. It is most notable preceding the rash in herpes virus infections (i.e., herpes simplex virus [HSV] or herpes zoster [HZ]).

What do associated symptoms tell me?

Key Questions
- Do you have a fever? Sore throat? Headache?
- How are you feeling in general?

Fever, sore throat, headache. Fever may be a common presenting complaint in infectious diseases accompanied by rash, such as herpes zoster, erythema infectio-

sum, scarlet fever, or Kawasaki disease. Similarly, malaise, sore throat, nausea, or vomiting may occur with mononucleosis.

General health. In a patient with a maculopapular eruption, the two most common causes are drug reaction and viral illness. Inquire about viral symptoms, such as fever, malaise, and upper respiratory or gastrointestinal symptoms.

Are there possible contacts or sources of contagion?

Key Questions
- Does anyone you live with or have close contact with have something similar? How long have they had it?
- Have you traveled recently? Where?
- What do you do for a living? Hobbies or leisure activities?
- Do you have any pets? Or been around animals?

Living situation. Explore the patient's living situation. The geographics of his or her daily activities may help provide diagnostic clues, particularly for rashes caused by infectious or infestation mechanisms. Children, in particular, may contract scabies, pediculosis (lice), or impetigo by direct contact in school or day care.

Travel. The significance of recent travel may be overlooked by a patient who develops a rash weeks or months after return.

Diseases endemic to other parts of the world may present with rash, such as erythema nodosum, common in southeast Asia, or leprosy, common in Africa, southeast Asia, or South America. Both eruptions may also occur secondary to tuberculosis. Camping trips to wooded areas may result in a bite by a deer tick, causing Lyme disease. The resultant skin eruption in Lyme disease is known as erythema chronicum migrans (ECM). ECM begins 4 to 20 days after the bite of the tick, but only a third of patients remember being bitten.

Other exposures. Outdoor occupations or leisure activities may potentially expose persons to a variety of rashes and lesions, including insect bites and allergic or contact dermatitis from poison ivy or chemical substances. Sun exposure can also worsen chronic eruptions, such as rosacea or the malar butterfly rash in systemic lupus erythmatosus (SLE). Ringworm is common in farmers who work with cattle.

Pets. Flea bites produce a urticarial lesion with a central punctum. The reaction is an immunological one, making it different in each individual. Bites are usually on the legs. New lesions may appear daily, and itching is variable but sometimes intense. Cat or dog fleas are usually the culprits. An atypical form of scabies may be transmitted from dogs to humans and usually presents only as a single lesion.

Is there anything that exacerbates or triggers the reaction?

Key Questions
- Does anything seem to make this worse?
- Do you have any known allergies?

Triggers. Aggravating factors are often easily identified by patients. Any rash involving vasodilation will become more vivid and likely more pruritic with heat exposure, whether via sunlight, sweating, or a hot shower. Localized eruptions, especially on the hands or forearms, prompt many patients to consider chemicals or other products as causes. Persons with eczema whose hands are frequently exposed to water are vulnerable to the development of irritant eczema on the exposed skin. Foods occasionally exacerbate skin lesions. Rosacea is a vasomotor instability disorder characterized by exacerbation with dietary consumption of vasodilators, such as coffee, tea, alcohol, or spicy foods. Stress, whether physiological (e.g., menstruation, pregnancy) or psychological, is widely believed to trigger or worsen many chronic rashes, especially eczema and psoriasis. Stress also may facilitate recurrent eruptions of HSV.

Could this rash be caused by a medication?

Key Questions
- Are you taking any medications (prescription or over the counter)?
- Do you have any medication allergies?

Medication. There are four types of dermatological effects of drugs: side effects (such as photodermatitis), allergic reactions (such as urticaria, fixed drug eruptions, or morbilliform eruptions), commensal skin eruptions (such as pityriasis versicolor in a patient on systemic corticosteroids), and worsening of existing skin eruptions (such as tinea eruptions mistakenly treated as eczema with topical corticosteroids). Medications used after the onset of a rash may be irritants or sensitizers and worsen the condition.

Is this inherited or is there a significant dermatological family history?

Key Question
- Does anyone else in your family have chronic skin problems?

Family history. A family history of dermatological problems may add insight to the diagnosis. Atopic disease (atopic dermatitis, asthma, hay fever) tends to cluster in families. Psoriasis, seborrheic dermatitis, and rosacea are also frequently noted to have a familial inheritance pattern. Multiple café-au-lait spots with a positive family history for neurofibromatosis can help identify children with this dominantly inherited disease.

DIAGNOSTIC REASONING: FOCUSED PHYSICAL EXAMINATION

Look at All the Skin and Mucous Membranes

"Peephole" diagnosis should be avoided; the whole organ should be examined. If the patient is not fully undressed, relevant lesions could be missed. The feet should always be examined in the presence of hand dermatitis in order not to miss an id (hypersensitivity) reaction to a tinea infection or a concomitant hand tinea.

Inspect for Distribution

Determine if the lesion is widespread or localized. Determine if it is unilateral or bilateral, symmetrical or asymmetrical. Symmetrical lesions commonly have internal causation (eczema, psoriasis, acne); asymmetrical lesions have external causation (bacterial or fungal infections, allergic contact eczema). Determine if the lesion is predominantly on the flexor (atopic eczema) or extensor (psoriasis) surfaces. Determine if the distribution is confined either to protected areas or to light-exposed areas, such as in collagen-vascular diseases, photosensitive reactions to drugs, and airborne contact dermatitis. Determine if the lesion is predominantly centrifugal (affecting the extremities), seen in erythema multiforme, Rocky Mountain spotted fever, insect bites, or centripetal (sparing the extremities and concentrated on the trunk). Determine if it has intertriginous distribution (neck, axilla, groin), such as is evidenced in candidiasis, some inflammatory fungal infections, and some forms of psoriasis.

Inspect the Mouth

Drug eruptions from sulfonamides, penicillin, streptomycin, quinine, and atropine often have associated mucosal erosions and crusts. Mucosal involvement is common in hand and foot lesions (e.g., hand-foot-and-mouth disease), herpes, and syphilis.

Inspect the Hair

In children, a triad of hair loss, scaling, and lymphadenopathy is considered diagnostic of tinea capitis until proven otherwise. A high index of suspicion is warranted in inner city areas where the condition is common.

Palpate the Skin

Palpation of the skin assesses its texture and consistency for softness, firmness, fluctuance, and depth. Smooth skin has no felt irregularity. Uneven skin has fine scaling or some warty lesions. Rough skin feels like sandpaper and is characteristic of keratin/horn or crusts. Palpation is also used to tell whether the lesion is tender.

Assessing the superficial skin for texture is done by palpation with the fingertips. Deeper palpation is done using the thumb and index fingers. Soft skin feels like the lips, normal skin like the cheeks, firm skin like the tip of the nose, hard skin like the forehead. The depth of the lesion determines if it is sitting on the surface or is situated within the dermis or the subcutaneous tissues. An indurated base is a thickening in the depths of the lesion rather than on the surface.

Palpate the Regional Lymph Glands

Many viral exanthems present with rash and lymphadenopathy. Palpation of the regional lymph glands may be of assistance in diagnosis if neoplasm is suspected.

Perform an Abdominal Examination

Detection of hepatic or splenic enlargement may assist in diagnosis of a systemic cause of skin disorders.

LABORATORY AND DIAGNOSTIC STUDIES

Diascopy

Diascopy is used to assess for blanching on pressure and is accomplished by pressing a glass or clear plastic slide on the lesion. Diascopy is most helpful in evaluating purpuric lesions: blood outside vessels (as in petechiae) will not blanch, while that entrapped within dilated vessels (as in telangiectasias) will demonstrate this phenomenon.

Wood's Light

Longwave ultraviolet (UV) light is used in the diagnosis of lesions suspected as fungal. Many, but not all, fungal rashes fluoresce. *Trichophyton* species, dermatophytes that are frequently identified in tinea eruptions, do fluoresce; *Microsporum* species, which may also be responsible for tinea eruptions, do not.

Skin Scraping and Potassium Hydroxide Preparation

Microscopically examine a sample of cells retrieved from a lesion, assessing for the presence of fungal or dermatophytic spores and hyphae. The lesion should be gently scraped using a scalpel (collect from an active area such as the border of the lesion), the cells treated with a drop of 20% potassium hydroxide (KOH), and then warmed or allowed to stand a few minutes to soften the keratin. Addition of DMSO (40% dimethylsulfoxide) to the KOH solution accelerates diagnosis. Chlorazol Black E stain highlights fungal hyphae as dark blue-black against a light gray background.

Tzanck Smear

In a Tzanck smear, an indirect test for herpes virus infections (HSV, HZ), cells are retrieved by swabbing the base of a lesion (usually a vesicle), smearing it onto a glass slide, and then staining it with Giemsa or Wright's solution. Examined microscopically, the presence of multinucleated giant cells confirms the diagnosis.

Bacterial Culture

In taking a bacterial culture, exudate from a lesion is collected on a sterile swab, then cultured for growth. Gram stain may also be done. Once a bacterial isolate is known, antibiotic sensitivity testing is also performed.

Viral Culture

For a viral culture, cells from the base of a lesion (usually a vesicle) are collected on a dacron swab and cultured for identification of viral infections, particularly herpesvirus (HSV or HZ).

Punch Biopsy

In a punch biopsy, a tissue sample is assessed histopathologically for identification. Select a punch size about 2 to 3 mm larger than the lesion or sample an active area if the lesion is large. Gently swirl while exerting slight downward pressure on the punch. When well into the dermis, remove the punch and excise the sample at its base. The defect may be closed with electrocautery, suture(s), or left open to heal by secondary intention. Place the sample in preservative (e.g., formaldehyde solution).

Excisional Biopsy

In excisional biopsy, a tissue sample is assessed histopathologically for identification. Excise the entire lesion, usually making an elliptical incision around the lesion beyond its margins. Excise the base and close the defect with sutures or cauterize bleeding vessels. Place the sample in preservative (e.g., formaldehyde solution).

DIFFERENTIAL DIAGNOSIS

Conditions discussed in the following sections represent many of the most common skin eruptions observed in primary care. Consult a dermatology text for a complete review.

FOLLICULAR ERUPTIONS

Acne Vulgaris

Acne presents as a chronic eruption of the pilosebaceous unit, with noninflammatory (open and closed comedones) and/or inflammatory (papules, pustules, cysts) lesions. Its distribution follows that of the sebaceous glands—face, neck, chest, back, upper arms. Neonatal acne first occurs between 2 to 4 weeks of age, lasting until 4 to 6 months. Persistence beyond 12 months may indicate endocrine dysfunction. African-Americans and other dark-skinned persons need aggressive treatment to prevent (even in mild acne) post-inflammatory hyperpigmentation.

Rosacea

Rosacea is a vasomotor instability disorder characterized by sebaceous gland hypertrophy, papules, pustules, persistent erythema, and telangiectasias. It shows a predilection for the face.

INFECTIOUS ERUPTIONS

Impetigo

Impetigo presents as a superficial pustular, bullous, or nonbullous eruption, followed by crusting (often honey colored). Causative organisms are usually staphylococcus or streptococcus. Contagion occurs by direct inoculation. It is typically a localized eruption that may occur anywhere on the body, with a predilection for the face and trunk.

Folliculitis

Folliculitis is a superficial pustular infection of the hair follicles. Causative organisms are usually staphylococcus, occasionally streptococcus or Gram-negative organisms, including *Pseudomonas, Klebsiella,* or *Proteus* species. It is typically a localized eruption that may occur anywhere on the body, with a predilection for hairy areas and flexural regions.

Furuncle

A furuncle, otherwise referred to as a "boil," is a larger infection from an antecedent folliculitis (see previous section).

Carbuncle

A carbuncle is an abscess of conjoined or adjacent furuncles (see previous section).

MACULAR/PAPULAR ERUPTIONS

Erythema Infectiosum (Fifth Disease)

Fifth disease, also known as "slapped cheek disease," presents as a systemic illness of sudden onset characterized by a coalescing, red, maculopapular eruption on the face. Two to three days later a reticular eruption on the extremities occurs. The causative organism is parvovirus B-19. This is a self-limiting condition.

Children with underlying hemolytic anemia may experience aplastic crisis.

Measles

Measles is caused by a viral exanthem, and the systemic illness that results is characterized by a fine, erythematous, morbilliform eruption on the face that spreads rapidly to the trunk and becomes confluent and reticulate. Cough, purulent coryza, photophobia, and fever precede the rash. This is a self-limiting condition.

Rubella

Rubella results from a viral exanthem similar to measles and starts as fine macules and papules on the face and progresses caudally. Lymphadenopathy of post-auricular nodes is characteristic of this disease.

Pityriasis Rosea

Pityriasis rosea presents with a rapidly evolving papulosquamous eruption of possible viral etiology. It is characterized by an initial "herald patch," followed within days by numerous faintly erythematous patches on the trunk and upper extremities ("T-shirt and shorts" distribution). The patches demonstrate fine scaling, and mild to severe pruritis may be present. It is more common in the spring and fall and among adolescents. In African-American children, the eruption may consist only of occasional oval lesions along the cleavage lines. The remaining lesions are discrete, scattered follicular or nonfollicular papules over the trunk and proximal extremities. The face may also be involved.

Scarlet Fever

Scarlet fever is a systemic illness associated with group A beta-hemolytic (GABHS) strep throat. It is characterized by a macular erythema of the face (flushing), except around the mouth (circumoral pallor), followed by a disseminated fine papular erythema (scarlatiniform), which may then desquamate. The rash is intensified in the flexor folds (Pastia's lines). Associated symptoms are sore throat, malaise, fever, circumoral pallor, and a white or strawberry tongue.

Roseola

Roseola is a viral infection thought to be caused by human herpes virus (HHV-6). It is characterized by 2 to 3 days of sustained fever in an irritable infant who otherwise appears well. Mild edema of the eyelids and posterior cervical lymphadenopathy are occasionally seen. Following the temperature fall, a pink, morbilliform, cutaneous eruption appears transiently and fades within 24 hours. This is a self-limiting condition.

VESICULAR AND BULLOUS ERUPTIONS

Hand-Foot-and-Mouth Disease

Coxsackie virus A-16 is the causative organism of this viral exanthem and systemic illness. The condition is characterized by painful mouth ulcers, followed by painful white vesicles with a surrounding erythema on the fingers, palms, toes, and soles. Patients usully have a low-grade fever, sore throat, and malaise for 1 to 2 days. Some develop submandibular or cervical lymphadenopathy. This is a self-limiting condition.

Insect Bites

Mosquito and horsefly bites can cause a common blistering reaction that is surrounded by faint erythema, central pallor if swollen, and usually a visible central punctum. The bites may be arranged in groups if they are multiple. The lesions are pruritic and/or sore; the condition is self-limiting.

Herpes Simplex Virus

Herpes simplex virus lesions have vesicles (solitary or grouped) that are surrounded by an erythematous base, with discrete, well-demarcated areas that later crust. The condition is associated with soreness and/or pain and may be preceded by tingling. There is a predilection for lips and genitalia. Recurrences (same location[s]) are common and usually milder.

Herpes Zoster (Shingles)

Zoster lesions present as vesicles that are grouped, surrounded by an erythematous base, with discrete, well-demarcated lesions that later crust. Intense burning and pain often precedes the eruption. There is a predilection for dermatomal distribution (especially face or trunk).

Varicella Zoster (Chickenpox)

Varicella lesions are discrete vesicles with a disseminated distribution; lesions develop in crops or in succession. Vesicles later crust, and occasionally secondary impetigo develops. The illness is associated with malaise and fever. This is a self-limiting condition.

FUNGAL INFECTIONS

Candidiasis

Candidiasis is caused by a yeast-like fungus that produces rashes in a variety of sites: vulvovaginitis, thrush, intertrigo (groin, axilla, gluteal), and diaper dermatitis. The lesion is an erythematous maculopapular eruption, well demarcated, occasionally with satellite lesions (pinpoint papules) at the periphery with maceration in moist areas. It is associated with mild to intense pruritis; the causative organism usually is *C. albicans*.

Tinea

Tinea is a fungal eruption that causes rashes in a variety of sites: body (corporis), foot (pedis), beard (barbae), groin (cruris), and scalp (capitis). Lesions have erythematous scaling areas with a discrete border and central clearing that is often associated with pruritis or soreness. The causative organisms are *Trichophyton, Microsporum*, and *Epidermophyton*.

Pityriasis (Tinea) Versicolor

Pityriasis versicolor is a yeast infection characterized by a macular eruption of many colors, hypo- to hyperpigmentation, and fine scaling. Macules begin insidiously, may take weeks to months to fully develop, and may coalesce. The condition is usually asymptomatic but occasionally pruritic. There is a predilection for a sebaceous gland distribution (neck, trunk). The causative organism is *Pityrosporum orbiculare (Malassezia furfur)*. Repigmentation may take years or never occur. Recurrences are common.

IMMUNOLOGICAL AND INFLAMMATORY ERUPTIONS

Eczema

Eczema is a chronic relapsing inflammatory condition that can take several forms (atopic, nummular, or dyshidrotic). It is characterized by erythematous, poorly demarcated macules, papules, and vesicles that occasionally weep and/or crust. When severe, eczema may be associated with fissuring and bleeding. It is associated with mild to intense pruritis. In dark-skinned persons, scaling and dryness associated with eczema gives an "ashy" appearance to the skin.

Contact/Allergic Dermatitis

Contact dermatitis is an inflammatory reaction to many substances (e.g., poison ivy, nettles). Papulovesicular or bullous eruption surrounded by erythema, with weeping of exudate (non-contagious), is characteristic of the condition. It may be associated with moderate to intense pruritis.

Psoriasis

Psoriasis is a chronic, relapsing auto-immune disorder characterized by well-demarcated erythematous plaques, patches, and papules, which typically present with silvery scale. There is a predilection for elbows, knees, hands, nails (pitting), scalp, and gluteal cleft. The condition may be pruritic or sore. An interesting note is that the lesions may demonstrate

Auspitz's sign: pinpoint bleeding when the surface is scraped.

Seborrheic Dermatitis

Seborrheic dermatitis is a chronic relapsing disorder characterized by erythematous scaling patches, which are poorly demarcated and may be pruritic. There is a predilection for scalp, face, central chest, and genitals. The condition is aggravated by cold weather, dry skin, and stress.

ALLERGIC REACTIONS

Erythema Multiforme

Erythema multiforme is an immune complex disorder involving the skin and occasionally the mucous membranes. It is characterized by iris (target) lesions on the extremities; desquamation often follows. Common causes include numerous medications (especially sulfonamides, penicillins, barbiturates, salicylates), histoplasmosis, mycoplasma, HSV, mononucleosis, hepatitis B, or malignancies. It is often self-limited. A severe form, Stevens-Johnson syndrome, is characterized by widespread involvement with vesicobullous lesions. It involves the mucous membranes, conjunctiva, urethra, and possibly the lungs, gastrointestinal tract, and kidneys.

Urticaria

Urticaria is characterized by a well-demarcated, usually disseminated, eruption that is evanescent over minutes to about 24 hours. The condition usually has an asymmetrical distribution.

NEOPLASTIC ERUPTIONS

Malignant Melanoma

Melanoma is an aggressive cancer with a tendency for rapid spread and early metastasis. Characterized by asymmetry (half of a mole or lesion doesn't look like the other half), melanoma has an irregular, scalloped, or not clearly defined border with a color that varies or is not uniform (whether the color is tan, brown, black, white, red, or blue). The diameter is usually larger than 6 mm. However, any change in the size of a mole should be viewed with suspicion. The three most significant risk factors for developing melanoma include history of melanoma in a first-degree relative, a large number of moles (more than 50 to 100), or atypical moles as designated by biopsy. Other factors that increase risk of melanoma include adulthood, blond or red hair, blue or light-colored eyes, changed or persistently changing mole, Caucasian race, fair complexion, freckles, personal history of melanoma, immunosuppression, inability to tan, severe sunburns in childhood, and presence of a congenital mole.

Basal Cell Carcinoma

Basal cell carcinoma usually appears as a small, fleshy bump or nodule on the head, neck, or hands. Occasionally, these nodules may appear on the trunk of the body, usually as flat growths. These basal cell tumors do not spread quickly. It may take many months or years for one to reach a diameter of one-half inch. Untreated, the cancer will begin to bleed, crust over, then repeat the cycle. Although this type of cancer rarely spreads to other parts of the body, it can extend below the skin to the bone and cause considerable local damage. The cure rate for basal cell carcinoma (sometimes referred to as non-melanoma carcinoma) is 95% when properly treated.

Squamous Cell Carcinoma

Squamous cell carcinoma presents as an indurated papule, plaque, or nodule with thick scale that is often eroded, crusted, or ulcerated. It can be found on sun-exposed skin surfaces, in areas of radiodermatitis, or on old burn scars. Although slow growing, squamous cell carcinomas arising on the lip, mouth, or ears may be associated with regional lymphadenopathy and metastasis. If promptly and properly treated, it has a cure rate of 95%.

Table 3-2

Differential Diagnosis of Common Causes of Rashes and Skin Lesions

Disorder	Characteristics	Distribution/Progression	Associations	Diagnostic Studies
Follicular Eruptions				
Acne vulgaris	Comedones and/or papules, pustules, cysts	Face, neck, back, chest, upper arms	Onset of puberty, topical steroids, anabolic steroids, systemic corticosteroids , lithium, phenytoin	Usually none
Rosacea	Flushing, persistent redness, sebaceous hyperplasia, erythematous papules, telangiectasias, ocular involvement in up to 40%	Symmetrical, usually face only; may involve eyes	Topical steroids, systemic corticosteroids	Usually none
Infectious Eruptions				
Impetigo	Vesicular infection; honey-colored crusts and erosions	Face; any area of the body with a minor wound, especially excoriated lesions	Scratching as a result of insect bites, atopic dermatitis, scabies	Bacterial culture
Folliculitis	Superficial perifollicular papules and pustules	Any hair-bearing body surface, but especially the scalp, beard, legs, axillae	Shaving, hot tubs, contact with mineral oils, occlusive dressings	Bacterial culture
Furuncle	Very tender, deep-seated inflammatory nodule that develops from a folliculitis	Same as folliculitis	May have fever	Incision and drainage for bacterial culture
Carbuncle	Multiple coalescing furuncles	Same as furuncle	Same as furuncle	Same as furuncle

Macular/Papular Eruptions

Erythema in-fectiosum	Bright red rash or "slapped cheeks," followed by a diffuse maculopapular rash on the trunk and extremities, leading to a lacy appearance as exanthem fades	Cheeks, then trunk and extremities	Aplastic anemia in children with underlying hemolytic anemias; fetal hydrops has been reported in pregnant women infected with parvovirus B-19	IgM, IgG can be measured
Measles	Patient develops the three Cs: cough, coryza, and conjunctivitis; Koplik spots are evident on buccal mucosa; rash begins with spike of fever; rash is centripetal in distribution, possibly becoming hemorrhagic in severe cases	Rash starts on neck and ears faintly, then covers face, arms, and chest; on second day rash covers the lower torso and legs; on third day rash is on the feet and the face rash begins to fade	Abdominal pain, otitis media, and broncho-pneumonia are commonly associated; severe cases can cause encephalomyelitis	IgM can be measured for measles as well as acute and convalescent IgG titers
Rubella	Tender lymphadenopathy of the postauricular, posterior occipital nodes; maculopapular and confluent rash that is lacy and not pruritic; rash lasts 3 days	Rash begins on face and spreads to trunk and extremities within the first 24 hours	Infection with virus while pregnant results in congenital rubella	Confirmation by acute and convalescent IgG titers or by direct measurement of rubella IgM antibody
Pityriasis rosea	Multiple oval erythematous lesions with an inner fine circle of scale; ovals line up along skin cleavage lines on the trunk, producing a Christmas tree-like pattern	Trunk, proximal extremities, rarely on face; rash is preceded by a "herald patch," appearing from a few days to 3 weeks before generalized eruption	More common in spring and fall	If present on palms and/or soles and history warrants, check RPR to rule out secondary syphilis

Continued

Table 3-2				
Differential Diagnosis of Common Causes of Rashes and Skin Lesions—cont'd				
Disorder	**Characteristics**	**Distribution/Progression**	**Associations**	**Diagnostic Studies**
Macular/Papular Eruptions—cont'd				
Scarlet fever	Fine, mildly erythematous papules and sandpaper-like rash found on the trunk	Rash begins in axillae, groin, and neck; it avoids the face, but there is circumoral pallor	Strawberry tongue; Pastia's lines: areas of linear hyperpigmentation in the deep creases	Culture for group A streptococcus
Roseola	High fever for 3–4 days in infants and young children; as fever returns to normal, a diffuse maculopapular rash erupts	Rash begins on trunk, quickly spreads to arms, face, neck, and legs	Posterior cervical lymphadenopathy	None
Vesicular and Bullous Eruptions				
Hand-foot-and-mouth disease	Systemic illness caused by coxsackie virus A-16; painful white vesicles with surrounding red halo	Painful mouth ulcers followed in 24 hours by painful vesicles on fingers, palms, toes, and soles	Low-grade fever, sore throat, and malaise; cervical and submandibular lymphadenopathy possible	Tzanck smear
Insect bites	Flea bites most common; intensely pruritic eruption, usually in groups of three	Lower legs, but may appear anywhere on body if pets allowed on furniture or beds	Exposure to dogs or cats or to carpeted areas previously in contact with infected animals	Confirmational biopsy occasionally needed
Herpes simplex virus	Primary infection with grouped vesicles on an erythematous base at the site of inoculation; regional lymphadenopathy; may be preceded by prodrome of tingling, itching, burning, or tenderness	Can occur anywhere on the body, but most common areas are the genitals and thighs, mouth, lips and chin; may be disseminated in patients who are immunocompromised	Other STDs, HIV; triggered by sun, stress, fatigue, fever, trauma	Tzanck smear, viral culture; screen for other STDs, HIV if history warrants

	Clinical Features	Risk Factors	Diagnosis
Herpes zoster	Unilateral pain, itching, or burning that precedes by 3-5 days an eruption of vesicles or bullae; followed by crusting and erosions	May occur anywhere on the body but is unilateral, following a dermatomal pattern; requires prompt referral to ophthalmologist if eye involved (note: see lesion on the tip or side of nose for indication)	Immunosuppression, older age, local trauma in children / Viral culture (not Tzanck smear)
Varicella zoster	Generalized pruritic vesicular lesions that are in different stages of healing; erythematous vesicles, ruptured vesicles, and crusted vesicles with scabs	Lesions usually begin on trunk and spread to the face and proximal extremities	Herpes zoster occurs with reactivation of the virus / ELISA titers can confirm the acute infection
Fungal Infections			
Candidiasis	Beefy-red, well-demarcated plaques, often with scaling edge and satellite lesions; intertriginous areas may also show erosions and maceration	Diaper area in infants, body folds, mucosal surfaces, nails, and nail folds	Immunocompromised, diabetes, steroid inhalants, pregnancy, oral contraceptives, antibiotics, systemic and topical steroids / KOH, culture
Tinea	Variable: depending on body part affected; hair: scaling, hair loss, pustules; skin: red, scaly patch that may develop central clearing; feet: vesicles or bullae	Skin, hair, feet, nails	Immunocompromised, systemic corticosteroids, farmers and others with animal contact, hot humid weather with tight clothing or occlusive footwear / KOH, culture

Continued

Table 3-2

Differential Diagnosis of Common Causes of Rashes and Skin Lesions—cont'd

Disorder	Characteristics	Distribution/Progression	Associations	Diagnostic Studies
Fungal infections—cont'd				
Pityriasis (tinea) versicolor	Variably colored white to pink to brown scaling, round or oval macules of varying sizes; often coalescing to form large areas of discoloration	Upper trunk, axillae, neck, upper arms, abdomen, thighs, genitals	Heat, humidity, tropical climates, exercise, systemic corticosteroids, seborrheic dermatitis	KOH shows hyphae and spores in "spaghetti and meatballs" pattern
Immunological/Inflammatory Eruptions				
Eczema/atopic dermatitis	Erythema, papules, vesicles, scaling, excoriations, crusts, pruritus always present	Symmetrical; infant: face, flexures; children: flexural creases; adults: may be discrete round patches or be regionalized to specific area	Personal or family history of asthma, seasonal allergies, and eczema, secondary colonization with S. aureus or HSV	Serum IgE; culture for bacteria or HSV if indicated
Contact/allergic dermatitis	Vesicles and erosions with edema and inflammation, giving way to crusts and lichenification; pruritus	Localized, often asymmetrical; may be generalized with airborne allergens/poison ivy; linear pattern with plant dermatitis	Occupational, recreational pursuits	Patch testing
Psoriasis	Well-demarcated, ham-colored plaques and papules with silvery scale; chronic, recurrent pruritus is common	Favors elbows and knees, scalp, intertriginous areas; may involve nails	Streptococcal infection, arthritis, HIV infection, medications, ETOH, family history	ASO titer or strep culture if indicated; HIV if indicated; biopsy
Seborrheic dermatitis	Chronic scaling, flaking, erythematous dermatitis; variable pruritus	Areas where sebaceous glands are most active: face, scalp, eyebrows, eyelashes, body folds, ear folds, presternal area, mid- and upper back, genitalia	Atopic history, HIV infection	HIV if indicated

Allergic Reactions

Erythema multiforme	Hypersensitivity reaction seen as annular target or iris lesions	Begins on upper extremities and trunk	Herpes virus, *Mycoplasma pneumoniae* infections, drugs especially sulfonamides	Skin biopsy may assist in diagnosis if caused by Stevens-Johnson syndrome; chest film for mycoplasma
Urticaria	Transient wheals that may be acute or chronic (lasting longer than 6 weeks); individual lesions tend to come and go within hours; pruritic	Localized, regional, or generalized	Angioedema may also be present, may be life threatening; chronic infection, SLE, lymphoma	Biopsy; general medical work-up to rule out underlying systemic disease in chronic urticaria

Neoplastic Eruptions

Malignant melanoma	Asymmetrical border, irregular, has a color variation within the lesion and is >6 mm	Anywhere on body, including scalp	Usually asymptomatic, unless bleeding, ulceration, discharge is present	Skin biopsy, excisional biopsy
Basal cell carcinoma	Papular or nodular lesions, with raised pearly borders and numerous superficial telangiectases	Sun-damaged areas; also seen in covered areas when there is genetic predisposition to basal cell carcinoma	Usually asymptomatic	Skin biopsy
Squamous cell carcinoma	Indurated papule, plaque, or nodule; may be eroded, crusted, or ulcerated	Sun-damaged areas, areas of radiodermatitis, old burn scars but can occur anywhere on body	Usually asymptomatic; can be associated with HPV, immunosuppression, topical nitrogen mustard, oral PUVA, chronic ulcers, industrial carcinogens, arsenic	Skin biopsy, excisional biopsy

Chapter 4

Common Problems of the Cardiovascular and Respiratory Systems

Chest Pain

The first task in evaluating a patient with chest pain is to determine if the pain is cardiac or noncardiac in origin and how emergent the condition is. Myocardial ischemia and infarct are life-threatening causes of chest pain and must be assessed rapidly in order that emergent treatment can be initiated. Aortic dissection is a rare but equally catastrophic cardiovascular cause of chest pain that must also be diagnosed quickly. A semi-emergent cause of cardiac pain is acute pericarditis caused by inflammation of the pericardium, usually from a viral infection. Valvular diseases such as aortic stenosis and mitral valve prolapse are less emergent causes of cardiac pain.

Pulmonary, gastrointestinal, musculoskeletal, neurological, and psychological conditions may cause chest pain. The cause of pain in any organ or system can be the result of inflammation, obstruction/restriction, or distention/dilation. Pain arising from the gastrointestinal, musculoskeletal, respiratory, cardiac, and pulmonary systems all transmit to the same spinal cord segments, T1 through T5, making identification of the specific origin of discomfort difficult. Over 30 causes of noncardiac chest pain relate to chest anatomy, specifically skin, muscle, ribs and cartilage, pleura, lung, esophagus, mediastinum, and thoracic vertebrae.

In children, chest pain is rarely associated with serious organic disease. The three most common causes of chest pain in children are costochondritis; trauma and muscle strain to the chest wall; and respiratory conditions often associated with cough. Chest pain from cardiac disease is relatively rare; less than 5% of chest pain in children is cardiac in origin. However, patients and families often associate chest pain with heart disease and can be anxious about the condition because of reports of sudden death in young athletes.

DIAGNOSTIC REASONING: FOCUSED HISTORY

Identification of potentially acute life-threatening situations must be determined immediately. Once you have determined that there is no immediate risk of severe oxygen deprivation to vital organs (e.g., myocardial infarction, aortic dissection, and pulmonary embolism), proceed with a focused history (Table 4-1).

Pulmonary thromboembolism is a pulmonary cause of chest pain, but the presenting sign is usually dyspnea (refer to Dyspnea, p. 107).

First, is this an emergency condition?

Key Questions

- How severe is the pain? On a scale of 1 to 10, 1 being no pain and 10 the worst pain you can imagine, how would you rank your pain?
- Where is the pain? Does it go any-where?
- What were you doing when the pain started?
- Are you short of breath? Nauseated? Dizzy?
- Do you have a history of heart disease? Angina?
- Are you HIV positive, on chemo-therapy, or do you have an autoim-mune disease?

Severity of pain and location. Remember that chest pain is subjective and prior experience, personal attitudes, and cultural values form the patient's perception of pain.

The severity of the chest pain may not be an indication of the severity of the condition.

Assessment of the severity of the pain is often made easier by the use of rating scales that use 1 to 10 or color scales ranging from pink to red or happy to sad faces. Scales can be especially useful with children who may not yet have language to describe pain (see Chapter 5, Figure 5-1, p. 150). Constant, frequent, or severe pain is likely to interrupt the child's daily activity.

Pain that is described as substernal heaviness, pressure, a squeezing sensation, or a feeling of discomfort is classic coronary ischemic pain. The substernal pain or discomfort may radiate up the left shoulder and down the left arm and may extend to the neck and lower jaw. Pain described as an abrupt tearing pain, located in the anterior or posterior chest, characterizes

Table 4-1		
Differentiating Ischemic from Non-Ischemic Chest Pain		
FACTORS	**ISCHEMIC ORIGIN**	**NON-ISCHEMIC ORIGIN**
Character of pain	Constricting, squeezing, burning, heavy feeling	Dull or sharp pain
Location of pain	Substernal, mid-thoracic; radiates to arms, shoulders, neck, teeth, forearms, fingers; interscapular	Left submammary and hemothorax areas
Precipitating factors	With exercise, excitement, stress, after meals	Pain after exercise; provoked by specific body movements or deep breaths

Modified from Selzer A: *Principles and practices of clinical cardiology,* ed 2, Philadelphia, 1983, WB Saunders, p 17.

aortic dissection. It may migrate to the arms, abdomen, back, or legs.

Chest pain arising from pulmonary origin is usually the most emergent cause of non-cardiac chest pain. Pulmonary embolus (PE), pneumothorax, and pneumonia may all present with chest pain. The patient with PE is able to point to the area of pain over the affected lung and usually describes a gripping, stabbing pain that is moderate to severe in intensity. The pain may radiate to the neck or shoulders.

Patients experiencing a pneumothorax most frequently report mild to severe chest pain of sudden onset located in the lateral thorax and radiating to the ipsilateral shoulder. The quality of pain is described as sharp or tearing. Chest pain of pneumonia is located over the area of infiltration and does not radiate. It frequently has a burning or stabbing quality and is associated with cough (see Cough, p. 127).

Onset. Determine if the onset of pain is sudden or gradual and what the patient's activity was at the time of onset. Typical onset of angina is during exercise, exertion, or emotional stress. It is relieved by rest or nitroglycerin. Chest pain of myocardial infarction (MI) may occur at any time and is not relieved by rest or nitroglycerin. Sudden onset of chest pain and dyspnea is common with PE. In a pneumothorax, the patient may report that severe coughing, exertion, or straining suddenly precipitated the chest pain. Chest pain caused by pneumonia occurs gradually over several hours or days. Chest pain in adolescents that occurs after activity but not at any other time may indicate organic cardiac disease.

Associated symptoms. The person experiencing an acute MI frequently reports nausea, vomiting, diaphoresis, shortness of breath, and syncope. PE is often associated with shortness of breath, apprehension, and hemoptysis. Chest pain from PE increases with deep breathing. Fever, cough, and thick sputum production usually accompany chest pain caused by pneumonia.

Other health conditions. Persons reporting a history of autoimmune disease are at risk for pericarditis.

Does the patient have risk factors for coronary artery disease?

Key Questions
- Do you have high blood pressure, diabetes, or heart disease?
- Has anyone in your family had a heart attack or stroke before the age of 60?
- Do you smoke? How many packs a day?
- Have you ever been told your cholesterol is high?

Risk factors. According to the Report of the U.S. Preventive Services Task Force, clinically significant coronary artery disease (CAD) is uncommon in men under 40 and premenopausal women, but risk increases with advancing age. The presence of risk factors such as smoking, hypertension, diabetes, high cholesterol, and family history of heart disease increase the risk of CAD.

If this is not an emergency, what does a description of the pain tell me?

Key Questions
- When did the pain begin?
- What were you doing when the pain first occurred?
- Point to where the pain is located. Does it spread to any other part of your body?
- What seems to bring on the pain?
- Does the pain awaken you from sleep?
- Describe the pain. What does it feel like? (e.g., dull, sore, stabbing, burning, squeezing)

Acute or chronic. The more chronic the pain, the less likely it is that a specific cause will be found. Intermittent chest pain that occurs frequently probably indicates a more serious problem such as angina than one episode of brief, mild pain.

Onset. In children, ask about recent choking episodes or swallowing a foreign body when the pain increases with attempts to swallow. Pain that usually occurs when lying down after eating is associated with gastroesophageal reflux disease (GERD). Trauma to the chest wall from a fall or strenuous activity may cause rib fractures or chest contusions.

Sleep. Distinguish between awakening with pain and awakening from pain. Awakening because of pain signals a more serious problem of organic origin such as cardiac ischemia. Psychogenic chest pain in adolescents commonly accompanies sleep disturbances.

Location and character of pain. Pain arising from the thoracic skin and other superficial tissues, such as that associated with furuncles, contusions, and abrasions, is sharply localized.

Irritation of the intercostal nerves can result in a neuritis that produces sudden onset of a stabbing, burning pain and tenderness that is easily located to the intercostal spaces and along inflamed nerves with three maximal pain points: adjacent to the vertebrae, in the axillary lines, and along the parasternal lines. Pain may be severe when the patient breathes deeply, coughs, or moves suddenly.

Dorsal root irritation associated with herpes zoster may present with intense burning or knifelike pain along the spine to the lateral thoracic wall and the anterior midline. This pain may restrict movement of the trunk and respirations. Generally this pain is continuous and increases in severity.

Nerve root pain is caused by mechanical irritation or edema of the nerve root.

This pain can be felt at the point of irritation but is frequently referred to points along the peripheral course of the nerve. If the dorsal root is involved, the dorsal radicles in the proximity of the spinal cord are implicated. Thoracic spinal segment root pain is often referred to the lateral and anterior chest wall and is seen with spinal diseases and thoracic deformities.

Costal cartilage that loosens from the fibrous attachment and curls upward off the end of the cartilage on the inner aspect of the rib causes localized pain and tenderness over the 8th, 9th, and 10th rib on either side. The pain is dull and aching but may be acute, paroxysmal, or stabbing.

Musculoskeletal pain is produced by irritation of tissues and transmitted through the sensory nerves. The stimulus travels through the nerve to the dorsal ganglion up the spinal afferent pathway to the central nervous system.

Bone pain results from irritation of sensory nerve endings in the periosteum and is intense and well localized. Chronic diseases affecting the bone marrow may cause a poorly localized pain of varying severity. Ribs are common sites for metastatic malignant deposits, probably because of their rich vascularity. When metastasis expands to the rib and involves the periosteum, pain results. Referred pain from a nerve dermatome is described as intense, aching, and boring back pain.

When tumors involve the mediastinum, chronic aching or dull substernal chest pain is produced by pressure of the tumor against the spine or ribs.

Lung pain is caused by involvement of adjacent structures. The trachea and large bronchus are innervated by the vagus nerve (CN X). The finer bronchi and lung parenchyma are free of pain innervation, and, therefore, extensive disease may occur in the periphery of the lungs without pain until the process extends to the parietal pleura. Pleural pain results from the loss of normal lubricating function and irritation of the serous membranes of the pleura. Pleuritic pain indicates that the thoracic pathology involves the pleural surfaces. It is a sharply localized, knifelike, cutting sensation that is accentuated with respiratory movement and is present all the time. Diaphragmatic pleural pain may be referred to the base of the neck or abdomen.

Children often report chest pain from tachydysrhythmias because they are unable to differentiate between true pain and the unusual sensation of the dysrhythmia. Cardiac causes of chest pain in children are usually associated with congenital anomalies or acquired diseases of the coronary artery such as Kawasaki disease.

What do associated symptoms tell me?

Key Questions

- Do you have a cough or a change in your usual cough?
- Do you bring up sputum? If so, how much and what color?
- Do you have a fever?
- Are you lightheaded or dizzy?
- Do you feel like your heart is racing?

Cough and sputum production. Chest pain associated with cough and colored sputum production is usually caused by an acute infection such as pneumonia. Pain results from a pleural effusion or the collection of fluid in the pleural space. Sputum associated with pneumonia can be dark green, rust, or red. Frequent lower respiratory tract infections can be caused by congenital heart disease with large left to right shunts and an increase in pulmonary blood flow. Children and older adults with persistent cough may experience chest pain related to the musculoskeletal strain associated with coughing. Asthmatic persons can develop chest pain from straining of the chest wall muscles caused by tachypnea, coughing, or retraction.

Fever. Fever may indicate pneumonia, myocarditis, or PE. Elderly and immunosuppressed persons may not have fever, even with bacterial infections.

Lightheadedness, dizziness, or fainting. Arrthymias caused by hypoxia, trauma, or electrical shock may cause insufficient coronary blood flow and chest pain. Premature atrial tachycardia (PAT) may cause lightheadedness. Diastole is shortened in PAT, and thus cardiac output is decreased.

Most cases of syncope in adults are caused by cardiac problems such as structural heart disease, arrhythmias, and coronary insufficiency. Most cases of syncope in children are benign and are the result of breath holding, orthostatic syncope, hyperventilation, or vasosyncopal episodes. **Fainting induced by exercise, preceded by chest pain, or recurrent with a family history of unexplained death requires careful investigation.**

Palpitations. Caffeine, stress, and hormonal changes may cause the sensation of a rapid or forceful heartbeat. Mitral valve prolapse may present with a history of palpitations. Beta-adrenergic agents or theophylline can cause dysrhythmias, including supraventricular tachycardia, which may be perceived as palpitations.

Is the pattern of pain related to activity and position change?

Key Questions

- Describe your recent physical activities.
- Have you had any injury to the chest?
- Does chest movement or position make the pain better or worse?

Recent activities. Recent strenuous exercise (especially weight lifting) or horseplay can strain the pectoral, trapezius, latissimus dorsi, serratus anterior, and shoulder muscles. Rib fractures and musculoskeletal strains and contusions can cause significant chest pain, especially with movement. Musculoskeletal causes are the most common cause of chest pain in children and younger adults.

Decreased exercise tolerance may result from significant heart disease such as shunts, arrhythmias, or coronary artery disease. In children, congenital coronary anomalies may arise abnormally (as from the pulmonary artery), take an abnormal course, or have fistula connections to other structures, resulting in exertional chest pain. These conditions are rare and difficult to diagnose.

Any episode of moderate to severe chest pain during or following exercise should be thoroughly investigated. The problem is usually cardiac disease in adults and cardiac abnormalities in children. In children, if no other noncardiac etiology (such as exercise-induced asthma) is found, referral to a pediatric cardiologist is indicated.

History of chest trauma. A careful history of preceding activities should be obtained to detect any recent muscle strain. Post-traumatic pericardial effusion may develop 1 to 3 months after chest compressions. Blunt injury, such as may occur with motor vehicle accidents, can cause hemothorax, pneumothorax, and soft tissue injury and rib fracture. A ruptured spleen can cause irritation of the phrenic nerve, producing shoulder pain.

Pain with movement. Pain of cardiac origin, except for pericarditis, is not affected by respiration. Pain on inspiration suggests pleural etiology. A sharp, pleuritic pain relieved by sitting upright and leaning forward suggests pericarditis. Pain, which is aggravated by chest wall movement, especially along the sternal border, is most frequently costochondritis. Adults and children may experience this inflammatory condition of the costal cartilage. Lying flat, alcohol, aspirin, spicy meals, and tight clothing often precipitate the pain of esophagitis. Frequently, patients report that this pain occurs after lying down following a meal.

Is there a gastrointestinal (GI) origin for the patient's chest pain?

Key Questions
- Does the pain get better or worse with food?
- Do you have blood in your stools?
- Have you vomited any blood?

Food association. Differentiating between esophageal and cardiac origin of chest pain can present a challenge because the character and location of the pain may be very similar. Nitroglycerin may relieve both the pain of angina and the pain of esophagitis. In these instances, electrocardiographic studies may be indicated.

Esophagitis is the most frequent GI cause of chest pain. Patients describe this pain as "heartburn" or a dull, burning sensation in the epigastric and retrosternal area. The esophagus is more pain sensitive in its proximal portion. Therefore chest pain that is temporally related to eating meals or particular foods should suggest esophagitis.

Associated symptoms of a sour taste in the mouth and mild nausea may or may not be associated with esophagitis. Esophageal tear or spasm causes more acute, severe chest pain, described as a "tearing" or "crushing" sensation. Frequently the patient experiencing pain of GI origin will report mild to moderate chest pain occurring intermittently over days to months.

Peptic ulcer and cholecystitis may cause chest pain intermittently. Hematemesis (blood in the emesis) or hematochezia (blood in the stool) frequently accompany peptic ulceration. Cholecystitis is frequently reported as right anterior chest pain, which radiates to the shoulder or upper back.

Acute pancreatitis should be considered if the chest pain is excruciating, constant, and reported in the left upper quadrant of the abdomen radiating to the chest, shoulder, and arm. Pancreatitis is often accompanied by symptoms of severe hypotension. Physical examination and diagnostic tests are necessary to differentiate it from chest pain of cardiovascular origin.

Could this pain be from a systemic cause?

Key Questions

- Do you have any skin problems?
- Do you have any chronic health problems?

Skin symptoms. If the patient reports persistent unilateral chest pain of pruritic, burning, or stabbing quality, consider herpes zoster. This pain will follow the distribution of a cervical or thoracic nerve root. A vesicular rash in the area of pain is characteristic. This rash occurs several days after the occurrence of chest pain.

Systemic conditions. Chest muscle pain may be caused by localized inflammation of the muscles in collagen diseases such as polymyositis, fibromyalgia, or systemic lupus erythematosus. Arthritic inflammatory changes of the cervical and thoracic spine and shoulders may produce upper chest pain. This pain is aggravated by range of motion of the affected joints.

Sickle cell disease (SCD) may cause chest pain. In sickle cell anemia, the erythrocytes become rigid and "sickle," leading to capillary occlusion and sickle cell crisis. The heart increases the stroke volume to compensate for the anemia. The heart gradually dilates and heart failure ensues. Chest pain in a patient with SCD can also come from acute chest syndrome (ACS). In this condition, chest pain, fever, dyspnea, and cough are caused by infarction of lung tissue or an infectious agent.

Marfan's syndrome is a connective tissue disease. Cardiovascular involvement occurs in over 50% of persons by age 21. Mitral valve involvement is common, with auscultatory findings of mitral regurgitation and mitral valve prolapse.

What does the family history tell me?

Key Questions

- Has anyone in your family had heart disease, chest pain, or sudden death from cardiac arrest?
- Has anyone in your family been born with heart problems?

Family history. History of congenital heart disease in close relatives increases the chances of its occurrence in a child. When one child has the condition, the risk of siblings having it increases by one third. Essential hypertension and coronary artery disease show a strong family pattern. Hypertrophic cardiomyopathy has a positive family history with autosomal dominant transmission in one third of patients. Some hereditary diseases may be associated with certain forms of congenital heart disease, such as Marfan's syndrome.

DIAGNOSTIC REASONING: FOCUSED PHYSICAL EXAMINATION

A focused physical examination of the patient experiencing chest pain will provide objective data for the assessment. A thorough examination of the cardiovascular, pulmonary, upper gastrointestinal, and upper body musculoskeletal systems is essential.

Observe General Appearance

Initial observation of the patient will provide clues to the severity of the problem. Observe the patient for grimacing, diaphoresis, pallor, cyanosis, tachypnea, use of accessory muscles for breathing, splinting of chest wall, and unequal chest wall excursion. Persons experiencing an MI may be diaphoretic, pale, and anxious. Patients manifesting PE appear diaphoretic and anxious, respirations are rapid, splinting of the chest is common, and peripheral cyanosis may be present. Persons with fractured ribs or significant chest wall contusions splint their chest walls and take shallow breaths to avoid aggravating pain with respiratory expansion.

Observe height and weight of child. Abnormal findings for age may indicate chronic disease.

Measure Vital Signs and Respiratory Patterns

Vital signs for persons experiencing angina may be within normal ranges. Frequently, however, with acute MI, blood pressure is elevated and cardiac arrhythmias are present. If cardiogenic shock ensues, hypotension will occur.

The patient with aortic dissection may be hypotensive, with unequal peripheral pulses. Pericarditis may be accompanied by fever, rapid and shallow respirations, and hypertension. Myocarditis may present with fever, respiratory distress, and paradoxical pulse.

In heart failure, decreased stroke volume reduces the systolic blood pressure, and compensatory vasoconstriction maintains a constant diastolic pressure. This may result in a decreased pulse pressure.

Pneumothorax is manifested by tachypnea and unequal chest wall excursion. The patient with pneumonia may also be tachypneic, with signs of infection that include fever and a productive cough.

In children, chest pain with tachycardia and hypotension is generally caused by hypovolemia secondary to a hemothorax, hemopneumothorax, or vascular injury. Pain may also be caused by rhythm disturbance.

The rate, rhythm, and depth of respirations in patients experiencing costochondritis, GI disease, or herpes zoster are not usually altered.

Hyperventilation can cause chest pain as a result of hypercapnic alkalosis or coronary artery vasoconstriction. Most hyperventilation is associated with a stressful event or emotional upset; however, aspirin overdose, severe pain, and diabetic ketoacidosis may be organic causes.

Inspect Skin

Cool, pale, moist skin may accompany an acute MI, PE, or aortic dissection. Observe the skin overlying the area of chest pain for signs of a vesicular rash of herpes zoster. Petechial rash on the face and shoulders may be a sign of protracted coughing as a result of pneumonia, asthma, or upper respiratory infection. Bruises may indicate trauma or abuse.

Sweat on the forehead of an infant may indicate congenital heart disease (CHD). A decrease in cardiac output causes a compensatory sympathetic overactivity, resulting in a cold sweat on the forehead. Examine the color of the mucous membranes, conjunctiva, soft palate, lips, and tongue for central cyanosis.

Palpate Trachea/Chest

Tracheal shift can occur with pneumothorax and, in children, with atelectasis involving a significant portion of one lung. To assess the trachea for lateral displacement, position your index finger first on the right side of the suprasternal notch, then the left. If the trachea has shifted to the side, you'll feel the wall on one side but only soft tissue on the other. In a pneumothorax, the trachea is deviated to the opposite side during exhalation and toward the side of the pneumothorax during inspiration. The trachea is displaced toward a lung that is atelectatic, with the displacement exaggerated during inspiration.

Palpate the entire chest wall for tenderness, depressions, or bulges. Fractured ribs and contusions will result in tenderness to palpation and possible deformity. Palpate each costochondral and chondrosternal junction. Costochondritis will be manifested by pain with palpation over the cartilage between the sternum and the ribs. Palpation and range of joint motion may elicit arthritis pain in the shoulder or cervical spine. Musculoskeletal chest pain is usually reproduced with palpation or by moving the arms and chest through a variety of positions. Subcutaneous emphysema may be palpable at the neck or upper

Table 4-2

Normal Breath Sounds

BREATH SOUND	LOCATION	QUALITY	INSPIRATION/ EXPIRATION RATIO
Bronchial	Heard on the chest over the sternum and in the back between the scapulae	High pitched and loud	Expiration longer than inspiration
Bronchovesicular	Heard over the bronchi at the first and second intercostal spaces anteriorly and between the scapulae posteriorly	Loud, medium pitched	Equal inspiratory and expiratory phases
Vesicular	Heard over most of the peripheral lung fields	Soft, low pitched	Inspiration longer than expiration

chest wall. Rib pain on palpation in children without a reported history of trauma may indicate child abuse.

To check the chest wall for symmetry, first test for diaphragmatic excursion of both the anterior and posterior thorax between the 8th and 10th ribs. As the patient takes a deep breath, each hand should move the same distance from the spine. Pneumothorax, pneumonia, and fractured ribs may alter this finding.

Percuss the Chest

Percussion in the area of pneumothorax will result in a hyperresonant sound of an air-filled cavity. Areas of infiltration as in pneumonia will produce a dull or flat sound.

Auscultate Breath Sounds

Instruct the patient to breathe through the mouth slowly and deeply. Auscultate systematically from the lung apexes to the lower lobes anteriorly, posteriorly, and lat-

erally. Table 4-2 lists normal breath sounds.

Auscultation of bronchial or bronchovesicular breath sounds over the peripheral lungs may indicate consolidation. If breath sounds are diminished over all lung fields, suspect chronic obstructive pulmonary disease (COPD). Obese patients may have breath sounds that are difficult to auscultate. Breath sounds will be inaudible in areas of pneumothorax.

Auscultate for Adventitious Sounds

Adventitious lung sounds are superimposed on normal sounds and can be auscultated over any area of the lung field during inspiration or expiration. Documentation of abnormal lung sounds should include the type of sound heard, location, and changes during both inspiration and expiration phases of respiration.

Crackles or rales are discontinuous popping sounds heard most often during inspiration. Any disease process that increases peripheral airway resistance, obstructs the peripheral airway, or causes a loss of elastic recoil will produce crackles. They indicate the presence of fluid, mucus, or pus in the smaller airways. Fine crackles are soft and high pitched. Medium crackles are louder and lower pitched. Crackles may be heard over the site of a PE.

Wheezing is frequently described as a whistling sound and can be heard during inspiration, expiration, or both. The sound is high pitched and musical. Wheezing indicates that there is fluid in the large airways, such as in severe heart failure, or more often it is associated with bronchospasm as seen in asthma. Wheezing occurs on exhalation because that is when small airways collapse. During inhalation, the negative pressure in the chest tends to hold the airways open. However, during exhalation, positive pressure in the alveoli is conducted from the outside of the small airways and tends to collapse them. The sound is usually polyphonic. This means that multiple slightly different high-pitched sounds are heard at the same time. Most of the etiologies that cause wheezing affect many small airways at the same time; each one collapses at a slightly different time creating a slightly different tone. The presence of a single-tone wheeze suggests a single area of blockage, such as with a foreign body. A prolonged expiratory phase of respiration is produced by intrathoracic airway obstruction associated with lower respiratory tract involvement.

Rhonchi are continuous, deep-pitched, coarse breath sounds usually heard during expiration. They are generated by turbulent air passing through secretions in large airways. Rhonchi may be present when the patient has pneumonia.

Pleural friction rub is a grating or squeaking sound heard in the lateral lung fields during inspiration and expiration. It indicates that inflamed parietal and visceral pleural linings are rubbing together.

If abnormal lung sounds are detected, additional auscultation for bronchophony, egophony, and whispered pectoriloquy are indicated (see Dyspnea, p. 118).

Auscultate Heart Sounds

Auscultate for normal heart sounds in all positions, identifying S1, S2, rate, and rhythm. Identification of myocardial ischemia cannot be reliably done by physical examination alone. An ECG or stress ECG must be done to assess electrical conduction and the condition of myocardial function. Abnormal sounds, such as a new, transient, paradoxical S2 during pain, is a useful sign of coronary ischemia. It results from transient left ventricular dysfunction. It may also be seen in chronic heart failure and left bundle branch block. A transient S3 (ventricular gallop) or mitral regurgitation murmur at the apex can occur occasionally with myocardial ischemia or congestive heart failure. An S4 (atrial gallop) typically indicates a stressed heart, which may be the result of hypertension, myocardial infarction, or coronary artery disease causing heart failure. A summation gallop is the result of an S3, S4, and rapid rate. This may also occur with heart failure. Abnormal rhythms, including tachycardia, bradycardia, and irregular rhythms, are often heard during MI. ECGs are necessary to identify the specific rhythm.

Also note any murmurs, their location, grade, and radiation. Incompetent heart valves produce murmurs and may be the cause of heart failure. In children, a loud murmur, best audible at the upper right sternal border or upper left sternal border with a thrill, may indicate a congenital heart defect.

Aortic diastolic murmur may be present with a dissecting aorta.

Midsystolic click/late systolic murmur (honk) is heard with mitral valve prolapse. The patient must be examined in the supine and upright position to elicit the characteristic sounds.

Observe the Spine for Evidence of Scoliosis

Persons with scoliosis are at increased risk for pulmonary problems because of structural variations that may cause compression of intrathoracic contents.

Examine the Abdomen

Auscultate for bowel sounds. Palpate the abdomen for tenderness and masses. Epigastric pain with palpation may occur with esophagitis or peptic ulcer disease. Cholelithiasis or cholecystitis may be manifested by pain on palpation in the right upper quadrant. Pancreatitis may produce left upper quadrant tenderness.

Examine the Extremities

Clubbing of the fingers may be an indication of chronic hypoxia resulting from congenital heart disease in children or chronic obstructive pulmonary disease in adults. Peripheral cyanosis indicates hypoxia if accompanied by central cyanosis. If peripheral cyanosis is seen alone, consider exposure to a cold environment or anxiety. Lower extremity edema is a sign of heart failure or venous stasis. Note the progression of the edema or if there is pitting edema up the leg.

Absent peripheral pulse(s) may be a sign of atherosclerotic vessel disease or dissecting aortic aneurysm. Compare the quality of the pulses bilaterally.

LABORATORY AND DIAGNOSTIC STUDIES

Diagnostic tests are usually indicated when cardiovascular, pulmonary, or gastrointestinal pathology is the suspected cause of chest pain. Musculoskeletal and neurological causes of pain usually do not require diagnostic tests.

Electrocardiogram

An electrocardiogram (ECG) can add objective data to the diagnostic process in evaluating chest pain. ECGs are most valuable when there is a previous ECG with which to compare the findings or when serial ECGs are done. ST elevation or depression indicates the presence of injured myocardium. T-wave inversion will demonstrate the presence of ischemia. The appearance of both strongly supports ischemia but is not diagnostic of coronary artery disease (CAD). Arterial spasm, pericarditis, and electrolyte imbalance can also cause these variations from normal. Q waves are indicative of myocardial muscle loss but are not diagnostic of CAD.

Evidence of ischemia is not always obvious on an ECG even when the patient is reporting anginal pain.

Treadmill Exercise Testing

Persons experiencing intermittent chest pain who have a normal ECG and are not taking digoxin should have an exercise stress ECG for diagnostic and prognostic purposes. Treadmill exercise testing uses a standardized protocol of increasing workload with continuous ECG recording. Stress tests provide information on myocardial function determined by blood flow. An important objective of stress testing is to identify patients who have a high risk of severe (left main or three-vessel) coronary artery disease. The sensitivity of the test ranges from 65% to 70%.

Exercise Myocardial Perfusion Imaging

This imaging has greater accuracy than the standard treadmill test when the resting ECG is abnormal. Because of its higher sensitivity, the test is able to localize and characterize the extent of myocardial ischemia and provide direct measurement of other variables, such as left ventricular function. This test is more costly than a treadmill test.

Cardiac Enzymes

The isoenzyme that is specific to cardiac tissue is creatinine kinase MB (CK-MB).

After the onset of chest pain, the CK-MB will peak at around 24 hours. The patient who has had an MI will have a CK-MB result that is 5 or more times the normal value. The diagnosis of MI may be further confirmed by looking at lactic dehydrogenase (LDH) levels. The LDH level will start to rise at 12 to 48 hours postinfarction and peak within 48 to 72 hours. The LDH will remain elevated for up to 14 days. Recently Troponin I (tn-I) has been used in the diagnosis of acute MI. This enzyme is a cardiac-specific marker that is found in the circulation as a result of myocardial necrosis. It is less sensitive in the first 12 hours for acute myocardial infarction than the CK-MB but remains elevated for 7 to 10 days after the cardiac event.

Echocardiogram

An echocardiogram is a noninvasive test for examining the heart that provides information about the position, size, and movements of the valves and chambers as well as the velocity of blood flow by means of reflected ultrasound. This test is used to determine biological and prosthetic valve dysfunction and pericardial effusion, evaluate velocity and direction of blood flow, furnish direction for further diagnostic study, and monitor cardiac patients over an extended period.

Ventilation/Perfusion Scan

With PE, the blood supply distal to the embolus is restricted. Imaging will show poor or no visualization of the affected area. The ventilation scan demonstrates movement or lack of movement of air in the lungs. The perfusion scan demonstrates blood supply to the affected area of the lungs. The ventilation/perfusion scan is reported as one of three categories: normal, high probability, and non-diagnostic. A normal scan is characterized by even distribution of radiotracer throughout both lungs and rules out significant pulmonary emboli; no additional diagnostic tests are required. A high probability scan is represented by multiple segmental or larger defects with normal ventilation in at least one area of abnormal perfusion. This is also known as a ventilation/perfusion mismatch. When a scan does not fit into either the normal or high probability category, the study is considered to be nondiagnostic, and further investigation is required.

Pulmonary Angiography

A pulmonary angiogram (arteriogram) is necessary if an embolectomy is considered. A radiographic contrast material is injected into the pulmonary arteries, and the vasculature is visualized. This test can detect emboli as small as 3 mm in diameter. The test sensitivity is 98% and the specificity is 96%. The test is the gold standard for diagnosing PE, but it is expensive and carries a small risk of cardiac arrhythmias, anaphylaxis, and death.

Arterial Blood Gases

Arterial blood gases (ABGs) are done to detect respiratory alkalosis resulting from hyperventilation, decreased carbon dioxide pressure (pCO_2), and sometimes decreased oxygen (pO_2) (hypoxemia). Hypoxemia often correlates with the extent of the lung area occluded in PE.

X-Rays

Pneumothorax and pneumonia can be objectively identified by chest x-ray. Pneumothorax reveals evidence of pleural air while pneumonia is seen on x-ray as a parenchymal infiltrate. Chest x-ray with suspected PE is usually nonspecific; it may be normal or an elevated hemidiaphragm or pulmonary infiltrate may be present. Rib x-rays will confirm rib fracture.

Cervical and thoracic spine and shoulder x-rays may show degenerative joint changes.

Computed Tomography Scanning (CT Scan)

CT scans produce cross-sectional images of anatomical structures without superimposing tissues on each other. They show the different characteristics of tissue structures within solid organs. Aortic dissections and tumors of the lung and pancreas can be detected with CT scans.

Magnetic Resonance Imaging (MRI)

MRI is a noninvasive technique that produces cross-sectional images of the body through exposure to magnetic energy sources. It does not involve radiation and is used to differentiate healthy and diseased body tissues. It is useful in detecting tumors, infection sites, and diseased vessels.

Activated Partial Thromboplastin Time (APTT) and Prothrombin Time (PT)

APTT is a clotting test that screens for coagulation disorders and is used to monitor the effectiveness of heparin therapy. Prothrombin time (PT) measures a potential defect in stage II of the clotting mechanism through analysis of the clotting ability of five plasma coagulation factors. Prothrombin times are commonly ordered to measure the effects of oral anticoagulant therapies. Ineffective anticoagulation therapy puts persons at risk for PE. These tests may also be ordered to search for the cause of PE.

Serum Amylase and Lipase

Amylase is an enzyme that changes starch to sugar and is produced in the pancreas, liver, salivary glands, and fallopian tubes. If there is inflammation of the pancreas or salivary glands, increased levels of amylase enter the bloodstream. Lipase changes fats to fatty acids and glycerol. The pancreas is the main source of lipase. Pancreatic damage results in elevated serum lipase. Serum amylase and lipase are useful diagnostic tests for pancreatitis. Amylase levels return to normal before lipase levels.

Abdominal Ultrasound

Abdominal ultrasound is a noninvasive procedure to visualize solid organs. It is useful in detecting masses, fluid collections, and infection. Pancreatitis and gallbladder disease may be detected with ultrasound.

Bronchoscopy

Bronchoscopy permits visualization of the trachea, bronchi, and select bronchioles. It is useful to diagnose tumors, hemorrhage, and trauma; to obtain brushings for cytological examinations; and to remove foreign bodies from the lower respiratory system.

Complete Blood Count (CBC)

A CBC is done to detect an elevated white cell count that occurs with infection. A hemoglobin and hematocrit are useful if anemia is suspected as an underlying cause of chest pain.

Esophageal pH

Twenty-four hour esophageal pH monitoring is done when GERD is suspected to document pathological acid reflux.

Endoscopy

Upper endoscopy with biopsy is necessary to document the type and extent of tissue damage in GERD. A normal endoscopy, however, does not rule out mild gastric reflux disease.

Erythrocyte Sedimentation Rate (ESR)

The ESR value will be elevated with inflammation, such as in arthritis and pericarditis. The test is not specific for a particular disease.

DIFFERENTIAL DIAGNOSIS

COMMON CAUSES OF EMERGENT CHEST PAIN

Acute Myocardial Infarction

Assessment of the patient experiencing acute chest pain must first focus on the potential diagnosis of MI to facilitate prompt initiation of treatment to limit infarct size. The patient having an acute MI generally describes a sudden onset of pain at rest. It is a persistent, often severe, deep, central chest pain and may radiate, as angina does, to the throat or neck, across both sides of the chest to the shoulder and/or down the medial aspect of either or both arms. Rest or nitroglycerin does not relieve the pain. The chest pain is often associated with a number of other nonspecific noncardiac complaints, such as shortness of breath, nausea, vomiting, and diaphoresis.

The quality of the pain or discomfort may be similar but is generally more intense than any previously experienced anginal symptoms. Patients may also express a sense of impending doom. Quick review for positive risk factors (age >40 years for men and >50 years for women; cigarette smoker, hyperlipidemia, hypertension, diabetes, history of CAD, family history of CAD) is useful. There may be some objective evidence of an MI, including skin pallor, cool diaphoretic skin, and possible transient paradoxical S2. The patient may be hyper- or hypotensive.

The patient experiencing severe chest pain or suspected of having an MI should be placed on a cardiac monitor as soon as possible. Observe for premature ventricular contractions and classic ECG changes that indicate infarction, including ST-segment elevations, T wave inversions, and Q waves. A 12-lead ECG and cardiac isoenzymes will help confirm or rule out an MI.

Aortic Dissection

The patient usually presents in a great deal of distress, describing the unrelenting chest pain as ripping and tearing and possibly radiating to the back and abdomen. Physical examination reveals extreme hypertension and possible unequal or absent peripheral pulses. Chest x-ray demonstrates a wide mediastinum with extension of the aortic wall beyond the calcific border. CT scan or MRI may be ordered, but aortography remains the gold standard. Patients with suspect aortic dissection should be referred for emergent care.

Acute Coronary Insufficiency

Acute coronary insufficiency refers to those situations in which chest pain is caused by lack of oxygen to the myocardium, but evidence of infarct is not present. The patient reports severe, oppressive, constricting, retrosternal discomfort lasting longer than 30 minutes. The patient may report prior history of MI or angina. The ECG may show intermittent ischemic changes or be normal. Cardiac isoenzymes are normal.

Pulmonary Embolus

Patients presenting with PE usually report sudden onset of severe sharp, crushing, nonradiating chest pain if there is a large embolus impacted in a major artery. Infarction of the pulmonary parenchyma nearer the pleural surface will cause pleuritic chest pain. This pain is most often accompanied by sudden onset of dyspnea and hemoptysis. Patients frequently express feelings of impending doom.

Review of risk factors will likely reveal one or more of the following: older age, prior venous thromboembolism, prolonged immobility or paralysis, cancer, heart failure, other chronic disease, pelvic or lower extremity surgery, recent pregnancy or delivery, obesity, oral contraceptive use, or varicose veins. Physical findings include restlessness, tachycardia, tachypnea, fever, diminished breath sounds, crackles and/or wheezes, and possible pleural friction rub. There may be signs of thrombophlebitis of the extremities. Initial diagnostic tests should include chest x-ray and ECG. These may both be normal, but, if clinical signs still point to PE, referral for consultation and further tests including arterial blood gases, venous Doppler studies, ventilation/perfusion scans, and pulmonary angiography are indicated.

Pneumothorax

Pneumothorax can be a life-threatening event, especially if the patient has underlying COPD or asthma. The patient reports sharp or tearing chest pain that may radiate to the ipsilateral shoulder. Sudden onset of shortness of breath is also associated with spontaneous pneumothorax. Objective findings include decreased or absent breath sounds on the affected side, tachycardia, tachypnea, and possible deviated trachea. A chest x-ray is needed to evaluate the possible complete or partial collapse of the lung.

Dysrhythmias

Palpitations and/or forceful heart beats are noticed by the patient. These arrhythmias can be the result of myocardial ischemia or cocaine abuse or less emergent conditions such as prolapsed mitral valve or anxiety. Syncope associated with palpitations indicates a more serious cardiac arrhythmia.

Congenital Coronary Anomalies

The coronary arteries may arise abnormally, take an abnormal course, or have fistulous connections to other structures, resulting in exertional chest pain that may lead to sudden death in the young athlete. The child or adolescent may have a history of moderate to severe chest pain during or following exercise. Family history of sudden death at an early age, heart disease, seizures, a prior history of lightheadedness, or loss of consciousness during exercise and tall and lanky body type, with double-jointedness, are risk factors. Referral to a pediatric cardiologist is warranted.

COMMON CAUSES OF NON-EMERGENT CHEST PAIN

Stable Angina

Stable angina refers to chest pain typically described as substernal chest pressure or heaviness, radiating to the left shoulder and arm, neck, or jaw. It is associated with nausea, diaphoresis, and shortness of breath. It is usually brought on and exacerbated by exercise and stress and is alleviated with rest and/or nitroglycerin. It typically lasts 2 to 10 minutes. Physical examination is usually normal. An S4 gallop may be transiently present during an episode of pain. Tests for angina include an ECG during an episode of pain, which may show ST segment depression and T wave inversions, or the findings may be normal.

Myocarditis

Myocarditis is an inflammation of the myocardium and is commonly caused by viruses. The heart is unable to contract properly because the inflammatory process interferes with the contractile function of the myocardial cells and eventually leads to cell death. It is frequently accompanied by pericarditis. The chest pain is caused by ischemia or dysrhythmia. Patients have fever, dyspnea, and may have evidence of heart failure. Heart murmurs and friction rubs may be heard. Chest x-rays show cardiomegaly.

Pericarditis

The pain associated with pericarditis is described as sharp, located in the center of the chest, short-lived, episodic, and radiating to the back in the trapezial area. The pain is worse when the patient is supine and sitting, whereas leaning forward often reduces the intensity of the pain. Shallow breathing may be an associated symptom in effort to avoid pain. Dyspnea may be present with compression of the bronchial tree by a large pericardial effusion. Risk factors for pericarditis include recent viral or bacterial infection, recent MI, uremia, myxedema, and history of autoimmune disease. Objective signs include fever before the onset of pain, tachycardia, and pericardial friction rub. The rub is pathonomic for pericarditis but is found in only 60% to 70% of patients with pericarditis. Diagnostic tests show elevated WBC and ESR and diffuse ST segment elevation in the early stages. Chest x-ray may be normal or show effusion with increase in cardiac shadow.

Aortic Stenosis

Aortic stenosis may cause exertional chest pain. Associated symptoms include fatigue, palpitation, dyspnea on exertion (DOE), dizziness, and syncope. Physical examination will reveal a loud, harsh crescendo-decrescendo murmur best heard at the second right ICS with the patient leaning forward. The murmur may radiate to the neck and is often associated with a thrill. An echocardiogram will provide diagnostic evidence of aortic stenosis.

Mitral Regurgitation

Symptoms of mitral regurgitation are similar to those of aortic stenosis. They include exertional substernal chest pain, fatigue, palpitation, dizziness, DOE, and syncope. The murmur associated with mitral regurgitation is holosystolic, blowing, and often heard best at the apex in the left lateral position. The murmur decreases with inspiration and may radiate to the left axilla and occasionally to the back. Again, echocardiogram will provide evidence of mitral regurgitation.

Pneumonia

Signs and symptoms of pneumonia include pleuritic chest pain; a productive,

moist cough with dark sputum; shortness of breath; and fever and chills. Risk factors include ineffective cough reflex, inability to swallow, the elderly, or the very young. Auscultation of the lungs reveals diminished breath sounds over affected areas, and crackles and wheezes may be heard. Rales and rhonchi are frequently heard on auscultation of the lungs. Dullness with percussion is heard over areas of consolidation. Vocal fremitus is positive. In addition, physical findings may include tachycardia, tachypnea, bronchophony, and egophony. Chest x-ray, sputum culture, and arterial blood gases will further support the diagnosis of pneumonia. Follow-up chest x-rays are indicated after pneumonia because lung tumors can be hidden by pneumonia. The very young and very old are most often hospitalized for observation and treatment of pneumonia. Healthy adults are usually managed on an outpatient basis.

Mitral Valve Prolapse

Patients with chest pain from mitral valve prolapse report a range of symptoms, including dysrhythmias, palpitations, and anxiety. Physical examination may be normal or a midsystolic click can be heard over the apex while the patient is sitting or squatting. An echocardiogram will provide evidence of mitral valve prolapse.

Pleuritis

Pleuritic chest pain occurs suddenly and is worsened by deep breathing, coughing, and sneezing. Pleuritic chest pain may be a manifestation of pneumonia or may represent pleural inflammation, especially following a viral upper respiratory infection. Physical examination of the chest may be normal or a pleural friction rub may be heard over the area of inflammation. The patient's respiration rate is normal, but respirations are often shallow or guarded. Unless pneumonia is suspected, no diagnostic tests are indicated. If signs and symptoms of pneumonia are absent, the cause of pleuritic chest pain is more likely of viral etiology.

Esophagitis

Esophagitis or esophageal spasm symptoms often mimic angina. In fact, sublingual nitroglycerin may also relieve the symptoms, but usually relief takes longer than the 3 to 5 minutes for angina to be relieved. Patients frequently report that the pain is worse after eating spicy foods, large meals, or if they lie down after eating. They may report a sour taste in their mouth. Physical examination is normal except for possible epigastric tenderness with palpation. The most reliable way to detect reflux as the cause of chest pain is to correlate episodes of chest pain with results of 24-hour esophageal pH monitoring.

Chest Trauma

Rib fractures usually follow trauma. Pain is made worse by deep breathing. The patient's respirations are shallow, and pain is exacerbated by palpation in the area of the fracture. Chest or rib x-rays will confirm suspected rib fractures.

Costochondritis and Tietze's Syndrome

Costochondritis and Tietze's syndrome are both identified by severe pain with palpation along the anterior cartilage where the ribs meet the sternum. Deep breathing and movement of the chest wall intensifies the pain. In Tietze's syndrome, swelling along this border also occurs.

Herpes Zoster

Herpes zoster is manifested by unilateral chest pain that follows along a dermatome. The pain is usually described as burning, stabbing, or pruritic. Early in the course of the disease, no objective manifestations are present. As the course progresses, a vesicular rash appears in the area of pain.

Peptic Ulcer Disease

Subjective manifestations of peptic ulcer disease include episodes of pain 1 to 3 hours after eating. The pain may awaken a person at night and is frequently relieved by antacids or eating. The patient may report hematemesis and or melena. CBC may reveal iron deficiency anemia. Personal or family history of ulcer disease may be a risk factor as well as cigarette smoking and alcohol abuse. Upper GI x-ray and endoscopy are diagnostic tests to perform to confirm peptic ulcer disease.

Cholecystitis

Cholecystitis is reported as colicky, intermittent epigastric or right upper quadrant pain that often follows a high fat meal. Nausea and vomiting may accompany the pain, which often radiates to the right infrascapular area. Physical examination may show a positive Murphy's sign, as indicated by tenderness in the region of the gallbladder. The gallbladder may be distended and palpable. Gallbladder ultrasound is the most important diagnostic test in the evaluation of this problem.

Acute Pancreatitis

Acute pancreatitis occurs as sudden onset of severe, steady upper epigastric or left upper quadrant abdominal pain, which frequently radiates to the left anterior chest, shoulders, or back. The pain is worse in the supine position. The patient appears restless, and pain can be associated with nausea and severe vomiting, hypotension, and unexplained shock. Left upper abdominal pain with palpation is present. The laboratory test most frequently used is the serum amylase and lipase. A rise in amylase level is seen 2 to 12 hours following onset of symptoms. Lipase returns to normal slower than the amylase levels and thus is more useful in diagnosing pancreatitis later in its course. Pancreas ultrasound and CT scans are necessary to show positive evidence of pancreatitis.

Lung and Mediastinal Tumors

Lung and mediastinal tumors may be manifested by chest pain. Associated symptoms include shortness of breath, cough, and hemoptysis. Pneumonia is often the initial diagnosis, and persistence of symptoms following treatment may lead to further investigation for tumors. Risk factors include a smoking history and family history of cancer. Physical examination may be normal or reveal diminished breath sounds in the area of the tumor. Dull sounds on percussion of the chest may be an objective manifestation of a chest mass. Chest x-ray and CT scans of the chest are diagnostic tools to identify these lesions. Bronchoscopy is done to obtain a biopsy.

Cocaine Use

Cocaine increases the metabolic requirement of the heart for oxygen and decreases the supply of oxygen, producing myocardial ischemia and chest pain. Cocaine causes adrenergic stimulation, thus increasing heart rate, blood pressure, and left ventricular contractility. Concomitantly, myocardial oxygen supply declines because of cocaine-induced vasoconstric-

tion of the coronary arteries. ECGs, serial cardiac enzymes, and urine drug screens are useful diagnostic tools.

Psychogenic Origin

Adults and adolescents with history of a recent stressful situation may present with chest pain. Physical examination is negative.

Pleurodynia

Group B coxsackie viruses may cause pleurodynia. Presentation is usually sudden, severe onset of stabbing, paroxysmal pleuritic pain over the lower ribcage and substernal area. Deep breathing aggravates the pain. Fever, headache, malaise, and unproductive cough are usually present. The chest examination is negative except for pleuritic friction rub in 25% of cases. The condition lasts from 1 to 14 days.

Precordial Catch Syndrome

Recurrent brief episodes of sudden, sharp, but not distressing pain occurring at rest or during mild exercise may indicate precordial catch syndrome. It is localized near the apex of the heart and along the left sternal border or beneath the left breast. It is seen in adolescents and is benign in nature.

Table 4-3

Differential Diagnosis of Common Causes of Emergent Chest Pain

Condition	History	Physical Findings	Diagnostic Studies
Acute myocardial infarction	Severe, oppressive, constricting retrosternal discomfort, radiating to left or right arm, neck, and/or jaw, lasting >30 min;	Hyper- or hypotension, cardiac arrhythmia, paradoxical S2	Serial ECGs, serial cardiac enzymes, nuclear scan

Table 4-3

Differential Diagnosis of Common Causes of Emergent Chest Pain—cont'd

Condition	History	Physical Findings	Diagnostic Studies
Acute myocardial infarction—cont'd	diaphoresis, dyspnea, nausea; history of CAD, cigarette smoker, positive family history of CAD, history of elevated lipids		
Aortic dissection	Sudden, tearing pain in anterior or posterior chest, migrates to arms, abdomen, and legs	Pulse deficits, hypertension; possible neurological changes in the legs; aortic diastolic murmur	Echocardiogram, angiography; CT scan/MRI; emergency referral
Acute coronary artery insufficiency	Severe, constricting retrosternal chest pain lasting >30 min; anxiety, diaphoresis, dyspnea; prior history of angina or MI	Restlessness, cool and clammy skin, tachycardia	ECG, isoenzymes
Pulmonary embolus	Acute onset; sense of doom; pleuritic pain, restlessness; mild to severe pain; hemoptysis; history of DVT, recent trauma to lower extremity, surgery; oral contraceptives	Fever, dyspnea, cough, tachycardia, tachypnea, diminished breath sounds; crackles, wheezing	PT/APTT; ABGs; chest x-ray ventilation/ perfusion scans
Pneumothorax	Sharp or tearing pain, may radiate to ipsilateral shoulder; dyspnea; children with asthma, CF, or Marfan's syndrome are at risk	Tachycardia; diminished breath sounds; decreased tactile fremitus; hyperresonance over affected lung area; tracheal shift	Chest x-ray; ABGs

Continued

Table 4-3

Differential Diagnosis of Common Causes of Emergent Chest Pain—cont'd

Condition	History	Physical Findings	Diagnostic Studies
Dysrhythmias	Palpitations, dizziness, forceful heartbeats, history of CHD, fever, and medications (sympathomimetics and beta-adrenergic agents); history of cocaine abuse	SVT = tachycardia of 150-250 beats/min, sinus or ventricular tachycardia, irregular pulse	ECG during episode; Holter 24-hour ECG
Congenital coronary anomalies	In children and adolescents, a history of moderate-to-severe chest pain during or following exercise; family history of early sudden death	May have murmurs, clicks, decreased lower extremity pulses, irregular pulse, BP	ECG and referral to pediatric cardiologist

Table 4-4

Differential Diagnosis of Common Causes of Non-Emergent Chest Pain

Condition	History	Physical Findings	Diagnostic Studies
Stable angina	Substernal chest pressure following exercise or stress and relieved by rest or nitroglycerine; nausea, SOB, diaphoresis, sternal chest pressure	Normal exam; possible transient S4	ECG during episode of chest pain
Myocarditis	Chest pain, history of fever, dyspnea	Heart murmur, friction rub, fever	ECG, chest x-ray
Pericarditis	Sharp stabbing pain referred to left shoulder or trapezius ridge, usually worse during coughing or deep breathing; may be relieved by sitting	Fever before onset of pain, tachycardia, pericardial friction rub	WBC, ESR, ECG, chest x-ray

Table 4-4

Differential Diagnosis of Common Causes of Non-Emergent Chest Pain—cont'd

Condition	History	Physical Findings	Diagnostic Studies
Pericarditis—cont'd	forward; history of viral or bacterial infection, autoimmune disease		
Aortic stenosis	Chest pain on exertion, substernal and anginal in quality, fatigue, palpitations, DOE, dizziness, syncope	Radial pulse diminished; narrow pulse pressure; loud, harsh, crescendo-decrescendo murmur heard best at the second right ICS with patient leaning forward; thrill	Echocardiogram, ECG, chest x-ray
Mitral regurgitation	Exertional chest pain, fatigue, palpitations, dizziness, DOE, syncope	Holosystolic, blowing, often loud murmur heard best at the apex in the left lateral position, which decreases with inspiration; murmur may radiate to the axilla and possibly the back	Chest x-ray, ECG, echocardiogram
Pneumonia	Productive cough of yellow or green or rust sputum; dyspnea; pleuritic pain	Fever; tachycardia, tachypnea; inspiratory crackles; vocal fremitus; percussion dull or flat over area of consolidation; bronchophony, egophony	Chest x-ray; sputum cultures; ABGs
Mitral valve prolapse	Chest pain, varies in location and intensity; palpitations; anxiety; non-exertional pain of short duration, history of Marfan's syndrome	Dysrhythmias, possible midsystolic click heard over the apex, heard best while the patient is in the sitting or squatting position; thoracoskeletal deformity common in children	ECG, echocardiogram

Continued

Table 4-4

Differential Diagnosis of Common Causes of Non-Emergent Chest Pain—cont'd

Condition	History	Physical Findings	Diagnostic Studies
Pleuritis	Mild, localized chest pain, worse with deep breathing; recent URI	Shallow respirations, local tenderness, pleural friction rub	None initially
Esophagitis	Substernal pain worse after eating and lying down; sour taste in mouth	Epigastric pain with palpation	Esophageal pH
Chest trauma (rib fracture)	History of injury or trauma; pain with deep breaths; splinting of chest wall	Shallow respirations; chest wall pain on palpation	Chest x-ray
Costochondritis	Pain along sternal border, increases with deep breaths, history of exercise, URI, or physical activity	Pain with palpation over costochondral joints; normal breath sounds	None
Herpes zoster	Unilateral chest pain; painful rash	Normal breath sounds; vesicular rash along dermatome	None
Peptic ulcer disease	Epigastric pain 1-2 hours after eating, may be relieved by antacids; hematemesis and melena; risk factors include smoking and alcohol overuse	Tenderness to palpation in the epigastric area; signs of hypovolemia	Upper GI x-ray, upper endoscopy, CBC
Cholecystitis	Right upper quadrant abdominal pain radiating to the right chest, often following a high-fat meal; nausea and vomiting	Positive Murphy's sign; palpable gallbladder	Gallbladder ultrasound

Table 4-4

Differential Diagnosis of Common Causes of Non-Emergent Chest Pain—cont'd

Condition	History	Physical Findings	Diagnostic Studies
Acute pancreatitis	Severe left upper quadrant abdominal pain radiating into the left chest; pain worse in supine position; nausea, vomiting, fever	Left upper abdominal pain with palpation; hypotension	Serum amylase, pancreas ultrasound or CT scan
Lung tumors	Chest pain, SOB, cough, hemoptysis, history of cigarette smoking; history of pneumonia	Normal exam or diminished breath sounds over tumor and dull percussion sound over tumor	Chest x-ray, CT scan of chest, bronchoscopy
Cocaine use	Chest pain, SOB, diaphoresis, nausea; may relate substance use	Tachycardia, hypertension	ECG, serial cardiac enzymes, drug screen
Psychogenic origin	Precordial chest pain, history of stressful situations	Normal exam	ECG, chest x-ray
Pleurodynia	Severe, acute-onset, stabbing, paroxysmal, pleuritic pain over lower ribcage and substernal edge; headache, malaise, nonproductive cough	Pleural friction rub 25% of time; chest examination normal; fever usually present	None
Precordial catch syndrome	Sudden sharp not distressing pain near apex of heart; seen in adolescence	Normal exam	None

Dyspnea

Dyspnea is a subjective sensation of air hunger that results in labored breathing. It usually reflects an impairment in pulmonary ventilation, perfusion, metabolism, or central nervous system (CNS) drive. It is normally experienced by healthy individuals during periods of strenuous exercise. Children less than 3 years of age usually cannot express the sensation. It is recognized by caregivers as either tachypnea, retractions, stridor, nasal flaring, or feeding difficulty.

The causes of dyspnea can be divided into five broad classifications: (1) cardiovascular, (2) respiratory. (3) metabolic, (4) mechanical, and (5) other extrapulmonary disorders. Within each class are specific pathological processes responsible for the sensation of breathlessness. In disease states it is usually a result of pulmonary or cardiac pathology. When eliciting the history, it is helpful to determine if this is new-onset acute dyspnea, chronic progressive dyspnea, or chronic recurrent dyspnea. Carefully directed questioning will provide essential clues for identifying the differential diagnoses.

DIAGNOSTIC REASONING: FOCUSED HEALTH HISTORY

Is this a medical emergency?

Severe dyspnea is a medical emergency. If not treated immediately, respiratory failure and death may occur. Assess the adequacy of the airway first. Emergency measures should be instituted to establish ventilation. Once the patient is stabilized, search for the underlying cause of the dyspnea.

Key Questions

- Did this come on suddenly or has it been developing gradually? Over what period of time (hours, days, weeks)?
- What were you/the child doing just before having difficulty in breathing?
- Is this your first episode of breathing problems?

Onset. New-onset acute dyspnea reported by a patient in acute distress may signal a life-threatening problem. In the patient with no previous history of heart or lung disease, dyspnea may indicate several conditions that require immediate treatment, such as aspiration of a foreign body, anaphylaxis, pulmonary embolism, and pneumothorax.

Acute upper or lower airway obstruction in children has the greatest potential to cause serious morbidity or mortality and, therefore, must initially be ruled out. The most serious problem is hypoxemia caused by the inability to transport oxygen past a blocked upper airway, such as with epiglottitis, croup, or a foreign body.

Acute dyspnea requires that assessment of the airway and ventilatory status with oxygen and cardiac monitoring be initiated immediately. Often this must occur before definitive diagnostic evaluation has been completed.

Foreign body aspiration. The adult patient with foreign body aspiration may report that dyspnea occurred while eating solid foods or drinking large amounts of alcohol. Children who put small objects in their mouth are at risk for aspiration of the object into the airway and subsequent airway obstruction. A history of sudden onset of choking, coughing, or wheezing, without preceding upper respiratory tract infection, is given by the patient or the care provider. Many times the child has been playing on the floor or outside at the time of the onset of symptoms.

Anaphylaxis. Anaphylaxis may follow insect bites or ingestion of medication or other potential allergens (i.e., shellfish). Generally, primary symptoms include not feeling well, flushing, generalized pruritus, fear, faintness, and sneezing. In severe cases, allergic response may occur within minutes, followed by death from suffocation caused by edema of the larynx, epiglottis, and pharynx. Shock and cardiac arrhythmia ensue within a short time unless emergency measures are instituted.

The sooner the symptoms occur the more severe the reaction.

Is the dyspnea caused by a secondary obstruction in the lower respiratory tract?

Key Questions

- Have you had cough or cold symptoms recently?
- Do you have a history of asthma?
- Family history of asthma?

Cough. Secondary partial airway obstruction caused by small airway disease contributes to hypoxemia by intrapulmonary shunting. The pulmonary obstruction can be intraluminal (distal foreign objects, asthma), intramural (edema, bronchomalacia, bronchiolitis), or extramural (compression from tumor, lymph nodes). The narrowing increases both airway resistance and turbulence of air flow. The imbalance between pulmonary ventilation and perfusion affects oxygen exchange. This causes the patient to work harder to maintain adequate ventilation, resulting in dyspnea.

History of asthma. Both adults and children may experience airway obstruction caused by reactive airway disease or asthma. Personal or family history of asthma increases the risk of dyspnea from acute bronchospasm.

Is the dyspnea caused by trauma to the chest?

Key Question

• Have you experienced any trauma to the chest?

Trauma. Limitation of motion of the thoracic cage because of pain and/or trauma may be associated with the development of severe alveolar hypoventilation and subsequent dyspnea.

Pneumothorax occurs most frequently in young persons during strenuous activity. Spontaneous pneumothorax results in sudden loss of lung volume, hypoxia, hypercapnia, and significant shortness of breath.

Is the dyspnea caused by a pulmonary embolus?

Key Questions

• Have you been confined to bed recently? Had recent surgery? Had a recent fracture?
• Are you taking birth control pills? Do you smoke?
• Do you take any other medications?
The person with pulmonary embolism is usually in acute distress and reports signifi-

cant shortness of breath, localized pleuritic chest pain, apprehension, bloody sputum production, diaphoresis, fever, and history of conditions causing risk for emboli. These risk factors include age >60 years, pulmonary hypertension, congestive heart failure, chronic lung disease, ischemic heart disease, stroke, and cancer. Predisposing factors that can contribute to thrombus formation include (1) venous stasis, (2) hypercoagulability, and (3) endothelial injury with inflammation to the vessel lining. Trauma, muscle spasm, or clot dissolution may cause the thrombus to dislodge, creating an embolus. Emboli circulate in the blood to the right side of the heart and enter the lung via the pulmonary artery. If the clot is not dissolved within the lung, it occludes the pulmonary artery and obstructs blood flow and perfusion of the lung. Patients with suspected pulmonary embolism are referred for emergency pulmonary/vascular consultation.

Confinement, surgery, fracture. Pulmonary embolus (PE) is most likely to occur in persons with history of deep vein thrombosis or prolonged immobility. Vascular lung disease is characterized by a decrease in the size of the pulmonary vascular bed. When emboli reach the pulmonary artery, the reduced blood flow through the lungs results in arterial hypoxemia and hypercapnia, which in turn lead to symptoms of dyspnea. Dyspnea resulting from PE is usually accompanied by fever, chest pain, and restlessness.

Trauma to leg. There is an increased risk of pulmonary embolus in adolescents who have sustained traumatic injury to their lower limbs.

Anxiety. People with PE feel a sense of impending doom. There is no clear explanation for this sensation. Significant oxygen deprivation may contribute to the cause.

Birth control pills. Remember to question women, including adolescent girls, about their use of birth control pills, which may put them at risk for PE. Additionally, the risk of PE increases with the combination of smoking and oral contraceptives.

Medications. A complete medication history may provide clues to a possible hypercoagulability state. Patients taking anticoagulants and perhaps underdosed may be at risk for PE. Patients on medication for heart failure, such as digitalis or angiotensin-converting enzyme (ACE) inhibitors, are at risk because of chronic heart failure. In addition, be certain to ask about hormone replacement therapy because these drugs also increase the risk of PE.

Is the dyspnea a complication of a pre-existing disease?

Key Questions

- Do you have a history of heart problems? Lung problems (asthma)? Anemia?
- Are you taking any medications?
- Do you have any numbness or tingling in your body? Where?
- Have you noticed any other unusual symptoms besides shortness of breath?

Past history of disease. History of coronary artery disease (CAD), heart failure, valvular heart disease, chronic obstructive pulmonary disease (COPD), or asthma should raise the level of suspicion for recurrence or complications of that disease. Myocardial infarction (MI) may be the cause of severe sudden dyspnea in persons with or without prior history of CAD. Careful questioning regarding associated symptoms and risk factors may reveal characteristics of probable MI (see Chest Pain, p. 98).

Progressively increasing shortness of breath is frequently a symptom of worsening COPD. It is often associated with (1) frequent cough that is worse in the morning, (2) sputum production that is clear to yellow in color, (3) decreasing exercise tolerance, and (4) mild to moderate fatigue.

Chronic progressive dyspnea in the patient with a history of heart failure or cardiac valve disease is most frequently a symptom of heart failure. Associated symptoms include (1) peripheral edema, (2) ascites, (3) cough possibly with frothy sputum production, (4) chest pain, and (5) fatigue. Orthopnea (difficulty breathing when lying flat) and paroxysmal nocturnal dyspnea (PND) (a sudden onset of shortness of breath when lying flat) are most often associated with heart failure.

In children with heart disease, dyspnea occurs because of insufficient blood being pumped to the lungs as a result of congenital structural anomaly, pump failure, or secondary to pulmonary hypertension. Simple respiratory tract infections may cause severe respiratory insufficiency in the child who has cardiopulmonary disease. Associated symptoms include retractions (including abdominal muscles), tachypnea, nasal flaring and grunting, peripheral edema, ascites, cough, and fatigue.

Chronic progressive dyspnea because of lung involvement may also be present in patients with a history of systemic illnesses such as sarcoidosis, rheumatological disease (rheumatoid lungs), cystic fibrosis, or Goodpasture's syndrome, a rare syndrome of progressive glomerulonephritis, hemoptysis, and hemosiderosis.

Periodic recurrent dyspnea is most often the result of bronchospasm and inflamed bronchi caused by asthma. Persons with asthma may be relatively symptom-free between episodes and can often identify the cause of their shortness of breath with little prompting. Symptoms are frequently associated with recent respiratory infection, exercise, or exposure to allergens. Associated symptoms reported by the patient may include audible wheezes, decreased exercise tolerance, and frequent paroxysmal cough. Most children also have associated wheezing. Wheezing is extremely unusual in the neonatal period and generally signifies a structural or functional congenital abnormality. The symptom implies intrathoracic airway obstruction with one or more of the following causes: intraluminal obstruction, fixed airway narrowing, variable narrowing, or external compression. All these factors lead to turbulent expiratory flow and audible wheeze.

Hematological diseases can affect the oxygen-carrying capacity of the blood, resulting in tissue hypoxia and a decrease in arterial pH, which stimulates the CNS to cause the symptom of dyspnea. Severe anemia from any cause can result in this reaction. Also, whenever the oxygen-carrying capacity of the blood is decreased because of the inability of hemoglobin to bind oxygen, dyspnea can occur. Carbon monoxide poisoning, cyanide poisoning, and methemoglobinemia are examples.

The progressive dyspnea of anemia is usually associated with unusual fatigue, palpitations, lightheadedness, or dizziness.

Hyperventilation. Hyperventilation syndrome, a non-emergent but frightening experience, is usually accompanied by paresthesias around the mouth and of the distal extremities. Anxiety-related dyspnea should not be diagnosed until one has ruled out more serious causes.

When dyspnea is caused by pulmonary or cardiac conditions, the shortness of breath worsens with increasing activity and improves with rest. Dyspnea caused by anxiety does not improve, and may worsen, with rest.

Are there any exogenous factors that precipitate or aggravate the dyspnea?

Key Questions
- Is there anything that seems to make you more short of breath? Walking? Climbing stairs? Dressing? Eating? Talking?
- Have you missed any prescribed medication?

- Do you have any known allergies? Trees? Dust? Pollen? Animals? Have you been exposed to these recently?
- Is there anything you can do to help yourself feel less short of breath? Sit up? Stay indoors? Lie down? Use medication?

Precipitating factors. Chronic dyspnea of pulmonary origin is most frequently precipitated and aggravated by exposure to smoking. This is true for both progressive and recurrent dyspnea. Progressive dyspnea manifested in COPD is often exacerbated by exercise or exertion and is alleviated (or improved) with rest. As the disease progresses, less and less intense exercise can result in increased shortness of breath. In addition, respiratory infections are frequent causes of increased shortness of breath for these patients.

Medication use. The dyspnea related to asthma is relieved by use of bronchodilator agents and steroids.

Allergies. Exposure to cold and/or allergens, exercise, and viral respiratory infections frequently precipitate chronic recurrent dyspnea associated with asthma.

Recumbence, missed medications, high sodium intake, and exertion often precipitate chronic dyspnea associated with heart failure. This applies to both progressive and recurrent chronic dyspnea.

Alleviating factors. Alleviating factors for dyspnea include sitting upright, diuretic medication, and prolonged rest.

Is the dyspnea caused by a neuromuscular problem?

Key Questions
- Are the patient's immunizations up to date?
- Has the infant had any honey?
- Do you live on a farm?

- Is the child at risk for lead poisoning?
- Do you have a headache, muscle weakness, or visual changes?

Neuromuscular effects. Abnormalities of neural or neuromuscular transmission to the respiratory muscles may result in paresis or paralysis, leading to alveolar hypoventilation. Direct involvement of the respiratory muscles affected by systemic musculoskeletal diseases may lead to reduction of vital capacity and total lung capacity and result in hypercapnic hypoventilation and dyspnea. Examples of neuromuscular health problems leading to dyspnea include infections, such as poliomyelitis or tetanus, or a CNS insult.

Immunizations. Lack of childhood or adult immunizations for poliomyelitis or tetanus may lead to paralysis or tetany of the respiratory musculature, resulting in dyspnea and subsequent respiratory distress.

Honey. Honey is a common source of contamination of *Clostridium* botulism, which can cause respiratory distress in infants and small children. The incubation period is only a few hours. Nausea, vomiting, and diarrhea, followed by cranial nerve involvement, diplopia, weak suck, facial weakness, and absent gag reflex result. Generalized hypotonia and weakness then develop and may progress to respiratory failure.

Farm. Organophosphate chemicals that are commonly used as insecticides may cause a myasthenia-like syndrome in children exposed to these toxins. Children residing on farms are most at risk.

Primary causes. Primary changes in neuromuscular control of respiration are uncommon in children. Although rare, some causes that affect the primary respiratory center are myasthenia gravis, myopathies, insecticide poisoning, and lead (heavy metal) poisoning.

Secondary causes. Diseases that affect the CNS include respiratory distress from meningoencephalitis, seizures, or a CNS lesion.

Does the patient have any pertinent risk factors that will point me in the right direction?

Key Questions
- Do you or have you smoked? Are you exposed to cigarette smoke frequently?
- What type of work do you do?
- Have you had a recent change in weight?
- Have you ever had eczema?

Risk factors. Persons at risk for developing dyspnea are those with a history of pulmonary and/or heart disease, cigarette smokers, persons exposed to noxious environmental pollutants, and persons with predisposition to allergies.

Work. Occupational exposure to asbestos, silicon, and coal dust put the patient at risk for lung disease with resultant dyspnea.

Obesity. Physically deconditioned and obese persons report dyspnea on exertion more frequently than their counterparts. Obese persons may have a complaint of dyspnea, especially during exercise. This is caused by an increase in metabolic requirement for a given amount of work. In addition, the diaphragm moves against increased abdominal pressure, and the chest wall is heavier, resulting in more energy required to be expended to maintain ventilation.

Eczema history. Asthma occurs in 20% to 40% of children with a history of atopic dermatitis.

DIAGNOSTIC REASONING: FOCUSED PHYSICAL EXAMINATION

Note General Appearance and Observe Posture

Patients who appear in acute distress with manifestations of severe oxygen deprivation require emergent evaluation and treatment. Assess vital signs immediately. Tachypnea, eupnea, and hypopnea are critical clues to impending respiratory failure. Use of accessory muscles to breathe, posturing, and chest retraction all point to severe dyspnea. The severity of the dyspnea almost always correlates with the severity of the problem. In such situations consider pulmonary embolism, anaphylaxis, foreign body aspiration, pneumothorax, status asthmaticus, and severe heart failure. Persons presenting with COPD, anemia, mild asthma, and mild heart failure appear less acutely ill.

Determine if the patient has to lean forward or sit up to breathe comfortably. With severe respiratory distress or upper airway obstruction, an infant may adopt a posture of hyperextension of the trunk and neck. A child with epiglottitis prefers to sit up and lean forward.

Any child who is in acute respiratory distress, is sitting forward, and perhaps drooling with dysphasia may have epiglottitis and immediate assistance should be secured. Do not attempt to lie the child down as this may occlude the airway.

Assess Level of Consciousness

Diminished level of consciousness, confusion, and restlessness are manifestations of hypoxia in a patient experiencing respiratory problems. Frequently the patient with a PE expresses a sense of impending doom.

An acutely ill child may have an alteration in level of consciousness, restless-ness, mouth breathing, and flaring of the nostrils.

Observe Chest Movement

Place the patient in a sitting or side-lying position with the chest exposed. The chest cannot be adequately viewed through clothing. Many respiratory abnormalities are unilateral or localized, so compare findings on one side of the body with those on the other. Also compare front to back. Pneumothorax and PE may cause unequal expansion of the chest.

Inspect the Shape and Symmetry of the Chest

Cardinal features of restrictive pulmonary disease are deformities of the chest wall and reduction in lung volume and pulmonary compliance secondary to pathological changes in the lung parenchyma or pleura. Examples of deformities that cause decreased lung volume include kyphosis, scoliosis, and kyphoscoliosis. Decreased volume necessitates an increase in respiratory rate to maintain a normal volume. The work of breathing must be increased to overcome the reduced compliance.

Kyphoscoliosis is associated with marked structural abnormality of the thoracic cage, leading to abnormal positioning and functioning of the respiratory muscles. The lungs are compressed by the thoracic deformity, leading to a small lung volume. Breathing entails a high work and energy cost, and dyspnea can appear.

An increased anteroposterior (AP) diameter indicates air trapping. This is a frequent finding in persons with COPD. Other musculoskeletal chest abnormalities to note include pectus excavatum, pectus carinatum, severe scoliosis, and kyphoscoliosis. These conditions can contribute to chest infection and respiratory failure because of decreased lung volume and ability to cough. Also bronchomalacia, a softening of the bronchial tissue, is an abnormality associated with pectus excavatum. Pectus carinatum is associated with chronic lung disease such as asthma or with cystic fibrosis, heart disease, and idiopathic scoliosis. Harrison's sulci are exaggerated grooves running parallel to the subcostal margins, produced by prolonged diaphragmatic traction, and are associated with chronic airway disease or rickets.

In the presence of neuromuscular disease, chest movement in children should be examined in both the supine and sitting positions. Diaphragmatic weakness leads to paradoxical abdominal movements in the supine position, which may be missed if the child is examined only in the sitting position.

Respiratory distress brought on by placing the child in the supine position may be the only subtle abnormality in older children having mediastinal compression of the trachea.

Look for Retractions

In normal breathing, the work of inspiration is the sum of the work necessary to overcome the elastic forces of the lung, the tissue viscosity of the lung and chest wall, and airway resistance. When there is a problem with any of these, the work of breathing is increased and the accessory muscles (sternocleidomastoid, anterior serratus, and external intercostal muscles) are recruited to help. Contraction of these muscles causes forceful expansion of the thorax, resulting in an unusually large negative intrathoracic pressure. This negative pressure draws in the soft tissues of the chest wall resulting in retractions, which can be seen in children. Retractions occur in lower intercostal spaces first, then move up to the higher spaces. In an infant, head-bobbing in time with respirations reflects use of the accessory muscles of respiration.

Observe the Rate, Rhythm, and Depth of Respiration for One Full Minute

In children, the respiratory rate should be counted while the child sleeps if possible.

When tachypnea is present without other signs of respiratory disease, causes other than a primary respiratory disease should be considered. Tachypnea is an early sign of most pulmonary, parenchymal, cardiac, or systemic causes of respiratory distress. Hyperventilation can occur secondary to acidosis or CNS disease. Slow respirations may indicate CNS depression, hypoxemia, shock, or systemic infection.

Exhaling should take about twice as long as inhaling, but in COPD patients it may take up to four times longer. Rhythm should be even, with occasional sighs. Shallow respirations, which are rapid, indicate that restrictive forces must be overcome. Box 4-1 describes abnormal breathing patterns.

Listen for Stridor

Stridor is caused by extra-thoracic inspiratory dynamic narrowing of the airway in the oropharynx, glottis, or subglottic region, or mid-trachea. Any condition that causes further decrease in the lumen of the airway will obstruct airflow and produce stridor. Inspiratory stridor usually indicates a supraglottic obstruction. If the obstruction varies or is extrathoracic (i.e., above the vocal cords), inspiration is affected more because the negative intra-airway pressure during inspiration tends to collapse the extra-thoracic airway. If the obstruction varies and affects the intra-thoracic airways, expiration is prolonged because the positive intra-thoracic pressure tends to collapse these airways during expiration. Expiratory or biphasic respiratory stridor generally indicates an obstruction at or below the larynx.

With severe narrowing of the air passage, stridor may be audible both on inspiration and expiration but is worse during inspiration. Biphasic or expiratory stridor

Box 4-1

Abnormal Breathing Patterns

Cheyne-Stoke's respirations are manifested by rhythmic increase and decrease in depth, punctuated by regular episodes of apnea. This may be a sign of severe heart failure or neurological disease.

Tachypnea is rapid breathing with no change in depth and can be brought on by hypoxia, pain, fever, or anxiety. Consider pulmonary embolism, foreign body aspiration, anaphylaxis, pneumothorax, heart failure, asthma, or pneumonia.

Asymmetrical chest movement with respirations may be observed in lobar pneumonia, pleural effusion, or any condition that affects just one side of the chest.

Use of accessory muscles indicates respiratory distress. Observe for bulging or retraction of the intercostal, sternocleidomastoid, and/or trapezius muscles.

Nasal flaring is an objective manifestation of hypoxia.

anomalous vascular rings, laryngeal webs, laryngomalacia, or tracheomalacia. Stridor in older children may indicate foreign body aspiration, infection, inflammation (angioneurotic edema), trauma, or tumor.

Listen for Audible Wheeze

Expiratory wheezing is a high-pitched musical sound caused by partial airway obstruction. It is commonly associated with disorders of the lower respiratory tract that cause inflammation, infection, or bronchoconstriction such as asthma and bronchitis.

Increased inspiratory effort suggests disease in the upper airways, whereas increased expiratory effort suggests disease in the smaller airways or lower respiratory tract.

Listen for Voice Changes

Voice changes may occur in association with upper airway obstruction. Paralysis of the vocal cords results in dysphonia. Subglottic stenosis results in decreased volume of the voice because a much smaller column of air is making the vocal cords vibrate. Involvement of the supraglottic area, proximal to the vocal cords, can result in a hyponasal or muffled voice (seen in tonsillitis and epiglottitis). A normal voice with stridor may indicate the lesion is subglottic or tracheal.

Take Pulse, Temperature, and Blood Pressure

Palpate the radial, femoral, popliteal, and pedal pulses for rate and quality.

Tachycardia increases cardiac output. It occurs either as a result of primary heart disease, or as a secondary process in response to oxygen deprivation because of pulmonary embolism, pneumonia, fever, and/or heart failure. Tachycardia and drowsiness may indicate a metabolic acidosis. Bradycardia is usually seen late in respiratory disease.

Tachycardia may occur with an irregular pulse, signaling heart failure from atrial

alone usually indicates a more significant obstruction. Supraglottic stridor is usually quiet and wet and is associated with a muffled voice, dysphasia, and a preference to sit. Subglottic lesions produce a loud stridor, often causing a hoarse voice, barky cough, and possibly facial edema. Inspiratory stridor may be a sign of incomplete obstruction of the airway by a foreign body.

Infants less than 6 months of age who present with stridor may have an underlying anatomical abnormality that may now be symptomatic secondary to an acute illness. Common anomalies that predispose the infant to upper airway obstruction are fibrillation and/or heart block. Diminished peripheral pulses indicate possible atherosclerotic vessel disease or decreased cardiac output.

Fever may indicate epiglottitis or any other upper and/or lower respiratory tract infection.

Orthostatic hypotension may be a manifestation of hypovolemia, secondary to dehydration associated with pneumonia or status asthmaticus. Anaphylaxis is also manifested by a severe drop in blood pressure. Pulsus paradoxus, an inspiratory drop in systolic blood pressure of more than 10 mm Hg, is caused by greater inspiratory effort from increased airway resistance. Negative intra-thoracic pressure imposes a greater net transmural pressure on the left ventricle and aorta, increasing the afterload and lowering systolic blood pressure. In heart failure, decreased stroke volume reduces the systolic blood pressure. Compensatory vasoconstriction maintains a constant diastolic pressure and along with the decreased systolic pressure may produce a decreased pulse pressure.

Inspect the Oral Cavity

First observe the oral pharyngeal cavity for any evidence of a foreign body that may be obstructing the airway. Also evidence of vomitus may indicate possible aspiration. Note the color of the tongue and mucous membranes for signs of central cyanosis.

Inspect the posterior pharynx for peritonsillar cellulitis, a retropharyngeal abscess, or other intra-oral pathology that might be causing obstruction. Lift the jaw forward. Obstruction of the airway associated with micrognathia, depressed airway reflexes, or an enlarged tongue will diminish with this maneuver because the tongue will be lifted off the posterior pharynx.

Inspect the Nose

Assess the patency of the nares. Fifty percent of airway resistance comes from the nose.

Noisy, difficult breathing in an infant, especially while feeding, may signal choanal atresia. A deviated septum compromises the patency of one side of the nose when there is additional mucosal swelling.

Palpate the Neck

Neck masses caused by intraoral, paratracheal, or intrathoracic malignant disease may cause respiratory distress. Inspect the position of the trachea. To assess the trachea for lateral displacement, position your index finger first on the right side of the suprasternal notch, then the left. If the trachea has shifted to the side, you'll feel the wall on one side but only soft tissue on the other. This is most likely to occur with pneumothorax. Observe the neck for jugular venous distention. This is a sign of heart failure.

Examine the Skin/Extremities

Note cyanosis. Bluish color seen in the lips and mucous membranes of the mouth (central cyanosis) is associated with low arterial saturation and may result from inadequate gas exchange in the lungs or from cardiac shunting. Cyanosis implies >5 g/100 ml of desaturated hemoglobin, but its absence does not imply that hypoxemia is not present. Dark-skinned patients' mucous membranes may appear gray with central cyanosis. Central cyanosis may also be seen in persons with COPD. Bluish color of extremities (peripheral cyanosis) may be observed in Caucasian persons and is associated with low venous saturation, resulting from vasoconstriction, vascular occlusion, or reduced cardiac output.

Pallor may be a manifestation of severe anemia.

Note clubbing, which is characterized by the loss of the angle between the skin and nail bed. This is a manifestation of chronic tissue hypoxia that occurs with lung cancer and other chronic lung diseases. It is uncommon in children other than those with cystic fibrosis or cyanotic congenital heart disease. Clubbing develops rapidly with infective endocarditis.

Test for peripheral edema. Edema of the lower extremities may be a sign of increased right-heart filling pressure caused by primary lung disease or left-heart failure. Make note of how high the edema extends up the extremity. In children, the location of peripheral edema is age dependent. In young infants, edema occurs as hepatomegaly and periorbital or flank edema. In older children, lower extremity edema can occur.

Note any angioedema. The presence of generalized or local giant urticaria is objective evidence of probable anaphylaxis.

Check skin perfusion by pressing on the skin of a finger or sole of a foot and saying "capillary refill" after removing the pressure. A normal finding is that the color returns to the skin in 2 seconds or before you can finish saying the words.

Palpate the Chest

Using the palmar surface of the hands, palpate the entire chest for tenderness, depressions, bulges, and crepitus (presence of air in the subcutaneous tissues). Crepitus may indicate a chest injury, pneumothorax, or emphysema.

Pneumothorax, atelectasis, pneumonia, and partial paralysis of the diaphragm will result in reduced expansion of one side of the chest wall, and chest wall motion will be decreased.

Assess for Vocal Fremitus

Fremitus is diminished in pneumothorax, asthma, emphysema, and other conditions that trap air in the lung. Vocal fremitus intensity may be increased in pneumonia, heart failure, and tumor, all conditions that increase the lung density.

Percuss the Chest

Sounds produced by percussion indicate density of lung tissue (see Cough, p. 134).

In children, transmission of a percussion note and assessment of the quality of transmitted sound are useful to reveal an area of consolidation or effusion that would be difficult to auscultate with an uncooperative child.

Auscultate Breath Sounds

Auscultation of bronchial or bronchovesicular breath sounds over the peripheral lungs may indicate consolidation, which occurs when lungs fill with exudate. If breath sounds are diminished over all lung fields, suspect obesity or COPD. Breath sounds will be inaudible in areas of pneumothorax.

Abnormal lung sounds are superimposed on normal sounds and can be auscultated over any area of the lung field during inspiration or expiration. Documentation of abnormal lung sounds should include type of sound, location where it is heard, and the phase(s) of respiration in which it is noted.

Crackles or rales are discontinuous popping sounds heard most often during inspiration. They are caused by the explosive equalization of gas pressure between two compartments of the lung when a closed section of the airway separating them suddenly opens. They indicate the presence of fluid, mucus, or pus in the smaller airways. Fine crackles are soft and high-pitched. Medium crackles are louder and lower pitched. Coarse crackles are moist and more explosive.

The frequency and timing of crackles is the important part of assessment. In resolving pneumonia, crackling is heard on inspiration. This is caused by a mix between the aerated and non-aerated alveoli and bronchioles. In airways that are swollen and narrowed, such as in asthma bronchiolitis, generalized medium or coarse crackles are heard throughout both phases of respiration. Early inspiratory crackles are heard in COPD. Mid-to-late inspiratory crackles are more likely a sign of interstitial lung disease or heart failure. Crackles may be heard over the site of a pulmonary embolus.

Wheezing is frequently described as a whistling sound and can be heard during inspiration, expiration, or both. The sound is high pitched and musical. Wheezing indicates that there is fluid in the large airways such as in severe heart failure, or it more often heralds bronchospasm as seen in asthma. In addition, localized wheezing may accompany incomplete obstruction of the airway by a foreign body.

A wheeze of fixed pitch occurring with inspiration and expiration suggests a localized abnormality. Wheezes of varying pitch occurring predominantly throughout expiration reflect the narrowing of airways of different calibers.

Rhonchi are continuous, deep-pitched, coarse breath sounds usually heard during expiration. Rhonchi are frequently present when the patient has bronchitis or pneumonia.

Pleural friction rub is a grating or squeaking sound usually heard in the lateral lung fields during inspiration and expiration. It indicates that parietal and visceral pleural linings are inflamed and are rubbing together as may occur with pneumonia, pleural effusion, and tumors. It is often accompanied by limited chest expansion because of pain.

If abnormal lung sounds are detected, additional auscultation for bronchophony, egophony, and whispered pectoriloquy are indicated. Consolidation will produce positive findings for each of these tests. To test for bronchophony, instruct the patient to say "ninety-nine." The words sound louder and clearer than they usually do. In egophony, instruct the patient to say "ee." This sound is transmitted as "ay" if consolidation is present. To test whispered pectoriloquy, instruct the patient to whisper a sentence. Whispered sounds are louder and clearer than normal.

Auscultate Heart Sounds

In COPD, lung hyperinflation may muffle heart sounds. Poor tissue oxygenation may result in tachycardia. In children, muffled heart sounds may indicate pericarditis.

In heart failure, S1 and S2 may equal rapid pulse rate or may indicate a pulse deficit. An S3 (ventricular gallop) is an early sign of heart failure and is heard best at the apex of the heart. S4 (atrial gallop) typically indicates a stressed heart and is also pathonomic of heart failure in children. In adults it may be the result of hypertension, myocardial infarction, or coronary artery disease causing heart failure. A summation gallop may also occur with heart failure. This is the result of S3, S4, and rapid rate.

Listen for the presence of any murmurs and note their location, grade of loudness, timing, or radiation. Incompetent heart valves may be the cause of heart failure.

LABORATORY AND DIAGNOSTIC STUDIES

Diagnostic tests are indicated in almost all initial evaluations of the patient presenting with shortness of breath. Posteroanterior (PA) and lateral chest x-rays, hemoglobin level, and spirometry are useful preliminary tests.

Chest X-Ray

Chest x-ray should be observed for the following abnormal findings:

- Altered depth of lung inflation: depth less than 8 ribs suggests an interstitial fibrotic process, neuromuscular disease, or collagen disease; depth of 10 or more ribs suggests hyperinflation of obstructive airway disease.
- Parenchymal infiltrates may indicate acute pneumonia, pulmonary edema, or chronic interstitial lung disease.
- Abnormal pattern of pulmonary vasculature may indicate heart failure.
- Increased cardiac size may indicate heart failure.

- Deflated lung indicates a pneumothorax.
- Mass lesions suggest possible carcinoma.
- Cavernous lesions suggest tuberculosis.

Hemoglobin and Hematocrit

Significantly decreased hemoglobin and hematocrit suggest anemia as a possible cause of dyspnea. Erythrocytosis may indicate chronic hypoxia resulting from a number of causes, including COPD.

Spirometry

Spirometry is indicated if the dyspnea is related to obstructive or restrictive lung disease. Spirometry measures forced vital capacity (FVC), 1-second forced expiratory volume (FEV1), and the FEV1:FVC ratio. In obstructive lung disease (i.e., asthma and COPD), the FEV1 and the ratio are less than predicted. In restrictive lung disease (i.e., pneumonia, pneumothorax, pleural effusion), the FVC is reduced and the ratio is normal or elevated.

Additional Tests

Additional diagnostic tests may be indicated after the initial data gathering. These can include:

- Decubitus chest x-rays to assess pleural effusions. The patient is in the recumbent lateral position.
- CT or MRI to provide more detailed assessment of mass lesions.
- Pulmonary angiography to confirm pulmonary embolism.
- CBC with differential to determine the presence of bacterial infection.
- Blood urea nitrogen and creatinine to assess renal function. Renal insufficiency frequently presents with dyspnea as a result of combined effects of volume overload and anemia.
- Arterial blood gases (ABGs) in an acutely ill patient with dyspnea and tachypnea (see Chest Pain, p. 96).

- Sputum culture if sputum is present to determine the presence of an infectious agent.
- ECG and echocardiograms when heart failure is suspected as the cause of dyspnea (see Chest Pain, pp. 95 and 96).
- Exercise stress testing in situations where the cause of dyspnea is elusive and for those whose symptoms are precipitated or aggravated by exercise. It is indicated in situations where you need to differentiate cardiac and respiratory limitations, document deconditioning, and identify psychogenic dyspnea.

DIFFERENTIAL DIAGNOSIS

When patients report severe dyspnea and manifest significant oxygen deprivation, emergent assessment and referral are indicated. The following health problems may be the cause of the emergent situation.

EMERGENT CONDITIONS MANIFESTED BY DYSPNEA

Pulmonary Embolus

A patient reporting severe dyspnea, cough, fever, hemoptysis, chest pain, history of deep vein thrombosis, and/or history of recent immobilization should be evaluated for possible PE. Physical examination will reveal a restless patient with tachycardia, tachypnea, possible pleural friction rub, and/or crackles and wheezes. Chest x-ray, ABGs, and ECG should be done immediately (see Cough, p. 136).

Foreign Body Aspiration

Foreign body aspiration occurs most frequently in children and the elderly. If the event was witnessed, history of aspiration is usually clear. If the person is found after the event, the history may not be as revealing. A child or adult who aspirated a foreign body can have a varied presentation. Generally, the onset of cough is sudden and unexpected. If the foreign body (FB) is obstructing the airway, the patient is in acute respiratory distress and immediate intubation or bronchoscopy is indicated to remove the FB and open the airway. Partial obstruction of the airway may cause stridor, cyanosis, labored respirations, and/or wheezing. Lateral neck and chest x-rays may reveal the location and size of the obstructing object (see Cough, p. 140).

Anaphylaxis

Anaphylaxis is an emergent situation. History may include history of insect sting, drug ingestion, recent meal containing shellfish, or exposure to known allergens. Early symptoms include pruritic rash, feeling of warmth over body, wheezing, fatigue, lightheadedness, and increasing dyspnea. On examination, persons in anaphylaxis manifest angioedema, tachypnea, clammy skin, hypotension, wheezes, and tachycardia. Immediate treatment and support of ventilation may be necessary.

Pneumothorax

History of blunt chest trauma often seen following a motor vehicle accident or a fall may cause pneumothorax, hemothorax, or pulmonary contusion. Cystic fibrosis may cause a spontaneous pneumothorax from rupture of subpleural blebs located at the apex of the upper lobe or in the superior segment of the lower lobe. Spontaneous pneumothorax may also occur in males, with the highest incidence between ages 15 to 30 in tall, asthenic individuals. There is sudden severe chest pain and dyspnea aggravated by normal respiratory movement. Absence or decreased breath sounds are found on the side of the pneumothorax. Chest x-ray may be diagnostic.

Croup

Croup is a viral infection that is usually preceded by symptoms of an upper respiratory infection. The illness is usually gradual in onset and includes a hoarse, seal-bark cough and fever. The degree of respiratory distress can be variable (see Cough, p. 138).

Acute Epiglottitis

Acute epiglottitis is a serious, life-threatening bacterial infection of the epiglottis caused primarily by *H. influenzae*. It typically has a rapid onset with stridor, high fever, drooling, muffled voice, and sore throat. A child will appear anxious and may be sitting forward.

Bacterial Tracheitis

Bacterial tracheitis is usually a secondary infection caused by *Staphylococcus aureus* or *H. influenzae* that inflames the trachea after an antecedent viral infection. It is a subglottic lesion and mimics croup; however, a high fever and toxic appearance is present. Frequently there is a copious amount of purulent sputum present.

Status Asthmaticus

Acute bronchoconstriction in a patient with asthma can develop as a result of a respiratory infection, exposure to allergens, inhalation of fumes, airway irritants, and environmental factors. Airway obstruction is caused not only by bronchial smooth muscle constriction but also by mucosal edema and excessive mucus production. Predominant symptoms include breathlessness, wheezing, and coughing. Absence of wheezing in a child with asthma may indicate severe airway obstruction with poor air exchange.

Botulism

Botulism is poisoning that may occur after ingestion of the toxin in inadequately cooked or improperly canned food. Infant botulism is caused by ingestion of the spores of *C. botulinum* rather than the exotoxin. It occurs before the first year of life, and honey has been implicated in 20% of patients. Symptoms occur 1 to 2 days after ingestion of contaminated food. Weakness and respiratory dyspnea and failure often accompany visual problems. Infant botulism begins with constipation, and the infant becomes weaker and listless. Respiratory arrest may be sudden.

NON-EMERGENT CONDITIONS MANIFESTED BY DYSPNEA

Chronic progressive dyspnea is most often caused by chronic pulmonary disease, heart failure, and obesity. It is seen less often in severe anemia and carcinoma of the pulmonary system. These patients report gradual onset of shortness of breath over days or weeks.

Chronic Obstructive Pulmonary Disease (COPD)

COPD is often associated with frequent cough that is worse in the morning, sputum production that is clear to yellow in color, decreasing exercise tolerance, and mild to moderate fatigue. Symptoms of infectious processes may accompany increased dyspnea. History of smoking is present in most instances. Exposure to asbestos, coal dust, and other significant environmental pollutants may also be reported. Objective manifestations of COPD include rapid shallow respirations, reddish complexion, increased AP diameter, use of accessory muscles to breathe, pursed lip breathing, decreased tactile fremitus, decreased respiratory excursion bilaterally, hyperresonant lungs, distant breath sounds, prolonged expiration, occasional wheezes, and muffled heart sounds. Chest x-ray, pulmonary function tests, and possible exercise tests are indicated to confirm the diagnosis of COPD.

Heart Failure

Persons reporting history of heart disease or heart valve disease, dyspnea, orthopnea, paroxysmal nocturnal dyspnea (PND), peripheral edema, weight gain, cough with frothy sputum, fatigue, and palpitations must be further assessed for acute heart failure. Physical examination findings may include altered level of consciousness, anxiety, jugular venous distention, tachypnea, rales, rhonchi, tachycardia, displaced point of maximum impulse (PMI), S3, S4, and possible ascites. Symptoms in children also include sweating on the forehead or upper lip. An ECG and chest x-ray usually reveals increased heart size, arterial pO_2 that may be decreased, and ejection fractions that are significantly reduced on echocardiogram.

Anemia

Patients reporting dyspnea (especially on exertion), fatigue, lightheadedness, palpitations, and possible history of chronic disease should have blood tests to measure the oxygen-carrying capacity of their blood (hemoglobin and hematocrit). Hematological diseases affect the oxygen-carrying capacity of the blood, with resulting tissue hypoxia. A decrease in arterial pH stimulates the CNS and dyspnea is seen. Objective signs of anemia include tachycardia and pallor.

Poor Physical Conditioning

Poor physical conditioning can cause the patient to experience shortness of breath with exertion. Associated symptoms may include cardiac palpitations and history of weight gain and sedentary life style. The physical examination is often normal except for tachycardia and possible obesity. Exercise stress tests will provide evidence of tachycardia and tachypnea with increasing workload.

Asthma

Asthma is the most frequent cause of recurrent dyspnea. Persons usually report a history of asthma and possibly allergies and may be on inhaled bronchodilators and/or inhaled steroids. Paroxysmal cough and audible wheeze often accompany dyspnea. They may report recent respiratory infection, exposure to known allergens, or strenuous exercise. Objective manifestation on physical examination includes restlessness, tachypnea, use of accessory muscles to breathe, intercostal retraction, decreased vocal fremitus, decreased breath sounds, and inspiratory and possible expiratory wheezes. Spirometry testing will provide confirming evidence of asthma. ABGs are indicated in the patient manifesting acute O_2 deprivation, and chest x-rays are indicated if a lower respiratory infection is suspected. If the patient does not have a history of asthma and the spirometry is normal, a methacholine challenge test may be diagnostic (see Cough, p. 135).

The lessening or absence of wheezes in a person with asthma may indicate mucus plugging and an impending episode of status asthmaticus.

Pneumonia

Pneumonia is usually associated with dyspnea, pleuritic chest pain, and cough with greenish or rusty-colored sputum, fever, and chills. In children, irritability, feeding problems, and lack of playfulness may also be seen. Objective manifestations of pneumonia include fever, tachycardia, tachypnea, inspiratory crackles, asynchronous breathing, vocal fremitus, dull percussion sound over area of consolidation, and bronchophony. Pneumonia can be confirmed by chest x-ray and sputum cultures.

Hyperventilation Syndrome

Hyperventilation syndrome is a common cause of recurrent faintness without actual loss of consciousness. Dyspnea, lightheadedness, palpitations, paresthesias (perioral and extremities) occur. Restlessness, anxiety, and a normal cardiovascular examination are present. Recumbency does not relieve the symptoms. Chest x-ray is negative.

Laryngomalacia

Laryngomalacia is the most common cause of persistent stridor in infancy. Onset of the stridor is almost always within the first 4 weeks of life, commonly in the first week (with preterm neonates who were on ventilation at high risk). Occasionally parents become aware of the condition when a respiratory infection is present. Stridor is predominantly inspiratory, and the sound may change with change in position of the infant. The cry and cough are normal. Direct visualization of the larynx is done for diagnosis.

Vascular Ring

Tracheal compression from vascular anomalies may cause stridor and dyspnea in infants. The main symptom is soft inspiratory stridor with expiratory wheeze. Frequently a brassy cough and difficulty in swallowing may be present. Barium swallow followed by echocardiography is done to establish the diagnosis.

Table 4-5

Differential Diagnosis of Common Causes of Emergent Conditions Manifested by Dyspnea

Condition	History	Physical Findings	Diagnostic Studies
Pulmonary embolus	Acute-onset dyspnea, cough, mild to severe chest pain, sense of impending	Restlessness, fever, tachycardia, tachypnea, diminished breath sounds, crackles,	ABGs, chest x-ray, ECG, ventilation/ perfusion scans

Table 4-5

Differential Diagnosis of Common Causes of Emergent Conditions Manifested by Dyspnea—cont'd

Condition	History	Physical Findings	Diagnostic Studies
Pulmonary embolus—cont'd	doom; hemoptysis; history of DVT, recent surgery, oral contraceptive, smoker, hypercoagulability states	wheezing, pleural friction rub	
Foreign body aspiration	Acute-onset dyspnea; history of eating or drinking large amounts of alcohol; in children, history of putting small objects in the mouth; possible cough	Apnea or tachypnea, restlessness, suprasternal retractions, intoxication, inspiratory stridor, localized wheeze	Lateral neck x-ray, chest x-ray, bronchoscopy
Anaphylaxis	Acute-onset dyspnea; history of insect sting, ingestion of drug, or allergen	Angioedema, tachypnea, clammy skin, hypotension, bilateral wheezes, tachycardia	None; emergency measures necessary
Pneumothorax	Acute-onset dyspnea; sharp, tearing chest pain; pain may radiate to ipsilateral shoulder	Tachycardia, diminished breath sounds, decreased tactile fremitus, hyperresonance of lung area affected; possible hypertension and tracheal shift	Chest x-ray, ABGs
Croup	History of upper respiratory infection	Hoarse, seal-bark cough, fever (variable)	None initially; if respiratory distress increases, pulse oximeter and referral
Acute epiglottitis	Positional sitting forward; sore throat; anxious, toxic child	High fever, drooling, stridor, muffled voice	Admit; life threatening

Continued

Table 4-5

Differential Diagnosis of Common Causes of Emergent Conditions Manifested by Dyspnea—cont'd

Condition	History	Physical Findings	Diagnostic Studies
Bacterial tracheitis	Recent viral infection	Fever, stridor, purulent sputum	Radiography of airway, WBC increased, tracheal culture
Status asthmaticus	Recent URI, exposure to allergens, breathlessness	Wheezing, coughing, tachycardia, tachypnea	Peak flows, chest x-ray, ABGs
Botulism	Honey ingestion in infant, contaminated food ingestion	Hypoventilation, drooling, weak cry, ptosis, ophthalmoplegia, loss of head control	Pulmonary function testing, chest x-ray, fluoroscopy, stool culture

Table 4-6

Differential Diagnosis of Common Causes of Non-Emergent Conditions Manifested by Dyspnea

Condition	History	Physical Findings	Diagnostic Studies
COPD	Chronic progressive dyspnea, dyspnea on exertion, persistent cough, minimal sputum, easy fatigue, history of smoking	Rapid shallow respirations, reddish complexion, increased AP diameter of thorax, use of accessory muscles to breathe, pursed lip breathing, decreased tactile fremitus, decreased respiratory excursion bilaterally, lungs hyperresonant, distant breath sounds, prolonged expiration, occasional wheezes, possible tachycardia, muffled heart sounds	Chest x-ray, pulmonary function tests, exercise tests, ABGs

Table 4-6

Differential Diagnosis of Common Causes of Non-Emergent Conditions Manifested by Dyspnea—cont'd

Condition	History	Physical Findings	Diagnostic Studies
Heart failure	Chronic progressive dyspnea, cough, frothy sputum, fatigue, lightheadedness, syncope, weight gain, ankle swelling, palpitations, PND, orthopnea, history of heart disease; in children, chronic progressive dyspnea, sweating above lip and forehead, especially while eating	Altered level of consciousness, restlessness, jugular venous distention, tachypnea, use of accessory muscles to breathe, rales, rhonchi, wheezes, tachycardia, decreased peripheral pulses, cool extremities, displaced PMI, S3, S4, ascites, liver enlargement	ECG, chest x-ray, ABGs, echocardiogram
Anemia	Dyspnea on exertion, fatigue, palpitations, lightheadedness, history of chronic disease	Pallor, tachypnea, cool dry skin of extremities, possible orthostatic hypotension	CBC, iron studies
Poor physical conditioning	Dyspnea on exertion, weight gain, palpitation on exertion, sedentary lifestyle, cigarette smoker	Overweight, tachycardia	Cardiac stress test
Asthma	Dyspnea, paroxysmal cough, audible wheeze, history of asthma or allergies	Restlessness, tachypnea, use of accessory muscles to breathe, intercostal retractions, decreased vocal fremitus, decreased breath sounds, inspiratory and possibly expiratory wheezes	Spirometry, chest x-ray, ABGs

Continued

Table 4-6

Differential Diagnosis of Common Causes of Non-Emergent Conditions Manifested by Dyspnea—cont'd

Condition	History	Physical Findings	Diagnostic Studies
Pneumonia	Dyspnea, cough, sputum production (green, rust, or red), pleuritic chest pain, chills; in infants and children: irritability and feeding problems	Fever, tachycardia, tachypnea, inspiratory crackles, asynchronous breathing, vocal fremitus, percussion dull or flat over area of consolidation, bronchophony, egophony	Chest x-ray, sputum cultures, ABGs, WBC
Hyperventilation syndrome	Dyspnea, lightheadedness, palpitations, paresthesias (perioral and extremities)	Restlessness, anxiety, normal CV exam	Chest x-ray
Laryngomalacia	Neonate, infant: history of stridor, history of URI	Inspiratory stridor; normal cough, cry	Refer for visualization of larynx
Vascular ring	Infant: dyspnea, brassy cough, difficulty swallowing	Inspiratory stridor with expiratory wheeze	Barium swallow, echocardiography

≡ Cough

Cough occurs when inspiration is followed by an explosive expiration. Coughing promotes clearance of airways of secretions and foreign bodies. Cough is usually the result of a reflex initiated by stimulation of the sensory nerve endings beneath and between the epithelium of the larynx and tracheobronchial tree. The reflex stimulation follows the vagal nerve to the "cough center," which is located in the medulla oblongata of the brainstem. However, other anatomical locations may be stimulated and initiate the cough reflex, including the pleura, pericardium, ear canals, esophagus, and stomach. The cough reflex is absent in very young infants. Effective coughing may also be impossible in emaciated persons, in those whose respiratory musculature is weak or paralyzed, and in those with massive ascites.

Causes of cough can be characterized by duration. A cough of recent onset is most often the result of viral or bacterial infection in the respiratory system. Allergies can also precipitate acute onset of cough in both children and adults. Coughs of longer duration (greater than 3 to 4 weeks) are more likely caused by chronic lung or heart disease, such as chronic obstructive pulmonary disease (COPD), cystic fibrosis, chronic bronchitis, asthma, postnasal drainage, heart failure, pertussis, and chronic sinusitis. Gastroesophageal reflux disease (GERD) and foreign body in the ear canal should also be considered in both adults and children.

Most coughs are a symptom of minor upper respiratory infections such as the common cold. Keep in mind, however, that a cough in a patient in acute distress may signal a life-threatening problem (such as foreign body aspiration with occlusion of airway), severe asthma, escalating heart failure, or pneumonia.

DIAGNOSTIC REASONING: FOCUSED HISTORY

Is this cough related to an underlying emergent medical problem?

Key Questions
- Are you short of breath?
- Do you have a history of heart failure?
- Have you had a fever?
- Do you have a history of asthma?
- Have you noticed the child putting small objects in his or her mouth?

Shortness of breath. Cough associated with shortness of breath (SOB) usually suggests a physical obstruction of the airway. The most common obstruction is a foreign body or the effects of acute asthma. Persons with heart failure report orthopnea, paroxysmal nocturnal dyspnea (PND), cough with possible frothy sputum, possible weight gain with swollen feet and ankles, and often a history of heart disease. Cardiac failure of any kind results in decreased lung compliance and cough.

Fever. Bronchopneumonia is characterized by cough with sputum production as the prominent symptom when airway involvement occurs. Pneumonia with alveolar involvement presents with cough, tachypnea, fever, tachycardia, and possible shortness of breath.

Copious, thick, purulent secretions in children accompanied by high fever and increasing inspiratory stridor may indicate bacterial tracheitis, which can be life threatening.

History of asthma. Acute exacerbation of asthma is characterized by an irritating non-productive cough that can progress to tachypnea, dyspnea, wheezing, grunting, cyanosis, fatigue, and finally respiratory and cardiac failure. Viral infection, especially respiratory syncytial virus (RSV), parainfluenza viruses, and rhinoviruses are the most important triggers of asthma in children.

Foreign body. Consider a foreign body aspiration in any child. A child who has aspirated a foreign body can have a varied presentation. Generally the onset of cough is sudden and unexpected. A brief period of severe coughing, gagging, and choking occurs. Then a quiet period ensues of no coughing. This can last for hours, days, or even months. A foreign body in the lower airway can produce either emphysema caused by a ball-valve phenomenon or complete distal atelectasis because of absorption of the trapped gas. A mobile foreign body in the lower airway can also produce a paroxysmal cough, with cyanotic episodes and stridor as a result of proximal migration and subglottic impaction.

A foreign body in the esophagus can also produce airway obstruction and cough as well as dysphasia to solid foods because the posterior trachea is compliant and adjacent to the anterior esophagus. Coins are the most frequently found foreign bodies.

Is the cough acute or chronic?

Key Questions
- How long have you had the cough?
- Do you smoke? Are you exposed to smoke?
- Is the cough getting worse or more frequent?
- What time of day is the cough most bothersome? Early morning? Nighttime?
- Did the child have an episode of severe cough, gagging, and choking a few weeks ago?
- What type of work do you do?

Duration of cough. Acute coughs are most likely infectious in nature, lasting from 1 to 2 weeks. The most common cause of cough lasting longer than 3 weeks in nonsmoking, immunocompetent adults is postnasal drainage. Asthma, GERD, chronic bronchitis, and bronchiectasis are also common causes.

Cough in children occurs frequently. Determine if the symptom is the result of a rapid succession of unrelated acute respiratory tract infections or represents a chronic cough. Young preschool children normally contract as many as 7 to 8 respiratory infections a year. In general, in children a chronic cough is a cough that lasts more than 3 weeks.

A cough that occurs several times a minute with regularity may indicate a habit (tic) cough.

Smoke exposure. Chronic cough is not uncommon in persons who smoke. Smoke exposure can trigger cough in persons with allergies or asthma.

Getting better or worse. A change in the chronic cough of a smoker may indicate the development of a new and serious underlying problem (i.e., pneumonia or lung cancer).

Severity of cough. A cough in children or adults that becomes progressively worse may indicate pertussis. Pertussis has three stages. The first stage presents with a mild cough, rhinorrhea, conjunctivitis, and low-grade fever for 1 to 2 weeks. Then the cough becomes severe and comes in short paroxysms. There is a "whoop" on the inspiration effort at the end of the paroxysm. In the convalescent stage, the coughing and paroxysmal whooping decreases, but the cough may persist in a milder form for 3 months. **Young infants and older adults with pertussis do not "whoop".**

A cough in children that begins with a history of mild upper respiratory illness followed in 2 to 3 days with a cough that is brassy in sound may indicate croup. The cough is usually worse at night. Symptoms escalate from 3 to 4 nights as compromise of the upper airway continues from the viral agent (usually parainfluenza). Obstruction increases, stridor becomes continuous, and is associated with nasal flaring and suprasternal, infrasternal, and intracostal retraction. The child is agitated and sits up. In most children recovery is generally in a few hours. Any intensification of symptoms of respiratory obstruction requires hospitalization. Persistent paroxysmal coughing is often associated with asthma.

History of choking episode. Consider foreign body aspiration in any child with a cough lasting longer than 3 weeks. Frequently the caregivers report an episode of severe coughing and choking occurring 1 to 3 weeks before with a period of absence of cough (because the level of obstruction is in a lobar or segmental bronchus) and then sudden recurrence of coughing. This period of absence can last for hours, days, or even months. The cough may reappear when irritation of the foreign body or reaction to the foreign body occurs.

Occupation. An occupational and hobby review is warranted. Asbestos or coal dust exposure increases a person's risk of lung disease, including lung cancer. Aerosol sprays, insecticides, chemical exposures, and sawdust can cause cough.

Occurrence of cough. Coughs that awaken persons at night are frequently associated with respiratory problems in which bronchial irritation is a factor, such as in asthma, chronic bronchitis, or nonrespiratory conditions such as GERD or heart failure. A hallmark of asthma is coughing at night, usually between midnight and 2:00 a.m. This is because of the low level of glucocorisol in the body at this time. A severe cough in the early morning indicates postnasal drip, cystic fibrosis, or bronchiectasis. Secretions accumulate through the night and fits of coughing are followed by bronchorrhea. Cough that is worse at night indicates croup, postnasal drip, lower respiratory infection, and allergic reaction. A cough that disappears with sleep is a habit cough.

What does the nature of the sputum tell me?

Key Questions

- Do you cough up sputum or phlegm?
- Does it have an odor?
- How much?
- What color is the material?

Malodorous sputum suggests anaerobic infection of the lungs. Very thick, tenacious, dark sputum is characteristic of bronchiectasis. Cloudy thick sputum suggests lower respiratory tract infection but may also reflect increase in eosinophils from an asthmatic process. Viral bronchitis rarely causes more than 2 tablespoons of mucopurulent sputum per day. Bacterial bronchitis, however, is frequently associated with purulent sputum, often more than 2 tablespoons per day. Clear, mucoid sputum indicates allergic disorder. Hemoptysis, uncommon in children, usually indicates a more serious disease, such as bacterial pneumonia, an acute inflammatory bronchitis, cystic fibrosis, or a foreign body.

Children tend to swallow rather than expectorate sputum. Occasionally emesis will have mucus in it and can be used to identify the sputum. A child with a persistent cough and purulent sputum is likely to have an infectious lung disease.

Cough associated with bloody sputum (hemoptysis) must be investigated for pneumonia versus cancer.

What does the nature of the cough tell me?

Key Question

- What does the cough sound like?

A throat-clearing cough is indicative of postnasal drip caused by irritation of the cough receptors in the pharynx, which are sensitive to mechanical stimulation such as secretions. A dry, brassy cough indicates pharyngeal or tracheal irritation, allergy, or habit. A loose or moist cough may indicate lung disease such as cystic fibrosis or asthma.

A paroxysmal cough is seen with asthma, pertussis, and cystic fibrosis and occasionally following inhalation of a foreign body. A barking, croupy cough indicates an irritation in the glottic and subglottic area. A sudden short burst of a cough in infants, called a staccato cough, is indicative of *Chlamydia trachomatis*. A harsh, dry cough caused by airway compression from enlarged nodes in the perihilar or paratracheal region seems to occur with TB or fungal infection.

A loud, bizarre cough that seems to be attention seeking may have a psychogenic origin. The cough usually is vibrating, throaty, and dry. The severity can range from occasional clearing of the throat to spells lasting several minutes. The cough usually follows a respiratory infection. The cough disappears with sleep or when the child is distracted. School absences are common.

Is the cough related to any event that would help me narrow down the cause?

Key Questions

- Does eating affect your cough?
- Does your cough get worse during certain times of the year?
- Does exercise affect your cough?

Eating. Inhalation into the tracheobronchial tree may occur as a result of lack of esophageal motility, gastroesophageal reflux with regurgitation into the pharynx, as well as CNS and neuromuscular disorders. Difficulty with sucking and swallowing or coughing and choking during eating are highly suggestive of an underlying disorder such as congenital malformations, congenital heart disease (CHD), or pneumonia.

In the adult, gastroesophageal reflux probably causes cough by direct stimulation of cough receptors with acid or by inflammation from aspiration of stomach contents into the airway.

Season. Chronic cough during winter months suggests viral infections. Exacerbation of cough during spring, summer, and fall is suggestive of allergic disease with increased pollen counts. Croup occurs most commonly in the fall from the parainfluenza virus type I. Smaller peaks of croup are seen with influenza B outbreaks in the winter months. Respiratory syncytial virus (RSV) is common in infants during the winter months. In the warmer months parainfluenza type 3 is the agent frequently isolated.

Exercise. The hyperpnea of exercise causes bronchospasm because of heat loss from the airway surface and is more pronounced in cold dry air. Asthma attacks are frequently exercise related, as is cough resulting from heart disease or airway compression.

Are there any associations of the cough with other symptoms?

Key Questions
- Do you have nasal congestion? Sore throat?
- Do you have or have you had a fever? Chills?
- Do you have a headache?

Nasal congestion. Nasal congestion occurs as a result of a cascade of events. First the offending organism invades the epithelial cells of the upper respiratory tract. Inflammatory mediators are released, resulting in altered vascular permeability, edema, and nasal stuffiness. Stimulation of cholinergic nerves in the nose and upper respiratory tract leads to increased mucus production (rhinorrhea) and occasionally to bronchoconstriction, which causes cough. It is hypothesized that cellular damage to the nasopharynx is probably what causes the sore and scratchy throat.

Runny nose with cough and mild fever for a few days, then persistent cough alone for over 1 week with some clear to thick off-white mucus greater in the morning suggests bronchitis.

Nasal congestion or a sensation of postnasal discharge, especially associated with facial pain or pressure, suggests sinusitis. A history of bloody nasal discharge may also be present.

Infants with nasal congestion 3 days to 8 weeks after birth with cough, but afebrile, may have *Chlamydia trachomatis,* contracted from the mother during childbirth. Older children and adolescents and adults who have a sore throat, fever, headache, and malaise progressing to a cough may have mycoplasmic pneumonia.

Fever. In adults, normal temperature or fever of $<38.3°$ C ($101°$ F), small amounts of clear to yellow sputum production, nasal congestion, sore throat, and generalized malaise most frequently accompanies acute cough caused by viral etiology. Acute coughs of a more serious nature (i.e., bacterial pneumonia) are usually accompanied by fever $>38.3°$ C ($>101°$ F), chest pain, shortness of breath, and purulent or dark sputum. Acute cough resulting from non-infectious processes (heart failure or pulmonary embolism) lack the signs of infectious disease such as fever, chills, and purulent sputum.

Headache. Headache pain may signal sinusitis causing the cough (see Chapter 2, Nasal Symptoms and Sinus Congestion).

Is this something that is going around?
Key Questions
- Anyone else at home ill?
- Anyone else ill in day care, school, workplace?

Exposure to respiratory viruses is very common in day care, school, and the workplace. Viruses that cause the common cold are shed in nasal secretions. Contacts acquire the virus by being sneezed on or by touching a sneezed on object, then touching their own nose or conjunctivae. Incubation period is 2 to 5 days. Mycoplasmic pneumonia tends to spread through school/households slowly as the incubation period is 21 days.

Is there anything that would lead me to suspect allergies or reactive airway disease?

Key Questions
- Does anyone in your family have allergies or asthma?
- Is there anything you do or take which stops the cough?
- Do you have pets?

Family history. Allergy-prone individuals are at increased risk for coughs associated with postnasal drip and asthma. Allergy-prone adults and children are those persons with personal or family history of atopic dermatitis, asthma, and allergic rhinitis. Pets residing in the household are frequently the source of the allergen, especially cats and dogs.

Environmental exposure. Frequently persons notice that the cough occurs following exposure to certain environmental irritants, such as smoke, pollen, dust, or animals. The cough may resolve spontaneously with withdrawal from these irritants. Ingestion of antihistamines or inhalation of bronchodilators may relieve a cough associated with allergies or asthma.

Does the patient have any risk factors for systemic disease that may present with cough?

Key Questions
- Do you have any chronic health problems? HIV, heart disease? High blood pressure?
- Are you receiving treatment for cancer?
- Have you ever been exposed to tuberculosis?

Chronic health problems. Chronic lung and heart disease may present with cough, indicating an exacerbation and/or complication of the disease. In addition, information about chronic health prob-

lems may indicate which medications patients take, placing them at risk for cough. ACE inhibitors may be given to treat hypertension or heart failure. Consider exacerbation of heart failure or consider an ACE inhibitor-induced dry, hacking cough, which can be eliminated by stopping the medication. In addition, a medication history may reveal use of drugs that treat or cause immunocompromise.

Immunocompromise. Cancer therapy, HIV, and administration of steroids should raise suspicion of immunocompromise. Adults and children who are immunocompromised are at high risk for infectious lung problems.

Tuberculosis. Inquiry should be made about potential exposure to tuberculosis. Family history of TB, incarceration, and inner city habitation put persons at risk for tuberculosis.

DIAGNOSTIC REASONING: FOCUSED PHYSICAL EXAMINATION

Note General Appearance

In those situations in which the patient appears in acute distress with manifestations of oxygen deprivation, dehydration, and fever, think first of bacterial pneumonia. If a patient has significant oxygen deprivation, but it is not accompanied by fever, consider foreign body aspiration, acute heart failure, or pulmonary embolism. The setting in which the patient is encountered will influence your response to the situation of acute distress. In most instances, oxygen is started immediately, and, if obstruction by a foreign body is strongly suspected, emergency personnel should be summoned for removal if you are unable to accomplish this. Emergency chest x-rays may be needed to look for pulmonary infiltrates, and pulse oximetry may be ordered to assess oxygen saturation status. Adults and children in acute respiratory distress require specialized care by health care professionals, and their assistance should be requested immediately. Persons presenting with viral respiratory infections or chronic cough from postnasal drainage, GERD, and chronic bronchitis appear less acutely ill. They are able to participate in the interview process without difficulty. Those whose cough is caused by bronchospasm may present in varying degrees of distress.

Assess Mental Status

Diminished level of consciousness, confusion, and restlessness are likely manifestations of hypoxia in the patient experiencing respiratory problems. Frequently the patient with a pulmonary embolus expresses a sense of impending doom.

Restlessness and agitation in the child may indicate hypoxemia. A lethargic and somnolent child may have CO_2 retention.

Take Vital Signs

An elevated pulse and temperature may signal bacterial or viral infection.

Respiratory rate is the best indicator of pulmonary function in young infants. The respiratory rate and tidal volume work together to produce adequate alveolar ventilation. For any given level of alveolar ventilation, there is an optimum respiratory rate at which the muscular work of breathing is at a minimum. Airway resistance increases at higher flow rates. In children with decreased compliance (pneumonia, pulmonary edema), respirations are very rapid and shallow. Children with increased airway resistance (asthma) have respirations that are relatively slow and deep to minimize the high-resistance work. The most reliable and reproducible respiratory rate is the sleeping respiratory rate.

Examine the Head and Neck

Erythema of upper respiratory mucous membranes, accompanied by enlarged anterior cervical nodes, is a common finding in an upper respiratory infection.

Observe the neck for jugular venous distention. This may be a sign of heart failure.

The ororespiratory reflex is mediated by Arnold's nerve, the auricular branch of CN X, and is a rare cause of chronic cough. Careful examination of the ears with removal of cerumen and any hairs in contact with the tympanic membrane or the opposite wall of the external auditory canal should be done.

A cobblestoning of the posterior pharynx is caused by lymphoid hyperplasia secondary to chronic stimulation by postnasal drip.

Inspect the Chest for Shape, Symmetry, and Use of Accessory Muscles

To inspect the chest, place the patient in the sitting position or side-lying position. Note if the patient has to lean forward or sit up to breathe comfortably. Some respiratory abnormalities are unilateral or localized, such as pulmonary embolus. Compare findings on one side of the body with those on the other. Also compare front to back.

Upper airway obstruction causes suprasternal and supraclavicular retractions. Intercostal retractions and subcostal retractions occur with lower airway obstructive disease. Severe obstruction of either upper or lower airways causes retractions of all the accessory muscles. Retractions occur when increase in the work of breathing requires an increase in the negative pressure within the chest. Remember that the pediatric airway is much smaller in diameter than the adult, and, because resistance to flow is related inversely to the fourth power of the radius, decreased diameter of this airway causes enormous increases in resistance. The chest wall is pliable and the softest parts of the thorax are pulled inward on inspiration, giving rise to retractions of the intracostal, suprasternal, and infrasternal spaces. The degree of retraction is proportional to the negative pressure generated within the thorax and, therefore, correlates with the severity of the problem.

Normally the anteroposterior (AP) diameter is approximately one-third to one-half the lateral diameter. In children up to 6 months of age, the head circumference is larger than the chest circumference. After 6 months of age, chest circumference is larger than head circumference. A ratio of the AP diameter to the lateral diameter of the chest of greater than 1 is a sign of increased AP diameter. If the AP diameter is equal to the lateral diameter, the condition known as barrel chest is evident and indicates probable COPD. Children with chronic cough because of cystic fibrosis or severe asthma may have an increase in this diameter. Other musculoskeletal chest abnormalities to note include pectus excavatum, pectus carinatum, severe scoliosis, and kyphoscoliosis. These conditions can contribute to chest infection and respiratory failure because of decreased lung expansion.

Observe Respirations

Next, observe the rate, rhythm, and depth of the patient's breathing. The normal respiratory rate in adults is 12 to 20 breaths per minute; in the elderly, it is 16 to 25. Children less than 12 years may have respiratory rates up to 30 to 40. Exhaling should take about twice as long as inhaling, but in COPD patients it may take up to four times longer. Rhythm should be even, with occasional sighs. Note any abnormal breathing patterns (see Dyspnea, Box 4-1, p. 115).

Listen to the Respirations and Cough

Note any stridor in the child. Stridor in the first 3 years of life is generally considered to be an emergency. Inspiratory stridor usually indicates an extrathoracic lesion. Low-pitched stridor, especially if accompanied by salivation or snoring, indicates inflammation in the supraglottic area. Stridor associated with wheezing occurs with intrathoracic or extrathoracic lesions, such as tracheal inflammation, where it is both inspiratory and expiratory. Stridor during expiration is usually the result of lower respiratory tract obstruction.

Grunting is a sign of respiratory distress caused by exhaling against a partially closed glottis. It can also be a sign of interstitial and alveolar diseases, such as pneumonia or pulmonary edema, and usually indicates severe distress.

The nature of the cough may be indicative of the underlying pathology.

Palpate the Chest

Using the palmar surface of the hands, palpate the entire chest for tenderness, depressions, bulges, and crepitus (presence of air in the subcutaneous tissues). Crepitus may indicate a chest injury, pneumothorax, and emphysema.

To assess the strength of chest wall movement and further check for symmetry, position the palms of the hands on the patient's back in the area between the 8th and 10th ribs. As the patient takes a deep breath, each hand should move the same distance—about 3 to 5 cm—outwards from the spine. With COPD, less movement will be seen. Pneumonia and partial paralysis of the diaphragm will result in a reduction in expansion of one side of the chest wall.

Assess for vocal fremitus (the vibrations transmitted to the chest wall during speech) by placing the ball of the hand lightly on the chest and asking the patient to repeat the words "ninety-nine." Evaluate the intensity of the vibration over all lung fields, comparing side to side. Dense tissue conducts sound better than air does; thus, conditions such as pneumonia, heart failure, and tumors may increase intensity. Fremitus is diminished in pneumothorax, asthma, and emphysema, which are conditions that trap air in the lung.

Percuss the Chest

Sounds produced by percussion indicate density of lung tissue. Percussing the back is more useful than anterior chest percussion because the heart and breast interfere with percussion. Percuss systematically at 3- to 5-cm intervals, starting just above the scapulae and moving downward from side to side. Note any differences in volume and pitch. Resonance is a long, low-pitched sound that can normally be heard over most lung fields. Hyperresonance is an abnormally long, low sound that may signal emphysema or pneumothorax. Dullness or flatness may be heard with pleural effusion, pneumonia, or large tumors.

Auscultate Breath Sounds

Instruct the patient to breathe through the mouth slowly and deeply. Auscultate systematically from the lung apexes to the lower lobes anteriorly, posteriorly, and laterally. Determine the presence, type, and location of both normal and abnormal sounds. Normal lung sounds include bronchial breath sounds heard on the chest over the sternum and in the back between the scapulae, bronchovesicular breath sounds heard over the bronchi at the first and second intercostal spaces anteriorly and between the scapulae posteriorly, and vesicular breath sounds heard over most of the peripheral lung fields. Determine the presence, type, and location of both normal and abnormal breath sounds (see Dyspnea, pp. 117 and 118).

Auscultate Heart Sounds

Note the location of normal and abnormal heart sounds, the location of their greatest intensity, and the heart rate and rhythm. In heart failure, S1 and S2 may equal rapid pulse rate or may indicate a pulse deficit. An S3 (ventricular gallop) is an early sign of heart failure and is heard best at the apex of the heart. S4 (atrial gallop) typically indicates a stressed heart and is also pathonomic of heart failure in children. In adults, it may be the result of hyperten-

sion, myocardial infarction, or coronary artery disease causing heart failure. A summation gallop may also occur with heart failure. This is the result of S3, S4, and rapid rate.

Also note any murmurs, their location, grade, and radiation. Incompetent heart valves may be the cause of heart failure.

In COPD, lung hyperinflation may muffle heart sounds. Poor tissue oxygenation or fever may result in tachycardia.

Auscultate Blood Pressure

In heart failure, decreased stroke volume reduces the systolic blood pressure. Compensatory vasoconstriction maintains a constant diastolic pressure, and, thus, along with the decreased systolic pressure, you may note decreased pulse pressure.

Examine the Skin and Extremities

Note the presence of cyanosis of the oral cavity (central cyanosis). It is associated with low arterial saturation and may result from inadequate gas exchange in the lungs or from cardiac shunting. Mucous membranes in dark-skinned patients may appear gray with central cyanosis. This may also be seen in persons with COPD. Bluish color of the extremities (peripheral cyanosis) may be observed in Caucasian persons and is associated with low venous saturation, resulting in vasoconstriction, vascular occlusion, or reduced cardiac output.

Clubbing is a loss of the angle between the skin and nail bed. This is a manifestation of chronic tissue hypoxia, which occurs with chronic lung disease. Edema of the lower extremities may be a sign of increased right-heart filling pressure, caused by primary lung disease or left heart failure.

Palpate Peripheral Pulses

Palpate peripheral pulses for rate and quality. Tachycardia may occur with oxygen deprivation caused by pulmonary embolism, pneumonia, fever, or heart failure. Irregular pulse may signal heart failure resulting from atrial fibrillation and/or heart block. Diminished peripheral pulses indicate possible atherosclerotic vessel disease or decreased cardiac output as occurs with heart failure.

Examine the Abdomen

Epigastric tenderness to palpation may be elicited in the patient with GERD, or the abdominal examination may be entirely normal. In addition, if heart failure is the cause of cough, ascites or hepatojugular reflex may be present. To test for hepatojugular reflex, position the patient so that the jugular pulsation is evident in the midneck. Exert firm and sustained pressure with the hand over the patient's right upper quadrant for 30 to 60 seconds. An increase in the jugular venous pressure during this maneuver of more than 1 cm is abnormal.

LABORATORY AND DIAGNOSTIC STUDIES

Some authorities suggest all patients with a cough lasting longer than 3 weeks should have a chest x-ray. If the x-ray is abnormal and consistent with infectious or noninfectious inflammatory disease or malignancy, the provider should proceed to expectorated sputum studies, CT scan of the lungs, or bronchoscopy. If history, physical examination, and x-ray suggest heart failure, an ECG, echocardiogram, or both may be indicated (see Chest Pain, pp. 95 and 96).

If the patient's history and physical examination strongly suggest a specific etiology (i.e., postnasal drip, asthma, GERD), proceed to those studies initially. Keep in mind that there may be more than one cause for the cough. For those patients whose history and physical examination suggest postnasal drip syndrome, sinus x-ray or CT scan of the sinuses may be indicated. Also consider allergy testing for those individuals whose history indicates allergens may precipitate the syndrome.

In those situations where investigation of signs and symptoms leads to probable asthma or, if no likely cause is identified, a spirometry test (see Dyspnea, p. 119) should be performed. If the test is normal, but asthma is still suspected, a methacholine challenge test may be done. This test is performed in the laboratory and involves administering methacholine chloride by nebulizer and then repeating the spirometry test. If the patient's cough is likely related to reactive airway disease, the patient would exhibit a 20% decrease in FEV1.

Complete Blood Count (CBC)

A CBC may provide evidence of acute infection with an elevated white count. Eosinophilia indicates atopy.

Esophageal Probe

GERD is best diagnosed with 24-hour esophageal pH probe monitoring. A barium swallow is less sensitive, and a gastroscopy will verify ulcerative disease but not mild reflux.

Sputum Culture

Sputum culture is important for the diagnosis of a specific infectious agent in the pulmonary system. A sputum specimen must come from deep within the bronchi. Coughing usually enables the patient to produce a satisfactory specimen. Examination includes macroscopic appearance, cellular composition, and bacterial count.

Sweat Test

A sweat test is used to determine the presence of cystic fibrosis.

Tuberculin Skin Testing

The Mantoux test is used to detect tuberculosis. Mantoux test results should always be read by a health professional. A Mantoux test result is considered positive at three different levels (≥ 5, ≥ 10, and ≥ 15 mm) of induration (diameter transverse to the long axis of the arm measured and recorded), depending on the individual's degree of risk for tuberculosis. In adults, a <5-mm diameter is considered negative, a 5- to 9-mm diameter is considered a weak positive, a 10- to 14-mm diameter is considered an intermediate positive, and a ≥ 15-mm diameter with or without vesiculation is considered a strong positive. In a child who has no known risk for TB, only a large reaction (≥ 15 mm) is considered to be positive. If a child is very young (under 4 years of age), has other medical risk factors, or has some environmental exposure to TB, then an intermediate reaction (≥ 10 mm) is considered to be positive. If a child is at high risk (e.g., a child who lives in a household with someone who has TB), then a small reaction (≥ 5 mm) is considered to be positive.

DIFFERENTIAL DIAGNOSIS

EMERGENT RECENT ONSET COUGH

Pulmonary Embolus

Approximately 50% of persons with PE complain of cough, which may be the predominant clinical manifestation. When patients present with acute cough in association with risk factors for thromboembolic disease, keep PE in mind as a differential diagnosis. The history reveals cough with possible hemoptysis, dyspnea, chest pain, history of DVT, recent immobilization, use of oral contraceptives, or hypercoagulability states. The patient with pulmonary embolism is usually extremely restless and expresses a sense of impeding doom. Fever, tachycardia, tachypnea, diminished breath sounds, crackles, wheezes, and pleural friction rub may be present on physical examination.

Chest x-ray, arterial blood gases, coagulation studies, and ECG may be completed along with referral for ventilation/perfusion scans.

Heart Failure

Persons reporting history of heart disease, orthopnea, PND, peripheral edema, weight gain, frothy sputum, fatigue, and palpitations must be further assessed for acute heart failure. Infants with a large left-to-right shunt and subsequent congestive heart failure may present with a persistent, nonproductive cough as well as a history of failure to thrive and poor feeding. Parents may also report the child sweats on the forehead or lip, especially while feeding. Physical examination findings frequently include altered level of consciousness, anxiety, jugular venous distention, tachypnea, rales, rhonchi, tachycardia, displaced PMI, S3, S4, and possible ascites. An ECG and chest x-ray usually reveal increased heart size and pulmonary edema. Children also have examination cyanosis, tachypnea, and hepatomegaly with a murmur. Arterial O_2 may be decreased, and ejection fractions are significantly reduced on echocardiogram.

Bacterial Tracheitis (Laryngotracheobronchitis)

Bacterial tracheitis represents a secondary bacterial infection of viral laryngotracheitis, generally with coagulase-positive staphylococci. It most commonly occurs during the fall and winter and in children less than 2 years old. The onset can be sudden and present with severe respiratory distress. More commonly, the onset is over a period of 1 to 5 days with mild upper respiratory symptoms and prominent cough, stridor, and hoarseness. The patient develops a high fever, a toxic appearance, and a significant increase in respiratory rate. Leukocytosis is present, but blood cultures are negative.

Foreign Body

History may suggest a possible environmental hazard that was aspirated. Foreign body may be present if there is a sudden onset of coughing with acute respiratory distress or subsequent coughing, wheezing, or stridor. Physical examination should be directed to where the foreign body has lodged. The most frequent finding is wheezing, decreased air movement, and rhonchi over the lung having the involved airway. Chest film of inspiration and expiration shows persistent air trapping on expiration.

Asthma

Acute bronchoconstriction in a patient with asthma can develop as a result of respiratory infection, exposure to allergens, inhalation of fumes, airway irritants, and environmental factors. Predominant symptoms include wheezing, coughing, and breathlessness. Physical signs include anxiety, tachypnea, use of accessory muscles to breathe, intercostal retractions, decreased breath sounds, and inspiratory and possibly expiratory wheezes. Absence of wheezing in a child with asthma may indicate severe airway obstruction with poor air exchange. Laboratory studies should include spirometry, pulse oximetry, and chest x-ray.

NON-EMERGENT RECENT ONSET COUGH

Pneumonia

Pneumonia is usually associated with dyspnea, pleuritic chest pain, cough with greenish or rusty-colored sputum, fever, and chills. Infants and young children will not produce sputum. Anorexia, malaise, and posttussive vomiting is seen. Objective manifestations of pneumonia include fever, tachycardia and tachypnea, inspiratory crackles, asynchronous breathing and vocal fremitus, dull percussion sound over area of consolidation, and bron-chophony. Pneumonia can be confirmed by chest x-ray, CBC, and sputum and nasal cultures.

Fever is frequently absent in the elderly with pneumonia, and thus a new onset of cough, especially when accompanied by either tachypnea or altered mental status, should suggest pneumonia.

The majority of pediatric pulmonary infections are viral and usually caused by respiratory syncytial virus, parainfluenza viruses, or influenza viruses. In the infant and young child, acute nonbacterial pneumonia presents after a 1- to 2-day history of coryza, decreased appetite, and low-grade fever. Increasing fretfulness, respiratory congestion, vomiting, cough, and fever may occur. Objective manifestations include tachypnea, tachycardia, nasal flaring, and retractions.

Viral Upper Respiratory Infection

The cough associated with viral upper respiratory conditions is often associated with low-grade fever, nasal congestion, mild sore throat, and small amounts of clear to yellow sputum production. Physical examination findings include mild nasopharyngeal erythema, enlarged cervical lymph nodes, clear lung sounds, and normal heart sounds. No diagnostic tests are required at this point. The patient is advised to return if the cough persists for more than 3 weeks or symptoms such as fever >38.3° C (101° F), chest pain, or shortness of breath develops.

Nasopharyngitis

The common cold is a self-limiting viral infection of the upper respiratory tract that is generally caused by a rhinovirus. The virus invades the mucous membranes of the upper respiratory tract and causes swelling and hypersecretion of mucus. Fever is low grade, and rhinorrhea is clear, thin, and watery. Hypersecretion of mucus causes coughing, especially at night when secretions pool in the nasopharyngeal cavity. Physical examination findings may include red and swollen nasal mucosa with clear secretions present and mild pharyngeal erythema. Other physical examination findings are negative.

Chlamydial Pneumonia

Chlamydial pneumonia is a pulmonary disease caused by *C. trachomatis* transmitted during delivery. It is one of the most common causes of interstitial pneumonitis and presents between the first 3 to 11 weeks of age with tachypnea and a characteristic staccato cough in an afebrile child. Mucoid rhinorrhea may have been present 1 to 2 weeks before the onset of cough. Fine rales, usually without wheezes, are heard on auscultation. Chest x-ray shows hyperinflated lungs with diffuse interstitial or alveolar infiltrates.

Bronchiolitis

Respiratory syncytial virus is mainly responsible for bronchiolitis. It usually presents in children less than 2 years old with 1 to 2 days of fever, rhinorrhea, and cough, followed by wheezing, tachypnea, tachycardia, and respiratory distress. Nasal flaring and retractions with accessory muscle use is seen along with shallow, rapid respirations. Cough increases as inflammation increases. The infant appears lethargic and has circumoral cyanosis. Wheezes are predominant, with a long expiratory phase. Crackles and rhonchi may also be heard diffusely throughout the lung fields. The chest x-ray shows hyperinflation with mild interstitial infiltrates. Viral isolates from nasal washings are used for diagnosis.

Acute Bronchitis

Inflammation of the large airways causes bronchitis that begins with a dry, nonproductive cough usually seen in winter. Continued cough and nasal congestion produces a productive cough and fever. Chest pain may accompany the cough. Lung auscultation reveals diffuse rhonchi on expiration. White blood cell count is normal or mildly elevated.

Croup (Acute Laryngotracheobronchitis)

Inflammation or edema of the subglottic area causes obstruction of the airways of the larynx, trachea, or bronchi. Parainfluenza virus causes most inflammation. Generally the onset occurs after a few days of an upper respiratory infection. Hoarseness, inspiratory stridor, and a characteristic barking cough is heard, which is usually worse at night. A low-grade fever may be present. Inspiratory stridor, suprasternal and intercostal retractions, and an increased respiratory rate is seen. Lateral neck x-ray in croup shows a normal epiglottis, subglottic narrowing, and ballooning of the hypopharynx. The posteroanterior neck view shows a steeple sign (narrowing of the air column at the top).

CHRONIC COUGH

Postnasal Drainage Syndrome

Postnasal discharge syndrome has been identified as the most common cause of chronic cough. It is suggested that the cough results from stimulation of the afferent limb of the cough reflex in the upper respiratory tract. Causes of postnasal drip include allergic, perennial nonallergic, postinfectious, environmental irritant; vasomotor rhinitis; or sinusitis. Both children and adults report dry cough, throat clearing, sensation of something in the back of the throat, and nasal congestion. Physical examination may reveal mucus in the posterior pharynx or a cobblestone appearance of the posterior pharynx. Sinus x-rays, CT scan of the sinuses, and allergy testing may be indicated if this syndrome is suspected to be the cause of cough.

Asthma

Asthma is the most common cause of chronic cough in children. It initially produces a dry cough, commonly worse at night, characteristically exercise-related, and often triggered by respiratory infections. Physical examination findings depend on the severity of the disease. Prolonged expiratory phase of respiration may be heard. Lungs may have crackles that clear with coughing, and overt or latent wheeze may be produced with forced expiration. Use of neck muscles to facilitate inspiration (called tracheal tugging or chin lag) may be seen. Chest film may show hyperinflation during acute attacks. Pulmonary function testing with and without aerosolized sympathomimetic bronchodilator is positive.

Gastroesophageal Reflux Disease (GERD)

GERD should be considered when patients report heartburn, a sour taste in the mouth, or history of esophagitis. Often persons with GERD are cigarette smokers, overuse alcohol, and are overweight. Microaspiration into the airways or reflux of acid into the esophagus occurs. Young infants may also experience reflux with their cough, usually worsening after feeding, which may be the only symptom. A recurrent, effortless vomiting with failure to gain weight and irritability may also occur. The physical examination of persons with GERD is most often normal. The diagnostic test of most significance is esophageal pH monitoring. Values outside the normal physiological range indicate reflux.

Chronic Bronchitis

Chronic bronchitis should be considered when the patient expectorates sputum on most days during a period spanning at least 3 consecutive months, and such periods have occurred for more than 2 successive years. In addition, exposure to smoke, irritating dust, or fumes is highly likely.

Cigarette smoking as well as fumes and dust stimulate the afferent limb of the cough reflex as irritants, inducing inflammatory changes in the mucosa of the respiratory tract, causing hypersecretion of mucus and slowing of mucociliary clearance. Persons with chronic bronchitis exhibit a rasping, hacking cough, possible rhonchi that clear with coughing, resonant to dull chest, possible barrel chest, prolonged expiration, and possible wheezing. Chest x-ray and pulmonary function tests are indicated.

Angiotensin-Converting Enzyme Inhibitor (ACEI)-Induced Cough

This cough occurs hours to months after beginning an ACEI. Persons report a nonproductive cough associated with an irritating, tickling, or scratching sensation in the throat. Physical examination is normal. The cough resolves within days to weeks after the drug is discontinued.

Bronchogenic Carcinoma

Hemoptysis reported by a cigarette smoker, accompanied by weight loss and/or shortness of breath, are frequent health concerns reported by the patient with bronchogenic cancer. Physical findings may include enlarged supraclavicular nodes, dull chest percussion over the tumor, and increased breath sounds distal to the tumor. Hemoptysis should be evaluated with a chest x-ray and a CT scan if indicated.

Cystic Fibrosis

A chronic cough is associated with cystic fibrosis. The cough is productive, and the child has signs of failure to thrive with poor weight gain. The child may have a family history of the disease. The cough is initially dry and hacking but eventually becomes loose and productive of purulent material. Physical examination often shows an increased anteroposterior diameter of the chest. Scattered or localized coarse rales and rhonchi are audible. Digital clubbing is often present. Sweat chloride test is positive.

Pertussis

Pertussis begins with mild upper respiratory tract symptoms associated with coryza and a cough, progressing to severe paroxysms of coughing. Fever is usually absent or minimal. The cough is paroxysmal and frightening to parents. Immunization history is helpful, yet the immunity provided by the pertussis vaccine in children with complete dosing may diminish over time. Vomiting and cyanosis with or without an inspiratory "whoop" may be present. Physical examination may be within normal limits. Nasopharyngeal secretions for *B. pertussis* may confirm the diagnosis.

Foreign Body in Ear Canal

Dry cough with no significant history may be indicative of a foreign body in the ear. Physical examination is negative except for cerumen in ears or hairs that are in contact with the TM or opposite wall of the external auditory canal, thus stimulating the auricular branch of the vagus nerve (Arnold's nerve).

Foreign Body Aspiration

Foreign body aspiration occurs most frequently in children and the elderly. A child or adult who aspirates a foreign body can have a varied presentation. Generally the onset of cough is sudden and unexpected. A brief period of severe coughing, gagging, and choking occurs. If the foreign body does not completely obstruct the airway, an asymptomatic period ensues. This period can last for hours, days, or even months. A foreign body in the lower airway can present with emphysema because of the ball-valve phenomenon or can occur as a complete distal atelectasis created by ab-

sorption of the trapped gas. A mobile foreign body in the lower airway can also produce a paroxysmal cough, with cyanotic episodes and stridor because of proximal migration and subglottic impaction. A foreign body in the esophagus can also produce airway obstruction and cough as well as dysphasia for solid foods because the posterior trachea is compliant and opposed to the anterior esophagus. Coins are the most frequent culprit.

Allergy

Upper airway allergy and vasomotor rhinitis can cause a reflex cough secondary to postnasal drip and irritation of the cough receptors. Such a cough is generally seasonal in nature, with a history of sneezing. Allergic shiners, allergic salute, and eczema may be present. Rhinorrhea with clear watery drainage is seen. Skin testing for allergies is positive.

Chronic Sinusitis

Chronic sinusitis produces a recurrent, fairly loose cough that is especially worse at night because of trickling of infected mucus from the nasopharynx down the posterior pharyngeal wall. History of symptoms is similar to cold-like symptoms that become persistent or recurrent. Noisy breathing and snoring with sleep may also be present. Physical examination reveals mucopurulent secretion in the posterior throat. Purulent rhinorrhea may be present. Sinus tenderness is less frequently present than in acute sinusitis. An x-ray using the Waters view of the head is positive.

Mycoplasmic Pneumonia

Mycoplasmic pneumonia is the most common cause of infection of the lower respiratory tract in the school-age group. There is a slow onset of symptoms with fever (39° C or 102.2° F), a cough that is usually dry at the onset, headache, malaise, and sore throat. The child does not look particularly ill, but on auscultation rales and rhonchi are frequently present. A chest x-ray may show interstitial or broncho-pneumonic infiltrates in the middle or lower lobes. WBC is usually normal, and cold hemagglutinin titer may be elevated during the acute presentation. A titer of 1:64 or higher supports the diagnosis.

Tuberculosis

Brassy cough is the most common symptom of tuberculosis but is often ascribed to smoking, a recent cold, or a bout of influenza several weeks before. At first, it is minimally productive of yellow or green mucus, usually on arising in the morning. As the disease progresses, the cough becomes more productive. In adults, a multi-nodular infiltrate above or behind the clavicle (the most characteristic location) suggests reoccurrence of an old TB infection. In younger persons in whom recent infection is more common, infiltration may be found in any part of the lung, and unilateral pleural effusion is often seen. In sputum examination, the finding of acid-fast bacilli (AFB) in a sputum smear is strong presumptive evidence of TB, but a definitive diagnosis is made only on results of a culture.

Smoking

Smoking is on the rise in female adolescents, and many smoke in closed rooms, increasing their respiratory irritation. History of a mildly productive hacking cough may be indicative of smoking. Infants exposed to passive cigarette smoke inhalation have increased bronchial reactivity. Physical examination may reveal yellow stains on the fingers, teeth, or tongue. Mild chronic conjunctivitis may also be present. Chest x-ray may be positive with interstitial markings.

Psychogenic Origin

School-age children or adolescents with a history of a loud, brassy, disturbing cough that is non-productive and explosive may indicate a psychogenic etiology. The child usually has missed many school days. The cough is not heard while sleeping, and the child is afebrile with no weight loss. The physical examination is negative.

Table 4-7

Differential Diagnosis of Common Causes of Recent Onset of Cough

Condition	History	Physical Findings	Diagnostic Studies
Emergent Causes			
Pulmonary embolus	Acute onset, cough, dyspnea, mild to severe chest pain, hemoptysis, history of DVT, recent surgery, oral contraceptive, hypercoagulability states	Restlessness, fever, tachycardia, tachypnea, diminished breath sounds, crackles, wheezing, pleural friction rub, sense of impending doom	ABGs, PT/APTT, chest x-ray, ECG, ventilation/perfusion scans

Continued

Table 4-7

Differential Diagnosis of Common Causes of Recent Onset of Cough—cont'd

Condition	History	Physical Findings	Diagnostic Studies
Heart failure	Cough, frothy sputum, fatigue, lightheaded-ness, syncope, weight gain, swelling of ankles, palpita-tions, PND, orthopnea, history of heart disease; also in children is seen failure to thrive, respiratory dis-tress, sweating on forehead or above the lip, especially when feeding	Altered level of consciousness, anxiety, jugular venous disten-tion, tachypnea, use of accessory muscles to breathe, rales, rhonchi/ wheezes, tachy-cardia, de-creased periph-eral pulses, cool extremities, displaced PMI, S3, S4, ascites	ECG, chest x-ray, ABGs, echocar-diogram
Bacterial tracheitis (laryngotra-cheobronchitis)	Child less than 2 years, fall, winter; sudden onset with severe respira-tory distress, appears toxic	High fever, stridor, hoarseness, in-creased respira-tory rate	WBC increases, blood cultures negative
Foreign body	Sudden onset of coughing, respi-ratory distress; environmental hazards present	Asymmetrical phys-ical findings of decreased breath sounds, localized wheez-ing; complete obstruction apho-nia, cyanosis	Chest x-rays com-paring inspira-tion and expiration, asymmetrical x-ray with forced expira-tory view
Asthma	Paroxysmal cough, audible wheeze, dyspnea, history of asthma or allergies	Anxiety, tachy-pnea, use of accessory muscles to breathe, inter-costal retrac-tions, decreased vocal fremitus, decreased breath sound, inspiratory and possibly expira-tory wheezes	Spirometry, chest x-ray, ABGs

Table 4-7

Differential Diagnosis of Common Causes of Recent Onset of Cough—cont'd

Condition	History	Physical Findings	Diagnostic Studies
Non-Emergent Causes			
Pneumonia*	Noisy cough, dyspnea, pleuritic chest pain, sputum production (yellow, green, red color) chills; in children also seen poor feeding and irritability	Fever, tachycardia, tachypnea, inspiratory crackles, asynchronous breathing, vocal fremitus, percussion dull or flat over area of consolidation, bronchophony, egophony	Chest x-ray, CBC, sputum and nasal cultures, O_2 saturation
Viral URI	Cough, nasal congestion, sore throat, fever, chills, myalgias	Fever, pharyngitis, enlarged anterior cervical nodes, normal TMs, nasal mucosa erythema, normal chest exam	None
Nasopharyngitis	Acute onset, low-grade fever, rhinorrhea, cough especially at night	Nasal mucosa red and swollen, pharynx mildly red; otherwise negative	None
Chlamydial pneumonia	Paroxysmal staccato cough in an infant 4-12 weeks	Afebrile, conjunctivitis in 50% of infants, tachypnea of 40-80/min, crackles, no wheezing	X-ray shows hyperexpansion of lungs with diffuse interstitial infiltrates
Bronchiolitis (RSV)*	Grunting, sneezing, cough, anoxia, exposure to passive smoke	Fever, wheezing on auscultation, prolonged expiratory phase, tachypnea of 60-80/min, tachycardia >200	WBC 5-24,000 with increased PMN; chest x-ray shows hyperinflation; infants less than 2 months refer; progressive respiratory distress refer

Continued

Table 4-7

Differential Diagnosis of Common Causes of Recent Onset of Cough—cont'd

Condition	History	Physical Findings	Diagnostic Studies
Acute bronchitis	Duration <3 months, winter months, URI for 3-4 days, loose hacking, cough that becomes productive, afebrile	Coarse, fine crackles on auscultation; low-grade fever or afebrile	Chest x-ray negative
Croup (acute laryngo-tracheobronchitis)*	History of URI, brassy, barking cough usually at night	Low-grade fever, inspiratory stridor, flaring of nares, prolonged expiratory phase, may see retraction of accessory muscles, breath sounds diminished	None

*Because of the possible rapid change in condition in infants and children, non-emergent causes of cough may become emergent.

Table 4-8

Differential Diagnosis of Common Causes of Chronic Cough

Condition	History	Physical Findings	Diagnostic Studies
Postnasal drainage	Cough, sore throat	Mucoid secretions in the posterior pharynx, cobblestone appearance of posterior pharynx, tenderness to palpation of sinuses, normal chest exam	Sinus x-rays, sinus CT scan, allergy testing

Table 4-8

Differential Diagnosis of Common Causes of Chronic Cough—cont'd

Condition	History	Physical Findings	Diagnostic Studies
Asthma	Dry hacking cough, especially at night, and with feeding and laughter	End-expiratory wheeze, prolonged expiratory phase	Pulmonary function testing
GERD	Cough worse at night, sour taste in mouth, heartburn, history of esophagitis, cigarette smoker, alcohol abuse, overweight; in children, seen at 0-18 months, failure to thrive, dysphagia, cough after eating and lying down, vomiting	Normal chest exam, normal upper respiratory exam, possible epigastric pain with palpation or normal abdominal exam	Esophageal pH monitoring, blood count for anemia, x-ray for aspiration pneumonia
Chronic bronchitis	Cough, mild dyspnea, history of COPD, history of cigarette smoking, yellow sputum	Hacking, rasping cough; normal breath sounds or rhonchi that clear with coughing; resonant to dull chest, possible barrel chest, prolonged expiration, possible wheezing	Chest x-ray, pulmonary function tests
ACEI-induced cough	Begin hours to months after starting ACEI, nonproductive, dry cough, scratching sensation in throat	Normal exam	Trial off ACEI
Bronchogenic carcinoma	Cough with hemoptysis, history cigarette smoking, weight loss, shortness of breath	Enlarged supraclavicular nodes, dull chest percussion over tumor, increased breath sounds distal to tumor	Chest x-ray, CT scan of chest

Continued

Table 4-8

Differential Diagnosis of Common Causes of Chronic Cough—cont'd

Condition	History	Physical Findings	Diagnostic Studies
Cystic fibrosis	Failure to thrive, chronic cough, bulky stools, family history	Nasal polyps, clubbing of fingernails, sputum	Sweat test positive
Pertussis	Persistent hacking cough, may have inspiratory whoop, vomiting	Fever absent, coryza	Nasopharyngeal aspirate positive, chest x-ray to rule out pneumonia
Foreign body in ear canal	Cough	Cerumen in ears, hairs in contact with TM or opposite wall of the external auditory canal	None
Foreign body aspiration	History of environmental hazard, choking episode	Asymmetrical physical findings of decreased breath sounds, wheezing	Asymmetrical x-ray with forced expiratory view
Allergy	History of sneezing, cough	Allergic shiners, allergic salute, rhinorrhea clear and watery	Chest x-ray negative, allergy testing positive
Chronic sinusitis	Rhinorrhea >7-10 days	Mucopurulent rhinorrhea	Waters x-ray
Mycoplasmic pneumonia	School-age child, gradual onset, headache, malaise, sore throat, hacking cough	Reddened pharynx, slightly enlarged lymph nodes, rales often fine and crackling	X-ray shows interstitial pneumonia; cold agglutinins positive, ESR elevated
Tuberculosis	History of exposure, high-risk group, weakness, malaise, weight loss	Brassy cough, weight loss, may have fever, night sweats	Mantoux test, chest x-ray shows abnormalities in apical and hyaline, sputum culture positive for *M. tuberculosis*
Smoking (passive/active)	History of smoking or being around a smoker	Yellow teeth, fingers; odor of smoke, productive sputum	X-ray may be positive with interstitial markings
Psychogenic origin	School age or adolescent, dry hacking cough present only during waking hours	None	As indicated to rule out other causes

Chapter 5

Common Problems of the Abdomen and Gastrointestinal System

≡ Abdominal Pain

Abdominal pain is a subjective feeling of discomfort in the abdomen that can be caused by a variety of problems. The goal of initial clinical assessment is to distinguish acute life-threatening conditions from chronic/recurrent or acute mild, self-limiting ones. Assessment is complicated by the dynamic rather than static nature of acute abdominal pain, which can produce a changing clinical picture, often over a short period of time. Additionally, both children and older adults tend not to follow the usual and anticipated clinical pattern of abdominal pain.

Three processes produce abdominal pain: tension in the GI tract wall from muscle contraction or distention, ischemia, or inflammation of the peritoneum. Pain can also be referred from within or outside the abdomen.

Colic is a type of tension pain. It is associated with forceful peristaltic contractions and is the most characteristic type of pain arising from the viscera. Colicky pain can be produced by an irritant substance, infection with a virus or bacteria, or from the body's attempt to force its luminal contents through an obstruction. Another type of tension pain is caused by acute stretching of the capsule of an organ, such as the liver, spleen, or kidney. The patient with this visceral pain is restless, moves about, and has difficulty getting comfortable.

Ischemia produces an intense, continuous pain. The most common cause of intestinal ischemic pain is strangulation of the bowel from obstruction.

Inflammation of the peritoneum usually begins at the serosa covering the affected and inflamed organ, causing visceral peritonitis. The pain is a poorly

---

Box 5-1

Some Causes of Pain Perceived in Anatomical Regions

Right Upper Quadrant	**Periumbilical**	**Left Upper Quadrant**
Duodenal ulcer	Intestinal obstruction	Ruptured spleen
Hepatitis	Acute pancreatitis	Gastric ulcer
Hepatomegaly	Early appendicitis	Aortic aneurysm
Pneumonia	Mesenteric thrombosis	Perforated colon
Cholecystitis	Aortic aneurysm	Pneumonia
	Diverticulitis	

Right Lower Quadrant	**Left Lower Quadrant**
Appendicitis	Sigmoid diverticulitis
Salpingitis	Salpingitis
Ovarian cyst	Ovarian cyst
Ruptured ectopic pregnancy	Ruptured ectopic pregnancy
Renal/ureteral stone	Renal/ureteral stone
Strangulated hernia	Strangulated hernia
Meckel's diverticulitis	Perforated colon
Regional ileitis	Regional ileitis
Perforated cecum	Ulcerative colitis

From Seidel HM et al: *Mosby's guide to physical examination*, ed 4, St. Louis, 1998, Mosby. Modified from Judge R, Zuidema G, Fitzgerald F: *Clinical diagnosis*, ed 5, Boston, 1988, Little, Brown.

localized aching. As the inflammatory process spreads to the adjacent parietal peritoneum, it produces localized parietal peritonitis. The pain of parietal peritonitis is more severe and is perceived in the area of the abdomen corresponding to the inflammation. The patient with parietal pain usually lies still and does not want to move.

Pain may be referred from within the abdomen or from other parts of the body. (Box 5-1). Referral of pain occurs as tissues supplied by the same or adjacent neural segments have the same common pathways inside the CNS. Thus, stimulation of these neural segments gives rise to the sensation of pain. For example, nerves that supply the appendix are derived from the same source as those that supply the small intestine, resulting in onset of appendicitis pain in the epigastric area.

Abdominal pain in adults can be classified as acute, chronic, or recurrent. The term "acute abdomen" refers to any acute condition within the abdomen that re-

quires immediate surgical attention. Not all acute abdominal pain, however, requires surgical intervention. Acute abdominal pain refers to a relatively sudden onset of pain that is severe or increasing in severity and that has been present for a short duration. Chronic pain is characterized by its persistent duration or recurrence. Recurrent episodes of pain may be either acute or chronic in nature.

In adults, acute pain requiring surgical intervention is commonly caused by appendicitis, perforated peptic ulcer, intestinal obstruction, peritonitis, perforate diverticulitis, ectopic pregnancy, or dissection of aortic aneurysm. Common causes of acute pain not requiring surgical intervention include cholelithiasis, gastroenteritis, peptic gastroduodenal syndrome, pelvic inflammatory disease (PID), or urinary tract infection (UTI). Chronic or recurrent pain can be caused by gastrointestinal disorders such as irritable bowel syndrome (IBS) or esophagitis, pelvic disorders such as dysmenorrhea or uterine fibroids, genitourinary disorders such as recurrent UTI or chronic prostatitis, or conditions outside the abdomen such as costochondritis, hip disease, or hernia.

In children, abdominal pain can be classified as acute or recurrent. Common causes of acute pain include appendicitis, food poisoning, UTI, viral gastroenteritis, and bacterial enterocolitis. Recurrent abdominal pain (RAP) is defined as more than three episodes of pain in 3 months in children older than 3 years. It affects 10% to 15% of children between the ages of 3 and 14; 90% of these children will not have an organic etiology.

DIAGNOSTIC REASONING: FOCUSED HISTORY

Is this an acute condition?

Key Questions

- How long ago did your pain start?
- Was the onset sudden or gradual?
- How severe is the pain (scale of 1 to 10)? In a child: what is the child's level of activity?
- Does the pain wake you up from sleep?
- What has been the course of the pain since it started? Getting worse? Getting better?
- Have you ever had this pain before?

Onset/duration. Acute onset of pain that is getting progressively worse may signal a surgical emergency. In general, patients who present with severe pain 6 to 24 hours from the onset are probably suffering from an acute surgical condition. Acute abdominal pain may signal a few potentially life-threatening conditions that must be considered first. These may be surgical emergencies that require immediate evaluation and intervention:

- Perforation: look for signs and symptoms of peritonitis (Box 5-2)
- Ectopic pregnancy: in any woman of childbearing age
- Obstruction: in the elderly

Box 5-2

Features of Peritonitis

P	Pain: front back, sides, shoulders
E	Electrolytes fall, shock ensues
R	Rigidity or rebound of anterior abdominal wall
I	Immobile abdomen and patient
T	Tenderness with involuntary guarding
O	Obstruction
N	Nausea and vomiting
I	Increasing pulse, decreasing blood pressure
T	Temperature falls then rises; Tachypnea
I	Increasing girth of abdomen
S	Silent abdomen (no bowel sounds)

From Seidel HM et al: *Mosby's guide to physical examination*, ed 4, St. Louis, 1998, Mosby. Modified from Shipman JJ: *Mnemonics and tactics in surgery and medicine*, ed 2, Chicago, 1984, Mosby.

- Ruptured abdominal aortic aneurysm: when back pain is present
- Intussusception: in infants
- Malrotation: in infants usually less than 1 month of age

Pain of sudden onset is more likely associated with colic, perforation, or acute ischemia (torsion, volvulus). Slower onset of pain generally is associated with inflammatory conditions, such as appendicitis, pancreatitis, and cholecystitis.

Acute pain that comes and goes may be related to intestinal peristalsis. The onset of pain in relation to food ingestion provides diagnostic clues: pain occurring several hours after a meal suggests a duodenal ulcer (pain with stomach empty), whereas pain right after eating occurs with esophagitis.

In children, recurrent abdominal pain (RAP) occurs in attacks lasting less than 1 hour and rarely longer than 3 hours

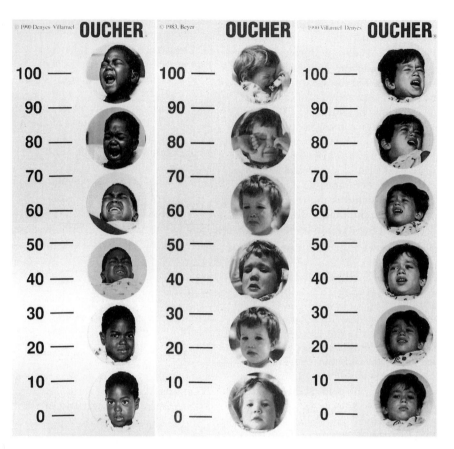

Figure 5-1 The Oucher Pain Scale illustrated with African-American, Caucasian, and Hispanic children to best fit the child's cultural identity. (From Seidel HM et al: *Mosby's guide to physical examination,* ed 4, St. Louis, 1998, Mosby.)

and frequently interferes with daily routines. Between episodes, the pain resolves completely. When interviewing a child, remember that he or she may not be old enough to have a clear sense of time.

Severity and progression. Severity is the most difficult symptom to evaluate because of its subjective quality. It is helpful to use a 1 to 10 scale in adults. Children may respond to the use of the pain faces or the Oucher Scale (Figure 5-1).

Determine if the pain is an acute episode or if it is chronic or recurrent. Acute abdominal pain requires immediate attention, as it may signal an acute surgical abdomen. Chronic or recurrent episodes of pain can be handled in a more temperate manner.

Pain that is steady, severe, and progressive is worrisome. Pain that causes one to awake from sleep is serious. A sudden pain severe enough to cause fainting suggests perforated ulcer, ruptured aneurysm, or ectopic pregnancy. A severe knifelike pain usually indicates an emergency. Tearing pain is characteristic of an aortic aneurysm. Appendicitis is often described as an ache. Colicky pain that becomes steady can indicate appendicitis or strangulating intestinal obstruction.

Children are poor historians as to the

severity of pain. The caregiver should indicate how severe the child's pain is by a description of the activity level of the child. The child's activity level helps to indicate pain. Generally, avoidance of favorite activities indicates an organic problem, as does avoidance of motion. Organic disease awakens the child from sleep.

Previous pain. Chronic pain may result when a potential surgical event is brought into check but is not totally resolved. Chronic pain that has been present for longer than a year generally is not caused by a neoplasm. Consider instead irritable bowel syndrome (IBS) or colorectal, endometrial, or inflammatory causes.

Recurrent attacks of acute pain may be caused by inflammation and exacerbation of a chronic condition, such as functional colonic pain, IBS, cholecystitis, chronic pancreatitis, or ulcer disease. Acute pain may also be caused by recurrent infection, such as pyelonephritis or cystitis. Urinary tract stones can also cause acute attacks of recurrent pain.

Will the location of pain give me any clues?

Key Questions
- Where is the pain? (point to it)
- Does it travel (radiate) anywhere?

Location of the pain. The viscera is innervated bilaterally so that pain is perceived in the midline. It is often described as a deep, dull, diffuse pain. Visceral pain originates from epigastric, periumbilical, and hypogastric causes; from intra-abdominal extraperitoneal organs (pancreas, kidneys, ureters, great vessels, pelvic organs); or from a referred source.

Parietal (also known as peritoneal or somatic) pain is more localized and is described as a sharp pain. Peritoneal pain originates from intra-abdominal and intra-peritoneal organs.

Inflammation, such as occurs with appendicitis, can produce either visceral or parietal peritonitis. Initially the inflammation is limited to the serosa covering an inflamed organ. The pain is visceral and is felt diffusely. As the inflammation progresses to the adjacent parietal peritoneum, it produces a more severe localized pain that is perceived in the corresponding area of the abdomen. Children have a poor ability to localize pain and in general are not helpful in the majority of cases.

Apley rule: The further the localization of pain from the umbilicus, the more likely there is an underlying organic disorder.

When the peritoneal cavity is flooded suddenly by either blood, pus, or gastric fluid, the pain is frequently reported as "all over the abdomen" at first. However, the maximum intensity of pain at the onset is likely to be in the upper abdomen with gastric problems and in the lower abdomen with tubal and appendix rupture. Irritating fluid from a perforated duodenal ulcer produces pain in the right hypochondrium, lumbar, and iliac regions.

Pain arising from the small intestine is always felt in the epigastric and umbilical areas of the abdomen. The 9th and 11th thoracic nerves supply the small intestine via the common mesentery. Appendicular nerves are derived from the same source as those that supply the small intestine, resulting in onset of pain in the epigastric area with appendicitis.

Table 5-1 describes the structures involved in specific pain locations.

Radiation of pain. Radiation of pain can help in diagnosis. Pain that radiates will do so to the area of distribution of the nerves coming from that segment of the spinal cord that supplies the affected area. Biliary colic pain is frequently referred to the region just under the right scapula (8th dorsal segment), while renal colic in males is frequently felt in the testicle of the same side. Pain from a ruptured spleen is often referred to the top of the left shoulder.

Table 5-1

Pain Location and Involved Structures

PAIN LOCATION	STRUCTURES
Epigastric	Esophagus, stomach, duodenum, liver, GB, pancreas, spleen
Upper abdominal	Esophagus, stomach, duodenum, pancreas, liver, gallbladder, or thorax
Right UQ*	Usually the esophagus, stomach, duodenum, pancreas, liver, gallbladder, or thorax; often indicates acute cholecystitis
Left UQ*	Spleen
Periumbilical	Jejunum, midgut, ileum, appendix, ascending colon; pain caused by inflammation, ischemic spasm, or abnormal distention
Lower abdominal	Colon, sigmoid colon, rectum, and GU structures—bladder, uterus, prostate
Right LQ*	Commonly caused by PID, appendicitis, ectopic pregnancy, or an ovarian cyst; establish the date of last normal menstrual period
Left LQ*	Sigmoid colon
Flanks	Kidney(s)
Localized	Occurs from local inflammation of the skin or peritoneum, as with appendicitis; lateralized pain occurs in the paired organs—kidneys, ureters, fallopian tubes, gonads
Generalized	Produced by diffuse inflammation of GI tract, peritoneum, or abdomen wall

*UQ, upper quadrant; LQ, lower quadrant.

What do the pain characteristics tell me?

Key Questions
- Describe the pain. (e.g., burning, sharp, achy, crampy)
- What makes it worse/better?

Character of pain. Colicky or cramping pain occurs with obstruction of a hollow viscus that produces distention. Generally there are pain-free intervals when the pain is much less intense but subtly still present. During the painful episodes, the patient is exceedingly agitated and restless, often pale and diaphoretic. The pain from obstruction of the small intestine is rhythmic, peristaltic pain with intermittent cramping. When the obstruction site is in the proximal small intestine rather than in the more distal portion, the paroxysms of cramping occur with greater frequency.

Steady pain is associated with perforation, ischemia, inflammation, and blood in the peritoneal cavity. Burning pain is characteristic of esophagitis. Pain from a duodenal ulcer has been described as burning or "gnawing." Pain of pancreatic origin is steady, epigastric, and prostrating. Pricking or itching pain comes from superficial causes such as herpes zoster. Dull, aching pain indicates deeper pain. In children, abdominal pain is generally characterized as colicky or inflammatory.

Remember, however, that despite descriptions of characteristic or typical abdominal pain, presentation in children and the elderly is often atypical and may not fit any pattern.

Precipitating or aggravating factors.
Lying down or bending forward often produces pain from esophagitis. Alcohol may aggravate gastritis or an ulcer.

Pain that is made worse by deep inspiration and is stopped or diminished by a respiratory pause indicates pleuritic origin. If the cause is peritonitis, intraperitoneal abscess, or abdominal distention from intestinal obstruction, pain will increase on deep inspiration. Biliary colic is made worse by forced inspiration. The pain from biliary colic often causes inhibition of movement of the diaphragm.

The patient with visceral pain is restless, moves about, and has difficulty getting comfortable. The patient with parietal pain usually lies still and does not want to move. Children with inflammatory pain secondary to peritoneal irritation usually present as quiet and motionless because movement exacerbates the pain.

Relieving factors. Food or antacids may relieve pain caused by an ulcer or gastritis. Both colicky and inflammatory pain are alleviated significantly with analgesics. However, the pain of a vascular accident will not respond to analgesics.

Are there any precipitating events that will help me narrow my diagnosis?

Key Questions
- Is the pain related to any other activity? (e.g., eating, lying down)
- Can you identify any trigger?

Relation to other events. Pain that is relieved by defecation, flatus, laxatives, or diet changes implicates the intestine. Pain associated with meals implicates the gastrointestinal (GI) tract.

Pain with sexual activity (dyspareunia) suggests a pelvic origin. Pain that occurs with position changes may be referred from the spine, hips, sacroiliac joint, pelvic bones, or abdominal musculature. Exertional pain may be of cardiac origin.

What does the presence of vomiting and diarrhea tell me?

Key Questions
- Are you vomiting? What does it look like?
- What do your stools look like?
- How frequent are your stools?

Vomiting. Vomiting in adults that precedes the onset of abdominal pain is unlikely to signal a problem requiring surgery. Vomiting suggests that the pain is visceral in origin. Anorexia is a nonspecific symptom, but its absence makes serious disease less likely.

Vomiting associated with acute abdomen may be from one of three causes:
- Severe irritation of the nerves of the peritoneum or mesentery: sudden stimulation of many sympathetic nerves causes vomiting to occur early and to be persistent.
- Obstruction of an involuntary muscular tube: obstruction of any of the muscular tubes causes peristaltic contraction and consequent stretching of the muscle wall and vomiting occurs. The area behind the obstruction becomes dilated, and, as each peristaltic wave occurs, the tension and stretching of the muscular fibers are temporarily increased so that the pain of colic comes usually in spasms. Vomiting usually occurs at the height of the pain.
- The action of absorbed toxins on the medullary centers: the chemoreceptor trigger zone is stimulated by drugs such as cardiac glycosides, ergot alkaloids, and morphine or by uremia, diabetic ketoacidosis, and general anesthetics. Impulses to the medullary vomiting center then activate the vomiting process.

Pain with vomiting. In sudden and severe stimulation of the peritoneum or mesentery, vomiting comes soon after the pain. In acute obstruction of the urethra or bile duct, vomiting is early, sudden, and intense. In intestinal obstruction, the timing of the vomiting indicates how high in the gut the obstruction is. If the duodenum is obstructed, vomiting occurs with the onset of pain. Obstruction of the large bowel has very late or infrequent vomiting.

Vomiting is not seen in ectopic pregnancy, gastric or duodenal perforation, or intussusception. Vomiting occurring before pain indicates gastroenteritis. In appendicitis, pain almost always precedes the vomiting.

Vomit appearance. Clear vomitus suggests gastric fluid; bile-colored vomitus is from upper gastrointestinal contents. Feculent vomitus occurs with distal intestinal obstruction. Patients with gastric outlet obstruction vomit fluid that contains food particles if the patient has eaten recently, but later the vomitus becomes clear. Infants with duodenal atresia will vomit bilious fluid, but in pyloric stenosis no bile is seen.

Stool characteristics. Diarrhea is associated with inflammatory bowel disease, diverticulitis, or early obstruction. The presence of blood in the stool suggests that the pain originates in the intestinal tract. Blood may indicate neoplasm, intussusception, or inflammatory lesions.

Diarrhea may precede perforation of the appendix as a result of irritation of the sigmoid colon by an inflammatory mass. Some patients will complain of gas stoppage symptoms: the sensation of fullness that suggests the need for a bowel movement. With appendicitis, the patient may attempt to defecate but without relief.

In children, mild diarrhea associated with onset of pain suggests acute gastroenteritis but may also occur with early appendicitis. A low-lying appendix, close to the sigmoid colon and rectum, may induce an inflammatory process of the muscle wall of the sigmoid colon. Any distention of the sigmoid by fluid or gas signals the child to pass gas and small amounts of stool. The

cycle repeats a few minutes later. In gastroenteritis, typically the child will have large liquid stools. Children can also have abdominal pain from chronic constipation. Constipation that precedes pain suggests disease of the colon or rectum.

Are there any clues to implicate a particular organ system?

If the patient gives a positive response to these history questions, refer to the topic or chapter indicated for additional discussion. Pain that is not abdominal in origin may be referred to or perceived to be in the abdomen. Accompanying symptoms of headache, sore throat, and general aches and pains suggest a viral, flu-like cause.

Key Questions
Gastrointestinal (Constipation, p. 195, Diarrhea, p. 176)
- Do you have any GI symptoms? (e.g., gas, diarrhea, constipation, vomiting, heartburn)
- Have you had any changes in your bowel habits, stools, eating pattern?
- Is the pain relieved by defecation? By burping?

Gas, bloating, diarrhea, constipation, and rectal bleeding may occur with pain that is intestinal in origin. Heartburn and dysphagia are characteristic of esophagitis. Changes in bowel habits may signal obstruction or neoplasm. Constipation alternating with diarrhea is characteristic of IBS. The patient may also complain of distention, bloating, belching, gas, and mucus in the stools.

Pain relieved by defecation or the passage of gas suggests IBS or gas entrapment in the large intestine. Pain relieved by burping suggests distention of the stomach by gas.

Genitourinary (Chapters 6 and 7)
- When was your last menstrual period (LMP)? Was it normal for you? Could you be pregnant?

- Do you have any vaginal symptoms or problems: unusual discharge, unusual bleeding, pain with sexual intercourse?
- Do you have any menstrual irregularity or unusual bleeding? (Sexual history may provide information relevant to the possibility of sexually transmitted diseases [STDs], pelvic inflammatory disease [PID], and pregnancy)
- Do you have any urinary symptoms? (frequency, urgency, dysuria, blood in urine, change in urine color)
- Do you have pain in the back (flank)? Point to it.

Menstrual irregularities, vaginal discharge, unusual bleeding, or dyspareunia indicate a pelvic origin of the pain. Sexually active adolescent girls are at the highest risk for contracting PID. Patients with PID may complain of both vaginal discharge and abnormal vaginal bleeding, although pain is often the only presenting symptom. The pain is usually severe and progressive. Pain just before the onset of menses may indicate endometriosis. Pain related to ovulation (mittelschmerz) occurs mid-cycle. In women of childbearing age, always consider ectopic pregnancy.

Urinary symptoms (dysuria, hematuria, hesitancy, or frequency) point to a urinary tract cause of the pain. Flank pain is usually associated with renal calculi or pyelonephritis. Upper abdominal pain that radiates to the groin signals ureterolithiasis.

Musculoskeletal (Chapter 9)

- Does the pain occur with change of position or movement?
- Do you have any joint pain, heat, swelling, noises, limitation in range of motion (ROM)?
- Do you have any difficulty walking?

Pain produced by musculoskeletal problems and referred to the abdomen may be provoked by position changes or walking. Costochondritis can produce pain with vigorous respiration. Symptoms of joint involvement point to either a local cause with referred pain or a systemic cause such as rheumatoid arthritis.

Cardiovascular (Chapter 4)

- Does the pain occur with exertion or at rest?
- Do you have any chest pain, palpitations, fast heartbeat, or pain that goes to the arm or jaw?

Referred pain from the chest is not uncommon. Pain on exertion signals coronary artery disease and angina. Right upper quadrant pain can be caused by congestive heart failure. Myocardial infarction and pericarditis can also cause abdominal pain.

Respiratory (Chapter 4)

- Do you have a cough or difficulty breathing?
- Do you have any shortness of breath?

Pneumonia, especially of a lower lobe, is a common cause of pain perceived in the abdomen, especially in children. Pleurisy can produce pain on deep inspiration. Persistent coughing can produce musculoskeletal soreness that may be referred to the abdomen.

Is the pain of psychogenic origin? Is it organic or functional pain?

Key Questions

- Do you feel unhappy, sad, depressed?
- Are you able to eat, sleep, engage in usual activities?
- Have you had recent problems with diarrhea or constipation?
- How is your energy level?
- Have you ever been diagnosed with or treated for a mental health or psychiatric problem?

Abdominal pain can be functional or psychogenic in origin and presents somewhat differently from organic pain (Table 5-2). The presence of vegetative symptoms suggests depression.

Table 5-2

Organic Versus Functional Pain

HISTORY	ORGANIC PAIN	FUNCTIONAL PAIN
Pain character	Acute, persistent pain increasing in intensity	Less likely to change or get more severe
Pain localization	Sharply localized	Various locations
Pain in relation to sleep	Awakens at night	Does not affect sleep
Pain in relation to umbilicus	Further away	At umbilicus
Associated symptoms	Fever, anorexia, vomiting, weight loss, anemia, elevated ESR	Headache, dizziness, and multiple system complaints
Psychological stress	None reported	Present

What else do I need to consider?

Key Questions

- What medications are you taking? What are you taking them for?
- Have you had any surgeries? What were they?
- Have you had an involuntary weight loss recently?
- Have you been camping?
- Is the child in a day care setting?

Medications. Erythromycin and tetracycline are commonly associated with abdominal pain. Gastrointestinal distress is a common adverse reaction to many medications.

Surgeries. Prior surgery can produce adhesions that cause intestinal obstruction. Adhesion of organs to the abdominal wall can also produce pain. Prior appendectomy does not preclude appendicitis, as the stump may become inflamed.

Involuntary weight loss. Involuntary weight loss raises the index of suspicion for colon cancer. Identify other factors that would lead you to suspect neoplasms, such as recent change in bowel habits in the middle aged, family history of colorectal or gynecological cancer, and the presence of blood in the stool.

Camping or day care. Ingestion of untreated water can result in intestinal parasites. Transmission of intestinal parasites is also common in day care settings. Intestinal parasites may cause only abdominal pain in children; therefore, stools should be evaluated for ova and parasites.

DIAGNOSTIC REASONING: FOCUSED PHYSICAL EXAMINATION

Note General Appearance

Patients with visceral pain are restless, move about, and have difficulty getting comfortable. These are patients with colicky type pain, often indicative of biliary obstruction, ureterolithiasis, obstruction, gastroenteritis, or early peritonitis.

Patients with parietal pain usually lie still and do not want to move. These are patients with localized peritonitis indicative of appendicitis, rupture, or perforation.

In children, note if the child looks sick (see Chapter 12, Yale Observation Scale). Children may react to pain differently from adults. With peritoneal irritation, they are typically quiet and motionless with their knees flexed and drawn up. Children who are septic or have serious diseases such as perforation or intussusception generally lie still and look lethargic, withdrawn, and apprehensive. A child with colicky pain frequently writhes in discomfort, occasionally rocking in a rhythmic fashion.

Assess Vital Signs

In patients who are tachycardic and tachypneic, suspect a serious thoracic, intra-abdominal, or pelvic disorder that is producing an acute abdomen. Shallow respirations may indicate pneumonia or pleurisy with referred pain. Orthostatic hypotension, an unusually low blood pressure or a "normal" blood pressure in someone who is usually hypertensive, may indicate an acute abdomen.

The presence of a fever suggests an acute inflammatory condition. Fever greater than 39.4° C (102.9° F) is associated more with pulmonary and renal infection than an abdominal problem and may indicate pneumonia or pyelonephritis.

In adults, look for documented recent involuntary weight loss, which may indicate a neoplasm. Weigh a child to determine weight loss and dehydration status.

Observe Abdominal Musculature

A rigid abdomen characterizes peritoneal irritation; whereas a soft abdomen suggests otherwise. A rigid abdomen may signal an acute abdomen that requires surgical intervention.

Note Coloring of Abdominal Skin

Ecchymosis around the umbilicus (Cullen's sign) is associated with hemoperitoneum caused either by pancreatitis or ruptured ectopic pregnancy. Ecchymosis of the flanks (Grey-Turner's sign) is associated with hemoperitoneum and pancreatitis. Look for skin rashes of viral exanthem.

In children a rash (palpable purpura) located on lower extremities, buttocks, and arms indicates Henoch-Schoenlein purpura.

Note Abdominal Distention

Generalized symmetrical distention may occur as the result of obesity, enlarged organs, fluid, or gas. Distention from the umbilicus to the symphysis can be caused by ovarian tumor, pregnancy, uterine fibroids, carcinoma, pancreatic cyst, or gastric dilation. Asymmetrical distention or protrusion may indicate hernia, tumor, cysts, bowel obstruction, or enlargement of abdominal organs. Remember the "Fs of distention": fat, fluid, feces, fetus, flatus, fibroid, full bladder, false pregnancy, fatal tumor.

To determine distention in children, stoop down by the child's side and sight across the abdomen. The skin is tense and taut with a distended abdomen, and, if the umbilicus is everted, ascites is often present. Superficial abdominal veins are often distended in children with peritonitis. The healthy child will usually have a flat abdominal profile. A flat abdomen is a straight line from the xiphoid to pelvis with no scaphoiding. A scaphoid abdomen may occur with marked dehydration or high intestinal obstruction.

Auscultate Bowel Sounds

If bowel sounds are absent, suspect peritonitis or ileus. Hyperactive bowel sounds suggest gastroenteritis, early pyloric or intestinal obstruction, or GI bleeding. High-pitched tinkling bowel sounds may indicate obstruction.

In children, use of the stethoscope can be helpful in palpation to determine abdominal pain. Begin listening to the chest; the child accepts this as painless. Then gently move the stethoscope down to the belly, slightly increasing the pressure, watching the child's face and feeling the resistance when painful.

Percuss for Tones and Guarding

In percussion, look for unexpected dullness. Guarding with percussion suggests peritoneal irritation. Tenderness can be elicited with gentle tapping. Tenderness is usually local and only rarely referred.

Palpate Entire Abdomen and Note Patient Response

Start with gentle palpation and palpate the area of pain last. Testing for rebound tenderness should be performed gently. Tenderness, guarding, and rebound tenderness suggest peritoneal irritation. The most reliable clinical indicator of parietal peritonitis is involuntary guarding, which must be distinguished from voluntary guarding because of pain or fear of worsening pain as a result of the examination. Guarding is determined with gentle palpation of the abdomen, not by deep palpation of the underlying organs.

You can induce guarding by having the patient place the chin on the chest, or cross arms on the chest and sit up. Palpate the painful area again. Note that intraperitoneal pain is made less severe by induced guarding. If the severity of pain is not decreased by induced guarding, consider other causes such as functional pain or abdominal wall pain.

Palpate for the liver, gallbladder, spleen, kidneys, aorta, and bladder to detect organ tenderness or involvement. Abrupt cessation of inspiration on palpation of the gallbladder (Murphy's sign) indicates acute cholecystitis.

Palpate for Masses

Palpation of a mass may indicate a neoplasm, obstruction, hernia, or the presence of feces in the colon. Anatomical structures may be mistaken for an abdominal mass. A mass in the upper abdomen that pulsates laterally suggests an abdominal aortic aneurysm.

A sausage-shaped mass may be felt in the upper mid-abdomen in 85% to 95% of infants with intussusception. An olive-shaped mass may be palpable in the right upper quadrant with pyloric stenosis.

Palpate the Groin

The groin must be examined in everyone who has abdominal pain to exclude an incarcerated hernia/ovary or torsion of the ovary or testicle (see Chapter 6, Penile Discharge, for testicular evaluation).

Palpate for Hernias

Palpate for inguinal, incisional, femoral, and umbilical hernias. Uncomplicated hernias will reduce; strangulated ones will not. Bowel sounds will be present in uncomplicated hernias.

Percuss for Flank Tenderness

Use of direct or indirect percussion over the costovertebral angle may elicit tenderness if the kidney is involved. Flank pain, especially with the occurrence of hematuria, may indicate a kidney stone.

Test for Peritoneal Irritation

Several maneuvers can be used to test for peritoneal irritation:
- *Obturator muscle test.* Perform this test when you suspect a ruptured appendix or pelvic abscess as these conditions can cause irritation of the obturator muscle. Pain in the hypogastric region is a positive sign, indicating obturator muscle irritation. With the patient supine, flex the right leg at the hips and knee to 90 degrees. Hold the leg just above the knee, grasp the ankle, and rotate the leg laterally and medially.
- *Iliopsoas muscle test.* Perform this test when you suspect appendicitis as an inflamed appendix may cause

irritation of the lateral iliopsoas muscle. Pain in the lower quadrant is a positive test. With the patient supine, place your hand over the lower thigh and have the patient raise the leg, flexing at the hip while you push downward against the leg.

- *Markle's (heel jar) test.* The patient stands with straightened knees, then raises up on the toes. The patient then relaxes and allows the heels to hit the floor, thus jarring the body. The maneuver will cause abdominal pain if positive.
- *Rovsing's test.* Perform this test if you suspect appendicitis. Press on the left lower quadrant. If pain in the right lower quadrant is intensified, the test is positive.

Perform a Pelvic Examination in Women

Perform a pelvic examination in women to rule out sexually transmitted disease (STD), pelvic inflammatory disease (PID), ovarian pain, ectopic pregnancy, and uterine fibroids. Vaginal discharge may or may not be present with STD or PID. Bleeding may accompany ectopic pregnancy.

Cervical motion tenderness (CMT) is the hallmark of PID. CMT plus adnexal pain (often bilateral) in the presence of abdominal pain and lower abdominal tenderness are criteria for a presumptive diagnosis of PID.

Adnexal tenderness in the region of pain may signal ectopic pregnancy. An adnexal mass may or may not be palpable, and its presence is not diagnostic. Vague adnexal tenderness may be present with STD. Bilateral, inflammatory ovarian pain and tenderness is usually related to salpingitis (PID), appendicitis, or peritonitis. A functional cyst may produce unilateral tenderness. Uterine fibroids may be palpable as masses in the uterus, or the entire uterus may be enlarged.

Perform Genital and Prostate Examinations in Men

Perform a genital and prostate examination in men to rule out STD and prostatitis. Look for penile discharge as an indicator of STD and perhaps prostatitis. A tender prostate signals prostatitis. In acute prostatitis, make sure the examination is gentle; vigorous examination or massage of the prostate can cause bacterial release and produce septicemia (see Chapter 6, Genitourinary Problems in Males).

Perform Digital Rectal Examination

Look for frank blood and test for occult blood. The presence of blood may indicate an acute process or carcinoma. Palpate for masses, polyps, and lesions. Occasionally patients with a rectocecal appendix and appendicitis may have a tender localized mass on rectal examination, even though the abdominal examination is normal.

Check Peripheral Pulses

Diminished femoral pulses in the presence of a pulsatile abdominal mass suggest ruptured abdominal aortic aneurysm.

Perform a Generalized Examination as Indicated

Because abdominal pain may be referred from other areas, examine the lungs, cardiovascular system, head and neck structures, and musculoskeletal system. Palpate for regional lymphadenopathy.

DIAGNOSTIC AND LABORATORY STUDIES

CBC with Differential

An elevated WBC greater than $12,000/\mu l$ indicates an inflammatory or infectious condition. The WBC is the total number of white blood cells in a cubic meter of blood. This is an absolute number. The other measure of white blood cells is the relative percentage of each of the types. Neutrophils are the body's first defense against bacterial infection and severe stress.

Normally the circulating neutrophils are in a mature form. The mature forms are known as "segs" because the nuclei of the cells are segmented. Immature forms are known as "bands" because the nuclei of the cells are not in segments but still in a band. An increased need for neutrophils will cause an increase in both the segs (mature cells) and the bands (immature cells).

Infection causes both leukocytosis (an increase in the absolute number of white blood cells) and an increase in neutrophils, both mature (segs) and immature (bands). This is also called a "shift to the left." When laboratory reports were written by hand, the bands were written first on the left-hand side of the page. Thus, a "shift to the left" means that the bands have increased, which is seen as an increase in the relative percent.

Qualitative Urine/Serum hCGs

Qualitative urine/serum hCG tests are monoclonal antibody tests using radioimmunoassay (RIA) to determine or exclude pregnancy. The serum hCG test is more sensitive than the urine hCG test. The serum test can be performed in about 2 hours, and hCG can be detected as early as 6 days after conception. The result is reported as either negative or positive. Since the beta-subunits are measured, it is highly specific and does not cross react with luteinizing hormone.

Depending on the specific test used, urine testing can detect pregnancy from before a missed period to several days after a missed period. The results are obtained in minutes. A positive test (usually a color change) indicates pregnancy.

Quantitative Serum hCG

Quantitative serum hCG is a fluorometric enzyme immunoassay that is highly spe-

cific for the beta receptors of hCG, with almost no cross-reactivity with other hormones. Results are provided as values. The reference ranges for determining an abnormal pregnancy are as follows:

Not significant	0-5.0 mIU/ml
Borderline significance	5.0-25 mIU/ml
Evaluate with serial determinations	>25 mIU/ml

Use this test if you are concerned about ectopic pregnancy. Ectopic pregnancy causes an increase in hCG levels at the same rate as a normal pregnancy, up to a certain point. In ectopic pregnancy that point is usually less than 4 to 6 weeks, at which time the hCG levels plateau or begin to fall. Therefore serial determinations are more useful than a single determination.

Erythrocyte Sedimentation Rate (ESR)

The ESR measures the speed with which red blood cells settle in a tube of anticoagulated blood. The results are expressed as millimeters in hours (mm/hr). An increase in plasma globulins or fibrinogen causes the cells to stick together and to fall faster than normal. Cells that are smaller than normal also fall faster; whereas, cells that are larger than normal fall more slowly. A marked increase in ESR during pregnancy is expected because there is an increase in globulins and in the fibrinogen level in pregnancy. Inflammation or tissue injury also causes an increase in globulins and fibrinogens and causes an increased rate. However, the test is non-specific, and, while it shows inflammation, it does not show the source. The ESR is often elevated as a result of PID, infectious states, or AIDS.

Urinalysis (U/A)

Evaluation of kidney infection, presence of a stone, renal failure, or systemic process is done with a urinalysis. Microscopic hematuria suggests urinary tract infection or stone. Glycosuria and ketonuria suggest metabolic disturbances. A positive nitrite test on a U/A dipstick indicates the presence of bacteria, which can be seen on microscopic examination. The finding of 20 or more bacteria/high-powered field (HPF) indicates a urinary tract infection. The presence of greater than 0 to 1 red blood cells/HPF or greater than 0 to 4 white blood cells/HPF on microscopic examination also suggests urinary tract infection. Red blood cells may also be present as a contaminant with vaginal bleeding. The presence of red cell casts suggests kidney disease or renal infarction. White cell casts indicate pyelonephritis.

Urine for Culture and Sensitivity (C & S)

If you suspect urinary tract infection, obtain a urine test for culture and sensitivity.

Culture for Sexually Transmitted Disease (STD)

Do a culture for STD. Collect a specimen of vaginal or penile discharge on a sterile swab and place in the medium provided for *gonorrhea, Chlamydia,* or mycoplasms. For penile discharge, use a sterile urethral swab to collect a specimen from the anterior urethra by gentle insertion and scraping of the mucosa (see Chapter 6, Penile Discharge).

DNA Probe for *Chlamydia* and *Neisseria gonorrhea*

Obtain a sample of vaginal or penile discharge with a sterile swab and place it in the medium provided. This test involves the construction of a nucleic acid sequence (called a probe) that will match to a sequence in the DNA or RNA of the target tissue. The results are rapid and sensitive.

Potassium Hydroxide (KOH)

The KOH test involves direct microscopic examination of material on a slide to deter-

mine whether fungus is present. Place a specimen of vaginal or penile discharge on a glass slide, apply a drop of aqueous 10% KOH, and put a coverslip in place. The potassium hydroxide dissolves epithelial cells and debris and facilitates visualization of the mycelia of a fungus. The presence of fishy odor (the "whiff test") suggests bacterial vaginosis. View under the microscope for presence of mycelial fragments, hyphae, and budding yeast cells (see Chapter 7, Vaginal Discharge and Itching).

Saline Wet Prep

In a female with vaginal discharge, this test can demonstrate the presence of *Trichomonas vaginalis* or *Gardnerella* organisms by microscopic examination. Place a specimen of vaginal discharge on a slide and add a drop of normal saline. Place a coverslip on the slide. The presence of trichomonads indicates *T. vaginalis.* The presence of bacteria-filled epithelial cells (clue cells) indicates bacterial vaginosis *(Gardnerella)* (see Chapter 7, Vaginal Discharge and Itching).

Gram Stain

Place a smear of vaginal or cervical discharge on a glass slide for Gram staining. Gram-positive organisms stain purple, whereas Gram-negative organisms stain red. *N. gonorrhea* is a Gram-negative organism.

Fecal Occult Blood Test (FOBT)

Perform this test to rule out GI bleeding. The test is positive if a stool smear on a prepared card turns color (usually blue or green) when a solution is applied. A 3-day series of samples provides more reliable results.

X-Rays

Abdominal x-rays are of limited value in evaluating abdominal pain. An AP x-ray of abdomen shows the kidneys, ureters, bladder (KUB) and adjacent structures. It can be used to exclude free air (perforation) and obstruction (e.g., renal calculi). A chest x-ray can reveal the presence of pneumonia or air under the diaphragm.

Abdominal/Pelvic Ultrasound

Abdominal ultrasound is useful if you are considering an ectopic pregnancy, abdominal aortic aneurysm, or acute cholecystitis.

Computed Tomography (CT)

CT scanning is appropriate if you suspect retroperitoneal bleeding or a pelvic abscess.

Other Tests as Indicated for GI Tract

Consider flexible sigmoidoscopy, proctoscopy, colonoscopy, upper GI series, or lower GI series if you suspect pain that is GI in origin.

DIFFERENTIAL DIAGNOSIS

When there is no worrisome history or physical findings, use the specific history questions as the "best test" to point you in the right direction. Then determine if the clinical findings are consistent. Review the history to see evolution over time, especially of an acute condition.

Identify physical findings that are worrisome as well, such as lower abdominal pain beginning at older age, involuntary

weight loss, abnormal bleeding in a perimenopausal or post-menopausal woman, palpable abdominal or pelvic mass, or stool that is positive for occult blood.

Look initially for surgical problems. Serial abdominal examinations are the best indicator of progression of an abdominal problem. Try to identify what organ seems to be involved and remember that extra-abdominal systems can cause abdominal pain (e.g., pneumonia). Try to determine if the pain is organic or functional in origin. Remember that common causes of acute pain differ from common causes of chronic pain. Box 5-3 lists indicators of abdominal emergencies.

ACUTE CONDITIONS THAT CAUSE ABDOMINAL PAIN

Appendicitis

Incidence of appendicitis peaks at age 10 to 20 years, although it can occur at any age. The patient complains of sudden onset of colicky pain that progresses to a constant pain. The pain may begin in the epigastrium or periumbilicus and later localize to the right lower quadrant (RLQ). The pain worsens with movement or coughing. Vomiting after the onset of pain sometimes occurs. On physical examination, the patient will be lying still and will demonstrate involuntary guarding. Classically, tenderness occurs in the RLQ. The other tests for peritoneal irritation will be positive. Rebound tenderness will be present. Variation in presentation is

---

Box 5-3

Indicators of Abdominal Emergencies

Subjective Findings
Progressive intractable vomiting
Lightheadedness on standing
Acute onset of pain
Pain that progresses in intensity over hours

Objective Findings
Involuntary guarding
Progressive abdomen distention
Orthostatic hypotension
Fever
Leukocytosis and granulocytosis
Decreased urine output

common, particularly with infants, children, and the elderly. Diagnostic testing includes CBC with differential to confirm or rule out infection and the use of either ultrasonography, CT scan, or laparoscopy.

Ectopic Pregnancy

Ectopic pregnancy can occur in any sexually active woman of childbearing age, especially those with a history of irregular menses. The patient experiences a sudden onset of spotting and persistent cramping in the lower quadrant that begins shortly after a missed period. On examination the patient shows signs of hemorrhage, shock, and lower abdominal peritoneal irritation that may be lateralized. On pelvic examination, the uterus is enlarged but smaller than anticipated from dates provided. The cervix is tender to motion, and a tender adnexal mass may be palpable. Diagnosis is confirmed by positive hCG and ultrasound. Serial quantitative serum hCGs may be useful. A ruptured ectopic pregnancy is a surgical emergency.

Peptic Ulcer Perforation

The patient complains of sudden onset of severe, intense, steady epigastric pain that radiates to the sides, back, or right shoulder. The patient may give a history of burning, gnawing pain that worsens with an empty stomach. The patient lies as still as possible. Epigastric tenderness will be present with palpation or percussion. Rebound tenderness is intense. The abdominal muscles are rigid, and bowel sounds may be absent. Diagnosis is confirmed by upright or lateral decubitus x-ray, showing air under the diaphragm or in the peritoneal cavity. Perforation is a surgical emergency.

Dissection of Aortic Aneurysm

This condition occurs more frequently in males and persons over 50 years of age, especially those with a history of uncon-

trolled hypertension. The patient experiences sudden onset of excruciating pain that may be felt in the chest or abdomen and may radiate to the legs and back. The patient will appear shocky. Vital signs will reflect impending shock, and there may be a deficit or difference in femoral pulses. Diagnosis can be made by CT or MRI. Additional tests include ECG and cardiac enzymes. This is a surgical emergency with a high mortality rate.

Peritonitis

The most common cause of peritonitis is perforation of the GI tract. It occurs more often in the elderly. The patient experiences sudden onset of severe pain that is diffuse and worsens with movement or coughing. On examination the patient will be guarding and have rebound tenderness. Bowel sounds will be decreased or absent. Diagnosis includes CBC with differential and abdominal x-rays.

Acute Pancreatitis

Acute pancreatitis is more common in patients with cholelithiasis or with a history of alcohol abuse. The pain is steady and boring in quality and is unrelieved by change of position. It is located in the LUQ and radiates to the back. The patient may also experience nausea, vomiting, diaphoresis, and will appear acutely ill. Abdominal distention, decreased bowel sounds, and diffuse rebound tenderness will be present on physical examination. The upper abdomen may show muscle rigidity. Examination of the lungs may reveal limited diaphragmatic excursion. Diagnostic testing includes CBC with differential, ultrasonography, x-rays, and serum amylase and lipase levels.

Mesenteric Adenitis

Adenovirus-induced (commonly *Yersinia*) adenopathy of the mesenteric lymph nodes may result in fever and RLQ abdominal pain that mimics appendicitis.

This condition is difficult to diagnose, but the white blood cell count is elevated and an abdominal x-ray will show abnormalities of the terminal ileus.

Cholecystitis/Lithiasis

Cholecystitis/lithiasis occurs more in adults than in children and more in females than in males. The pain is colicky in nature and progresses to a constant pain. The patient complains of pain in the RUQ, which may radiate to the right scapular area. The typical pain of cholelithiasis is constant, progressively rising to a plateau and falling gradually. The patient may also experience nausea and vomiting and give a history of dark urine and/or light stools. On physical examination, the patient will be tender to palpation or percussion in the RUQ. The gallbladder is palpable in about half the cases of cholecystitis. Painful splinting of respiration during deep inspiration (Murphy's sign) is frequently present with cholecystitis. Diagnostic testing includes CBC with differential, ultrasonography, x-rays, and serum amylase and lipase levels.

Ureterolithiasis

The patient complains of sudden onset of excruciating intermittent colicky pain that may progress to a constant pain. The pain is in the lower abdomen and flank and radiates to the groin. The patient may also experience nausea, vomiting, abdominal distention, chills, and fever. There is CVA tenderness on examination along with increased sensitivity in lumbar and groin areas. Hematuria and increased frequency of urination may be present. Diagnostic testing includes urinalysis, intravenous pyelography (IVP), or ultrasonography.

UTI/Pyelonephritis

Abdominal pain associated with urinary tract infection or pyelonephritis is common in children and may be the only presenting complaint. Urinalysis and culture and sensitivity is done to confirm the diagnosis (see Chapter 6, Common Problems of the Genitourinary System).

Pelvic Inflammatory Disease (PID/Salpingitis)

PID occurs most commonly in women under age 35 who are sexually active and have more than one sexual partner. Infection results from organisms transmitted by intercourse, by childbirth, or with abortion. PID is most often caused by *Chlamydia trachomatis* and *Neisseria gonorrhea*. Infection begins intravaginally in most cases and then spreads upward, causing salpingitis. The tubal infection produces an exudate, and, as it spreads, peritonitis can result. Onset is usually shortly after menses. Patients have lower abdominal pain that becomes progressively more severe. On examination, abdominal tenderness, cervical motion tenderness (CMT), and adnexal tenderness (usually bilateral) is present. With peritonitis, patients may also have guarding and rebound tenderness. Patients may also have a fever, irregular bleeding, vaginal discharge, or vomiting. WBC and ESR are usually elevated. Cultures and Gram staining can assist with diagnosis.

Obstruction

Obstruction occurs most often in the newborn, the elderly, and those with recent GI surgery. The patient presents with a sudden onset of crampy pain, usually in the umbilical area of epigastrium. Vomiting occurs early with small intestinal obstruction and late with large bowel obstruction. Obstipation (the absence of stools) occurs with complete obstruction, but diarrhea may be present with partial obstruction. Hyperactive, high-pitched bowel sounds may be present in small bowel obstruction. A fecal mass may be palpable in lower obstruction. Abdominal distention may be present. The rectum will be empty on digital examination. Diagnosis is confirmed with abdominal x-rays (supine and sitting).

Ileus

Ileus is associated with intra- or retroperitoneal infection, metabolic disturbances, and intra-abdominal surgery. The patient experiences abdominal distention, vomiting, obstipation, and cramps. On auscultation, there is minimal or absent peristalsis. Abdominal x-rays show gaseous distention of isolated segments of both the small and large intestine.

Intussusception

Bowel obstruction in children 2 months to 2 years of age usually occurs in the ileocecal region and classically presents with vomiting, colicky abdominal pain with drawing up of the legs, and eventual currant jelly stools. The onset is dramatic. The child is asleep or awake when suddenly he or she cries out with severe pain. The child twists and squirms; nothing gives any relief until, almost suddenly, there is a lull with absence of pain followed by a similar painful episode. The abdomen has a sausage-shaped mass that can be felt in the right upper quadrant. A positive fecal occult blood test (FOBT) is present.

Malrotation/Volvulus

Improper rotation and fixation of the duodenum and colon can cause an artery to obstruct, and the patient experiences ischemic necrosis. This disorder of the embryonic gut is usually seen in the first month of life. The infant presents with bilious emesis followed by abdominal distention and GI bleeding. Shock occurs from progression of the ischemia.

Henoch-Schoenlein Purpura

In Henoch-Schoenlein purpura, crampy, acute abdominal pain and bleeding are secondary to edema and hemorrhage of the intestinal wall. This disease is an IgA-mediated vasculitis that affects very small vessels. A urticarial rash occurring on the buttocks and lower extremities progresses to papular purpuric lesions. The laboratory findings show an elevated WBC count but normal platelet count. A mild increase in ESR, an increase in IgA concentration, and a negative ANA are also found.

Incarcerated Hernia

Incarcerated hernia occurs more commonly in the elderly. The patient complains of a constant severe pain in the RLQ or LLQ that worsens with coughing or straining. Physical examination reveals a hernia or mass that is non-reducible. Diagnosis is confirmed by UGI or x-ray. Surgical intervention is indicated.

Pneumonia

Pneumonia is a frequently overlooked etiology of abdominal pain in children. The pain is referred from right lower lobe pneumonia because of associated phrenic nerve irritation, which may cause muscular spasm, ileus, and pain referred to the right lower quadrant. The WBC count in pneumonia is typically higher than in early appendicitis.

CHRONIC CONDITIONS THAT CAUSE LOWER ABDOMINAL PAIN

Irritable Bowel Syndrome (IBS)

IBS begins in adolescent and young adult years. It produces crampy hypogastric pain that is of variable, infrequent duration. The pain is associated with bowel function, gas, bloating, and distention. Relief is often obtained with the passage of flatus or feces. The patient has a normal abdominal examination and is negative for FOBT (see Diarrhea, p. 187, and Constipation, p. 201). Consider a proctosigmoidoscopy or barium enema (BE) if onset is at middle age or older, the stool is positive for blood, there is a family history of colorectal cancer or polyps, or the patient fails to improve after 6 to 8 weeks of therapy.

Lactose Intolerance

Lactose intolerance produces crampy pain and diarrhea following consumption of milk or milk product foods (see Diarrhea, p. 188). It is caused by a deficiency in lactase, an enzyme that decreases in activity with increasing age. It is more common in Asians, Native Americans, and Blacks.

Diverticular Disease

Diverticular disease causes localized abdominal pain and tenderness. The patient will have a fever, elevated ESR, and leukocytosis. Perform a BE or proctoscopy/colonoscopy if there is rectal bleeding.

Simple Constipation

In adults, constipation is associated with infrequency or difficulty passing dry, hard stools and is associated with abdominal bloating.

Children with constipation frequently complain of abdominal pain. The pain is usually colicky in nature but may be dull and steady. The pain varies and is not persistent or progressively worsening. Mild, poorly localized periumbilical tenderness and, perhaps, guarding is reported. A fecal mass may be palpable.

Habitual Constipation

With habitual constipation, the patient presents with a lifelong history of constipation with onset as a young adult, has a normal physical examination, and does not have occult blood in the stool. Diet, activity, and bowel habits are often causally associated factors. Consider a proctoscopy or BE if you suspect a metabolic or systemic cause, the stool is heme-positive, or the patient is middle-aged or older or fails to respond to treatment.

Dysmenorrhea

Dysmenorrhea, a typically lower abdominal pain or cramping, occurs with menstruation. Dysmenorrhea can be classified as primary (no organic cause) or secondary (pathological cause). In primary dysmenorrhea, the onset is usually soon after menarche and gradually diminishes with age. The woman will have a normal pelvic examination. Secondary dysmenorrhea is associated with specific conditions and disorders such as endometriosis, pelvic inflammatory disease, cervical stenosis, and uterine fibroids. Obtain a gynecological consult and/or pelvic ultrasound for secondary dysmenorrhea, dysmenorrhea with increasing severity, or for abnormal findings on pelvic examination.

Uterine Fibroids

Fibroids produce pain related to the menstrual cycle and intercourse. The woman may experience dysfunctional uterine bleeding. On examination, palpable myomas are often present. Suspect this cause when there is no suspicion of other pelvic disorder. Order a pelvic ultrasound if ovarian or uterine neoplasm cannot be excluded. Obtain a gynecological consult for abnormal bleeding or severe symptoms.

Hernia

A hernia is a loop of intestine that has prolapsed through the inguinal wall or canal or through the abdominal musculature. The patient complains of intermittent localized pain that may be exacerbated with exertion or lifting. A physical examination will document the hernia, especially when the patient is instructed in maneuvers or positions to increase intra-abdominal pressure. Consider proctoscopy or BE if you suspect strangulation or bowel obstruction.

Ovarian Cysts

Ovarian cysts occur most commonly in young women and produce adnexal pain. The cysts may be palpable, late-cycle (corpus luteum) cysts. A pelvic ultrasound is indicated. Ovarian cysts can become quite large before producing symptoms.

Abdominal Wall Disorder

With abdominal wall disorder, the patient may present with a history of trauma. Ecchymosis or swelling may be visible. The patient may complain of pain with rectus muscle stress. GI/GU symptoms are absent. A hernia may be palpable. Obtain a CT scan if internal disease cannot be excluded.

CHRONIC CONDITIONS THAT CAUSE UPPER ABDOMINAL PAIN

Esophagitis/ Gastroesophageal Reflux Disease (GERD)

With GERD, the patient complains of a burning, gnawing pain in the mid-epigastrium ("heartburn") that worsens with recumbency. Regurgitation of gastric contents or water brash (hypersalivation secondary to acid stimulation of lower esophagus) may also be a complaint. The pain typically occurs after eating or when lying down and may be relieved with antacids. The physical examination is negative. Consider an upper GI, x-ray, or endoscopy if symptoms are severe or the patient does not respond to therapy.

Peptic Ulcer

The patient complains of a burning or gnawing pain that occurs most often with an empty stomach, stress, and alcohol. The pain is relieved by food intake. Some patients describe the pain as a soreness, empty feeling, or hunger. Typical pain is steady, mild, or severe and located in the epigastrium. Complaints may be atypical in children and minimal in the elderly. There may be epigastric tenderness on pal-

pation. Endoscopy, UGI, and gastric analysis can be used for diagnosis.

Gastritis

Gastritis pain is a constant burning pain in the epigastric area that may be accompanied by nausea, vomiting, diarrhea, or fever. Alcohol, NSAIDs, and salicylates make the pain worse. Physical examination results are negative. No diagnostic testing is necessary if the patient responds to therapy.

Gastroenteritis

Gastroenteritis may occur at any age and produces a diffuse, crampy pain that is accompanied by nausea, vomiting, diarrhea, and fever. Hyperactive bowel sounds will be heard on auscultation. The condition usually resolves on its own, and no diagnostic testing is needed.

Functional Dyspepsia

Functional dyspepsia refers to GI symptoms in which a pathological condition is not present or does not entirely explain the clinical presentation, although altered physiological activity may be present. The patient has vague complaints of indigestion, heartburn, gaseousness, or fullness. The patient also complains of belching, abdominal distention, and occasionally nausea. The physical examination results are negative. Do a CBC and FOBT. Consider an upper and lower GI series if the patient also has dysphagia, weight loss, vomiting, or a change in the pattern of the symptoms.

Recurrent Abdominal Pain (RAP)

RAP usually presents in children 5 to 10 years of age, rarely after age 14. The patient complains of dull, colicky periumbilical pain that is intermittent, occurs daily, and lasts from 1 to 3 hours with complete recovery between episodes. The pain does not awaken the child from sleep but may interfere with the ability to fall asleep. The child may have a low-grade fever, pallor, headache, and constipation. A history of stress associated with school social activi-

ties, parental conflicts, or loss is frequently elicited. Physical examination results are essentially negative. Initial laboratory tests are CBC, ESR, urinalysis, FOBT, and stool for ova and parasites (O & P).

Text continued on p. 176

Table 5-3

Differential Diagnosis of Common Causes of Acute Abdominal Pain

Condition	History	Physical Findings	Diagnostic Studies
Appendicitis	10-20 years although it can occur at any age; patient complains of sudden onset of colicky pain that progresses to constant pain; pain may begin in epigastrium or periumbilicus and then later localize in the RLQ; pain worsens with movement or coughing; vomiting after the onset of pain is sometimes present	Patient lying still; involuntary guarding; tenderness in RLQ; other tests for peritoneal irritation positive; rebound tenderness; variation in presentation common, particularly with infants, children, and the elderly	CBC with differential, ultrasonography, CT scan, laparoscopy
Ectopic pregnancy	Women of childbearing age; sudden onset of spotting and persistent cramping in the lower quadrant that begins shortly after a missed period	Signs of hemorrhage, shock, and lower abdominal peritoneal irritation that may be lateralized; enlarged uterus; cervical motion tenderness; tender adnexal mass	Positive hCG, ultrasound; ruptured ectopic pregnancy is a surgical emergency
Peptic ulcer perforation	Sudden onset of severe intense, steady epigastric	Patient lying still; epigastric tenderness; rebound	Diagnosis confirmed by upright or lateral

Table 5-3

Differential Diagnosis of Common Causes of Acute Abdominal Pain—cont'd

Condition	History	Physical Findings	Diagnostic Studies
Peptic ulcer perforation—cont'd	pain that radiates to the sides, back, or right shoulder; past history of burning, gnawing pain that worsens with an empty stomach	tenderness; abdominal muscles rigid; bowel sounds may be absent	decubitus x-ray showing air under the diaphragm or in the peritoneal cavity; perforation is a surgical emergency
Dissection of aortic aneurysm	More frequent in the elderly, especially if hypertensive; sudden onset of excruciating pain that may be felt in the chest or abdomen and may radiate to the legs and back	Patient appears shocky, VS reflect impending shock; deficit or difference in femoral pulses	CT or MRI; additional tests include ECG and cardiac enzymes; surgical emergency
Peritonitis	Occurs more often in the elderly; sudden onset of severe pain that is diffuse and worsens with movement or coughing	Guarding; rebound tenderness; bowel sounds decreased or absent	CBC with differential; abdominal x-rays
Acute pancreatitis	History of cholelithiasis or alcohol abuse; pain is steady and boring in quality and is unrelieved by change of position; located in the LUQ and radiates to the back; nausea, vomiting, and diaphoresis	Patient appears acutely ill; abdominal distention, decreased bowel sounds, diffuse rebound tenderness; upper abdomen may show muscle rigidity; may have limited diaphragmatic excursion of lungs	CBC with differential; ultrasonography; x-rays; serum amylase and lipase levels
Mesenteric adenitis	Fever, pain in RLQ, other symptoms suggestive of appendicitis	Pain on palpation in RLQ, there may be pharyngitis, cervical adenopathy	CBC with differential; adenovirus found in tissue of surgical specimen

Continued

Table 5-3

Differential Diagnosis of Common Causes of Acute Abdominal Pain—cont'd

Condition	History	Physical Findings	Diagnostic Studies
Cholecystitis/lithiasis	Appears in adults more than in children, females more than males; colicky pain with progression to a constant pain; pain in the RUQ that may radiate to the right scapular area; pain of cholelithiasis is constant, progressively rising to a plateau and falling gradually; nausea, vomiting, history of dark urine and/or light stools	Tender to palpation or percussion in the RUQ; gallbladder palpable in about half the cases of cholecystitis; positive Murphy's sign	CBC with differential; ultrasonography; x-rays; serum amylase and lipase levels
Ureterolithiasis	Sudden onset, excruciating intermittent colicky pain that may progress to a constant pain; pain in the lower abdomen and flank and radiates to the groin; nausea, vomiting, abdominal distention, chills, and fever; increased frequency of urination	CVA tenderness; increased sensitivity in lumbar and groin areas; hematuria	Urinalysis; IVP; ultrasonography

Table 5-3

Differential Diagnosis of Common Causes of Acute Abdominal Pain—cont'd

Condition	History	Physical Findings	Diagnostic Studies
Urinary tract infection/ pyelonephritis	Urinary symptoms with UTI, back pain with pyelo-nephritis; infants present with fever, failure to thrive, irritability, toddlers com-plain of pain in abdomen; may not complain of dysuria or fre-quency	Altered voiding pattern, mal-odorous urine, fever	Urinalysis and culture, IVP
PID	Lower abdominal pain that be-comes pro-gressively more severe; may have irregular bleed-ing, vaginal dis-charge and vomiting; most common in sexu-ally active women	Abdominal tender-ness, CMT and adnexal tender-ness (usually bilateral); with peritonitis may also have guard-ing and rebound tenderness; fever and vaginal dis-charge common	WBC and ESR are usually elevated; cultures and Gram staining
Obstruction	Sudden onset of crampy pain usually in the umbilical area of epigastrium; vomiting occurs early with small intestinal ob-struction and late with large bowel obstruc-tion; obstipation or diarrhea	Hyperactive, high-pitched bowel sounds; fecal mass may be palpable; ab-dominal disten-tion; empty rectum on digital examination	Diagnosis con-firmed with ab-dominal x-rays (supine and sitting)
Ileus	Abdominal disten-tion, vomiting, obstipation, and cramps	Minimal or absent peristalsis on auscultation	Gaseous distention of isolated seg-ments of both the small and large intestine shown on x-rays

Continued

Table 5-3

Differential Diagnosis of Common Causes of Acute Abdominal Pain—cont'd

Condition	History	Physical Findings	Diagnostic Studies
Intussusception	Sudden onset pain in infant; occurs with sudden relief, then pain again	Fever, vomiting, currant jelly stools	Abdominal films
Malrotation/ volvulus	Seen in infants up to 1 month of age, irritability, pain	Bilious emesis, abdominal distention	Abdominal films
Henoch-Schoenlein purpura	2-8 years old	Rash on lower extremities/ buttocks; arthralgias; hematuria	CBC; ESR; serum IgA
Incarcerated hernia	More common in elderly; is constant severe pain in the RLQ or LLQ that worsens with coughing or straining	Hernia or mass that is non-reducible	UGI or x-ray
Pneumonia	2-5 years of age, may present only with abdominal pain and fever	Tachypnea, retractions, pallor, nasal flaring, crackles	CBC; chest x-ray

Table 5-4

Differential Diagnosis of Common Causes Of Chronic Lower Abdominal Pain

Condition	History	Physical Findings	Diagnostic Studies
Irritable bowel syndrome (IBS)	Begins in adolescence, young adult years; hypogastric pain; crampy, variable, infrequent, duration; associated with bowel function;	Normal exam; heme-negative stool	Proctosigmoidoscopy, BE if onset middle age/ older, stool positive for blood, family history of colorectal cancer or polyps, failure to

Table 5-4

Differential Diagnosis of Common Causes Of Chronic Lower Abdominal Pain—cont'd

Condition	History	Physical Findings	Diagnostic Studies
Irritable bowel syndrome (IBS)—cont'd	associated with gas, bloating, distention; relief with passage of flatus, feces		improve after 6-8 weeks therapy
Lactose intolerance	Crampy pain after eating milk or milk products	Negative PE	Trial elimination of offending foods
Diverticular disease	Localized pain; older patient	Abdominal tenderness; fever	BE; elevated ESR; proctoscopy/colonoscopy if rectal bleeding
Simple constipation	Colicky or dull and steady pain that does not progress and worsen	Fecal mass palpable, stool in rectum	None
Habitual constipation	Lifelong history; younger patient	Normal exam; heme-negative stool	Proctoscopy, BE if metabolic or systemic cause suspected, heme-positive stool, onset in middle age or beyond, failure to respond to treatment
Dysmenorrhea	Typical premenstrual pain onset soon after menarche, gradually diminishing with age	Normal pelvic exam	GYN consult; pelvic USG if secondary dysmenorrhea, increasing disability, abnormal pelvic exam
Uterine fibroids	Pain related to menses, intercourse	Palpable myomas; no suspicion of other pelvic disorder	Pelvic USG if ovarian or uterine neoplasm cannot be excluded; GYN consult if abnormal bleeding or severe symptoms

Continued

Table 5-4

Differential Diagnosis of Common Causes Of Chronic Lower Abdominal Pain—cont'd

Condition	History	Physical Findings	Diagnostic Studies
Hernia	Localized pain that increases with exertion or lifting	PE documents hernia	Proctoscopy, BE if suspect strangulation or bowel obstruction
Ovarian cyst(s)	Young woman	Adnexal pain and palpable ovarian cysts especially in late cycle (corpus luteum)	Pelvic USG
Abdominal wall disorder	History of trauma	Visible ecchymosis or swelling; palpable hernia pain with rectus muscle stress; no GI/GU symptoms	CT scan if internal disease cannot be excluded

Table 5-5

Differential Diagnosis Of Common Causes Of Chronic Upper Abdominal Pain

Condition	History	Physical Findings	Diagnostic Studies
Esophagitis/GERD	Burning, gnawing pain in the mid-epigastrium that worsens with recumbency; water brash; pain occurs after eating and may be relieved with antacids; in infant, failure to thrive, irritability, postprandial spitting and vomiting	Physical exam negative; in infants, weight loss, in some cases aspiration pneumonia	Upper GI, x-ray, or endoscopy if symptoms are severe or do not respond to therapy
Peptic ulcer	Burning or gnawing pain; soreness, empty feeling or hunger; occurs most often with an empty stomach, stress, and alcohol, and relieved by food intake; pain steady, mild, or severe and located in the epigastrium; may be atypical in children and minimal in the elderly	May be epigastric tenderness on palpation	Endoscopy; UGI; gastric analysis

Table 5-5

Differential Diagnosis Of Common Causes Of Chronic Upper Abdominal Pain

Condition	History	Physical Findings	Diagnostic Studies
Gastritis	Constant burning pain in the epigastric area that may be accompanied by nausea, vomiting, diarrhea, or fever; alcohol, NSAIDs, and salicylates make pain worse	Physical exam negative	No diagnostic testing necessary if the patient responds to therapy
Gastroenteritis	Occurs at any age and produces a diffuse crampy pain accompanied by nausea, vomiting, diarrhea, and fever	Hyperactive bowel sounds will be heard on auscultation; dehydration if severe	No diagnostic testing needed
Functional dyspepsia	Vague complaints of indigestion, heartburn, gaseousness, or fullness; belching, abdominal distention, and occasionally nausea	Physical exam negative	CBC, FOBT; may consider upper and lower GI if patient also has dysphagia, weight loss, vomiting, or change in pattern of symptoms
Recurrent abdominal pain (RAP)	Children 5-10 years old, history of environmental or psychological stress	Physical exam negative	CBC; urinalysis; ESR; FOBT; stool for O & P

Diarrhea

Next to respiratory disease, acute gastro-enteritis is the most common illness in families in the United States. Most cases are of viral origin and are self-limiting. In children, 50% are of viral origin, approximately 25% are from bacterial causes, and another 25% are of undetermined etiology. Diarrhea can be classified according to its pathophysiological pattern (osmotic, secretory, or exudative), its cause (infectious or noninfectious), or its duration (acute or chronic).

Osmotic or malabsorptive diarrhea occurs when nonabsorbable water-soluble solutes remain in the bowel and retain water. This can occur through damage to the intestinal microvillus membrane. The result is malabsorption of luminal solute with osmotic loss of free water into the gut lumen. This is the most common cause of chronic diarrhea in children. Lactose intolerance is an example of this kind of diarrhea. Ingestion of large amounts of sugar substitutes in diet foods, drinks, candies, and chewing gum can cause osmotic diarrhea through a combination of slow absorption and rapid small bowel motility.

Secretory diarrhea occurs when the balance between fluid secretion and absorption across the intestinal mucosa is altered. When there is a change in this balance produced by physiological causes, diarrhea occurs. The loss of water and electrolytes can be rapid and massive. Diarrhea caused by *Vibrio cholera* is a classic example.

Exudative diarrhea occurs in the presence of mucosal inflammation or ulceration, which results in an outpouring of plasma, serum proteins, blood, and mucus. The consequence is an increase in fecal bulk and fluidity. Many mucosal diseases such as regional enteritis, ulcerative colitis, and carcinoma can cause this exudative enteropathy.

DIAGNOSTIC REASONING: FOCUSED HISTORY

What does this patient mean by "diarrhea"?

Key Questions
- How frequent is the stool?
- What is the volume of stools?
- Are the stools formed or liquid?
- At what intervals does the diarrhea occur?

Frequency of stools. In the United States, typical bowel frequency occurs from 1 to 3 times a day to 2 to 3 times per week and varies considerably from person to person. Changes in stool frequency, consistency, or volume may indicate disease.

Stool volume and consistency. Processes involving the small bowel tend to produce large-volume watery stools that are relatively infrequent. Large bowel involvement, usually resulting from a bacterially induced inflammatory process, tends to produce more frequent and less watery stools.

Intervals. A history of acute diarrhea followed by continued or intermittently occurring episodes of loose stools, suggests malabsorption commonly caused by lactase deficiency exacerbated by ingestion of lactose in milk or milk products. Intermittent diarrhea alternating with constipation suggests irritable bowel syndrome (IBS).

Proximal colon symptoms. Proximal colon symptoms include large-volume, less frequent, more homogenous stools, without urgency or tenesmus (painful defecation), and suggest food intolerance or infectious or inflammatory disease.

Distal colon symptoms. Symptoms of small volume, frequency, urgency, tenesmus, incontinence, and mucus suggests proctocolitis, colon cancer, diverticular disease, or IBS.

If this is an infant, is there a risk of dehydration?

Key Questions

- How many wet diapers has the child produced in the last 24 hours?
- Does the infant seem thirsty?
- Does the child have tears when crying?

Wet diapers. Dehydration in infants and young children can occur quickly and with fatal consequences, especially in infants. Diagnosis and treatment must be done in a timely manner. A general rule of thumb to determine signs of dehydration in infants is fewer than six wet diapers per 24 hours or a period of longer than 4 hours without urination.

Thirst. Infants demonstrate their thirst with irritability, crying, and eagerness to drink fluid that is offered to them. When dehydrated, some infants will suck on a wet towel, and toddlers may seek water in the toilet bowl. Test for thirst by offering fluids at the visit either in a bottle or on a spoon. The child with mild dehydration will exhibit increased thirst, the moderately dehydrated child will be very thirsty, and, with severe dehydration, the child will continue to be very thirsty. If left untreated, a child may become stuporous and unresponsive and, therefore, may be unable to manifest thirst.

Tears. In mild dehydration, tears are present; in moderate dehydration, tears may be present or not; in severe dehydration, no tears are present.

If this is an adult, is there risk for dehydration?

Key Questions

- How many times have you urinated in the past 24 hours?
- Are you thirsty?
- Do you notice a dry mouth? Dry eyes?

Dehydration. Symptoms of dehydration in an adult are more related to the rate of fluid loss rather than the absolute degree of fluid loss. The degree of dehydration can be estimated by symptoms of thirst, dry mouth, or dry eyes, and frequency and volume of urination. Patients may also experience weakness.

Is this an acute or chronic problem?

Key Questions

- How long have you had the diarrhea?
- Have you had this problem before?

Acute diarrhea in adults. An acute onset of diarrhea in a previously healthy patient without signs or symptoms or other organ involvement suggests an infectious cause. Acute diarrhea in adults is commonly viral in origin. The viral illnesses are self-limited, and an aggressive diagnostic workup is not indicated. Acute diarrhea in adults usually has an abrupt onset and lasts less than 3 weeks. Most of the disorders cause some combination of abdominal pain, diarrhea, nausea, vomiting, fever, and tenesmus.

Acute diarrhea in children. Acute diarrhea in children is characterized by loose or liquid stools. A large quantity of fluid and electrolytes that become pooled in the intestinal lumen are lost as stool is expelled. The number of stools is usually increased, but this is not an essential manifestation. Severe or protracted diarrhea may lead to metabolic acidosis, dehydration, azotemia, and oliguria.

Diarrhea in the neonate and young infant is considered more serious than in the older child because of lower tolerance to associated fluid shifts and greater likelihood of associated infection or congenital anomaly.

Chronic diarrhea in adults. Diarrhea is chronic when it lasts more than 4 weeks. Unless the diarrhea is bloody or the patient has a systemic illness, the most common causes of chronic diarrhea are parasites, medications, IBS, lactose intolerance, and inflammatory bowel disease.

Chronic diarrhea in children. Chronic diarrhea in children is defined as diarrhea for longer than 3 weeks. Malabsorption disorders are the most common cause. The diarrhea is the result of ingesting solutes that cannot be digested or absorbed, such as lactose products or excessive intake of sorbitol.

Does the presence or absence of blood help me narrow the cause?

Key Questions
- Is there any noticeable blood in the stool or tissue? How much?
- What color is the blood?
- What color are the stools?

Blood in the stools. Bright red blood limited to small spots on the toilet tissue suggest that the source of bleeding is from hemorrhoids and not from a diarrheal process higher in the gastrointestinal tract. Since diarrhea and repeated cleansing of the rectum produce local irritation, minor bleeding from hemorrhoids is not uncommon and must be distinguished from true blood in the stool. Reports of blood in stool in acute diarrhea are suggestive of a bacterial pathogen, notably *Shigella*. The blood is red in color. In infants less than 6 months of age, blood in the stool is most commonly caused by cow's milk intolerance or anal fissures. In adults and children, chronic bloody diarrhea may indicate inflammatory bowel disease, dysentery, colitis, or an invasive organism. Blood that is red in color usually indicates lower GI bleeding, whereas dark or black stools (melena) typically indicates upper GI bleeding. However, bleeding from the small bowel or right colon can also produce melena.

Color of stools. Some patients believe they have blood in their stool based on stool color. Sources of black stools are blood, iron, charcoal, bismuth, licorice,

huckleberries, and lead. Sources of red or pink stools include blood, food (beets, cranberries, tomatoes, peppers), food coloring (breakfast cereals, jello-water), and drugs (anticoagulants, salicylates, rifampin, Pyridium pamoate, diazepam syrup, phenothalein in alkaline stool). Green-black stools are caused by grape-flavored drinks and iron. Dark gray stools occur with cocoa and chocolate ingestion. Pale gray or white stools are caused by cholestasis, obstructive jaundice, malabsorption, excessive milk ingestion, and antacid ingestion. Green stools are produced by bile salts and chlorophyll-containing vegetables such as spinach.

What does the presence or absence of pain tell me?

Key Questions
- Are you having any abdominal pain or gas with the diarrhea?
- Where is the pain?
- What does the pain feel like?
- Is the pain constant or does it come and go?
- Does the pain awaken you at night?
- Does the pain interfere with your activities? (e.g., work, sleep, eating)

Occurrence of pain. Diarrhea, with abdominal pain and flatulent stools, is characteristic of a malabsorptive process. Most self-limiting viral diarrheas cause some combination of abdominal pain, diarrhea, nausea, vomiting, fever, and tenesmus.

Abdominal pain is common when diarrhea is caused by infective bacteria in the colon, such as ingestion associated with food poisoning. *Giardia lamblia,* introduced by ingestion of contaminated water or the oral-fecal route, produces crampy abdominal pain and is frequently seen in children and diapered infants in day care where handwashing may not be done between diapering.

Location of pain. Generalized abdominal pain is produced by diffuse inflammation of the GI tract as occurs with Crohn's disease or abdominal cramping from infective diarrhea. The pain from ulcerative colitis may be perceived over the entire abdomen or localized to the lower quadrants. The pain associated with IBS is usually confined to the lower quadrants or over the sigmoid colon. Large intestine pain is felt in the lower abdominal quadrants, whereas small intestine pain is felt in the epigastric and umbilical areas.

Severity of pain. Self-limited diarrhea usually presents with cramping but not severe abdominal pain. Other causes of abdominal pain should be investigated (see Abdominal Pain, p. 147).

Sleep-related. Persistent diarrhea that awakens the patient from sleep usually indicates a serious organic disease, such as diabetes enteropathy or HIV enteropathy. The symptoms associated with IBS occur during the waking hours.

What do associated symptoms tell me?

Key Questions
- Do you have any fever? What was the highest fever? Did you measure the temperature?
- Do you have any vomiting?
- What occurred first—the diarrhea or the vomiting?

Fever. Patients often report having a "fever" when they have symptoms such as facial flushing, shaking chills, headache, malaise or muscle aches, or a sensation of warmth. These symptoms are usually not validated by measuring body temperature with a thermometer. Fever is a cardinal manifestation of disease. Gastrointestinal and respiratory infections are responsible for 80% of febrile illnesses.

Vomiting. Vomiting is often present early in the course of viral gastroenteritis (especially the Norwalk virus), food poisoning, and food-borne bacterial infection. Vomiting is one of the main causes of dehydration in acute diarrhea. Also, small bowel processes commonly associated with viral agents cause delayed gastric emptying and luminal distention, which often induces vomiting before the onset of diarrhea.

Occurrence of vomiting and diarrhea. When diarrhea occurs before the vomiting, suspect a bacterial etiology.

Could this be caused by exposure to others or to contaminated food?

Key Questions
- Does the child attend day care?
- Are any of the other children in day care ill?
- Have you been around others who have similar symptoms?

Day care attendance. Children who attend day care are at greater risk to acquire many bacterial infections as the causes are transmitted through oral-fecal contamination and diapering.

Others with similar symptoms. Others who are ill with similar symptoms is common in food-borne infections acquired when food is served at social gatherings such as picnics. Patients may not always know if others were made ill, especially when onset of diarrhea occurs 1 to 2 hours after ingestion.

Could this be the result of exposure to animals?

Key Questions
- What pets do you have?
- Have you had contact with or have you handled dogs, cats, or turtles?

Exposure to infectious agents through animal contact. *Campylobacter jejuni* infection can be acquired from infected dogs or cats. Infected turtles are a source of *Salmonella*.

Could this be caused by exposure to contaminated water?

Key Question
• Have you traveled recently? Where?

Recent travel. Travel outside of the United States carries the potential to acquire enterotoxigenic *E. coli* or less commonly, *G. lamblia, Salmonella, Shigella, C. jejuni,* or *Entamoeba histolytica.* Camping exposes individuals to *Giardia* and *Campylobacter* through untreated water. Outbreaks of diarrhea caused by *Cryptosporidium* have been linked to contaminated water in urban areas of the United States.

Could sexual activities explain the diarrhea?

Key Question
• Do your sexual practices include anal sex? Suspect *Shigella* infection in patients who engage in anal sex, particularly homosexual males. Accompanying pain, tenesmus, and the passage of mucus suggest the presence of proctitis.

Could this be the result of an immune problem?

Key Questions
• Have you been diagnosed with a immune system problem?
• Do you have frequent colds or other illnesses?
• Are you receiving chemotherapy?

Immunocompromised host. IgA and IgG deficiencies are frequent causes of chronic diarrhea in children. Patients with a compromised immune system from AIDS or chemotherapy often develop enteropathy.

Could this be caused by medications?

Key Questions
• Have you taken any antibiotics recently? Which one(s)?
• What prescription medications are you currently taking?
• What over-the-counter medications/preparations are you currently using?

Recent treatment with antibiotics. Pseudomembranous enterocolitis caused by *Clostridium difficile* has been reported in persons who have been recently treated with antibiotics, most commonly ampicillin, clindamycin, or cephalosporins. Pseudomembranous enterocolitis a very serious disorder that can lead to paralytic ileus. More often antibiotics disturb the normal flora of the gut, leading to diarrhea.

Medications. Antacids that contain magnesium, antibiotics, methyldopa, digitalis, beta blockers, systemic anti-inflammatory agents, colchicine, quinidine, phenothiazine, high dose salicylates, and laxatives can cause diarrhea.

Could this be related to a surgical procedure?

Key Question
• Have you had any recent surgery?

Recent GI surgery. GI surgery can result in dumping syndrome following ingestion of meals. Inadequate mixing and digestion takes place in the stomach, resulting in rapid transit and diarrhea. Anatomical derangement from surgery can also cause stagnant loops of bowel. This stagnation leads to bacterial overgrowth and results in diarrhea. Extensive bowel resection can produce short bowel syndrome, which results in diarrhea from malabsorption.

Is this diet related?

Key Questions

- How much apple juice or how many sodas do you drink in a day?
- Do you drink milk or eat milk products?
- Do you eat wheat products?
- What have you had to eat in the last 3 days?

Excessive intake of high carbohydrate fluids. Ingestion of large amounts of apple juice and nonabsorbable fillers such as sorbitol may lead to malabsorptive diarrhea. Bacterial contamination of non-pasteurized apple juice can cause diarrhea.

Lactose intolerance. Ingestion of specific disaccharides, such as lactose, produces a malabsorptive osmotic diarrhea.

Cow's milk protein/soy protein hypersensitivity. Diarrhea, vomiting, colic, occult or grossly bloody stools, and white cells within the stools that begin within 2 to 3 weeks after starting either cow's milk or soy formulas may be caused by protein hypersensitivity.

Celiac sprue (gluten enteropathy). Gluten enteropathy is manifested by increasing frequency, looseness, paleness, and bulkiness of stool within 3 to 6 months of dietary intake of wheat, rye, barley, or oat products. Patients have a hypersensitivity reaction to the protein in these grains.

Starvation stools. History of this condition includes a diarrhea that persists for 2 to 3 weeks. Stools are loose because the liquid low-fiber diet used to ease symptoms of acute diarrhea is continued for too long. Health care providers may neglect to tell patients or parents to resume a regular diet once an acute diarrhea begins to resolve.

Could this be caused by food preparation problems?

Key Questions

- Have you eaten raw or undercooked poultry, shellfish, beef recently?
- Have you had unpasteurized milk recently?
- Do you prepare poultry and/or beef on the same surface as other foods?
- Is anyone else you know ill with similar symptoms?

Dietary exposure to infectious agents. Undercooked poultry is a potential cause of *Salmonella* or *C. jejuni* diarrhea. Undercooked beef or unpasteurized milk are food sources that contain *Escherichia coli* 0157:H7. Raw shellfish is a potential for source of Norwalk virus. Food can be contaminated through bacteria that remain on incompletely cleaned food preparation surfaces.

Other persons ill. Food poisoning should be considered if diarrhea develops in two or more persons following ingestion of the same food. Such multiple occurrences suggest ingestion of infected food or toxic substances (e.g., lead, mercury).

Is there any family predisposition that may point to a cause?

Key Questions

- Have you or anyone in your family been diagnosed with cystic fibrosis?
- Does anyone in the family have a history of chronic diarrhea, ulcerative colitis, or inflammatory bowel disease?

Family history of cystic fibrosis. Cystic fibrosis is the most common genetic disease in Caucasians. It has an autosomal recessive mode of inheritance. The condition leads to fat malabsorption and produces fatty, foul-smelling diarrhea.

Family history of diarrheal illnesses. Inflammatory bowel disease is genetically linked.

DIAGNOSTIC REASONING: FOCUSED PHYSICAL EXAMINATION

Inspect General Appearance

Observe the patient's general appearance. Diarrhea should be considered a symptom in all instances, and principal attention should be directed to determination and correction of the cause.

Assess Hydration Status (Table 5-6)

Assessment of hydration status is the most important aspect of physical examination in the child. Dehydration in otherwise healthy adults is uncommon unless the diarrhea is very severe. Hydration is also an important consideration in older adults and the chronically ill and in those persons who cannot replace fluid losses with oral intake. In the presence of hypernatremia, the state of dehydration may be found to be greater than suggested by physical examination because extracellular fluid volume tends to be preserved at the expense of intracellular volume.

Indicators of Hydration Status

Mucous membranes. The earliest clinical sign of dehydration is dryness of mu-

---

Table 5-6

Determining Hydration Status

SIGNS/SYMPTOMS	MILD DEHYDRATION	MODERATE DEHYDRATION	SEVERE DEHYDRATION
Estimated fluid deficit (% of body weight)*	<5	>6-9%	>10%
Estimated fluid deficit (mL/kg)	30-50 mL/kg	60-90 mL/kg	More than 100 mL/kg
Thirst	Increased	Marked increase	Very marked increase
Blood pressure (peripherally)	Normal	Postural drop only	Low or absent
Pulse (peripheral)	Normal	Rapid	Rapid, thready pulse
Heart rate	Mildly elevated	Elevated	Greatly elevated
Mucous membranes	Thick saliva	Dry	Very dry
Eyes	Normal	Sunken	Deeply sunken
Tears when crying	Present	Absent	Absent
Skin turgor	Normal	Tenting	None
Fontanel	Normal	Sunken	Very sunken
Urine output	Mildly decreased	Decreased	Markedly decreased or absent
Affect/sensorium	Normal	Restlessness/ irritability	Lethargy/coma

*% body weight loss = $\dfrac{(\text{normal weight} - \text{present weight})}{\text{normal weight}} \times 100$.

cous membranes. Hyperventilation with mouth-breathing may dry the mucous membranes of the mouth in the absence of dehydration. Recent vomiting makes the mucous membranes appear moist. The patient may also have halitosis.

Tissue turgor. Turgor reflects the amount of fluid in the interstitial spaces and is best assessed on the thigh, chest, and abdomen. Abdominal testing alone may be misleading because distention may mask the loss of turgor. Obese children may not appear to have loss of skin turgor because of the elasticity of their skin.

Fontanel. The fontanel, if still open, is best assessed with a child in an upright position. The normal fontanel may feel tense in the infant who is supine. In the crying child, physiological bulging occurs only during expiration; this bulging disappears when the child relaxes or inspires. The fontanel will be sunken in a dehydrated state.

Peripheral perfusion. Blanching of the nail bed with pressure and quick refill of capillary blood is normal. In dehydration, it takes longer for the blood to reappear in the tissue.

Urine output/specific gravity. In a mildly dehydrated child, the output decreases with slight increase in specific gravity. In a moderately dehydrated child, the output is decreased and the specific gravity is increased. In a severely dehydrated child, the urinary output is decreased to oliguria and the specific gravity is markedly increased, up to 1.030.

Take Temperature

An elevated temperature increases insensible water loss and may lead to more rapid dehydration. Presence of a fever in acute diarrhea indicates viral or bacterial infection. Fever in chronic diarrhea points to inflammatory causes.

The generally accepted normal basal body temperature is 37° C (98.6° F) determined orally or 0.6° C (1° F) higher rectally. Fever is generally accepted as any oral temperature above 37.8° C (100° F).

Weigh Patient and Note Persistent or Involuntary Weight Loss

Lactose intolerance, cystic fibrosis, intestinal malabsorption, infectious diarrhea, and inflammatory bowel disease can cause weight loss to occur. These persons have adequate or even increased food intake, but they cannot absorb enough nutrients to sustain normal nutrition. In children, this can cause failure to thrive and interruption of growth. In adults, colonic neoplasm can cause partial obstruction and diarrhea, and weight loss may be evident.

Observe Abdominal Contour

Abdominal distention may be associated with an ileus as in enteritis or gaseous dilation resulting from malabsorption. A scaphoid abdomen may be seen in children with severe dehydration.

Auscultate the Abdomen

The major objective is to detect the presence of bowel sounds anywhere in the abdomen. Listen in all four quadrants. The absence of bowel sounds is established only after 5 minutes of continuous listening. Bowel sounds that are high-pitched are heard with peristaltic rushes found in enteritis and secretory diarrhea. Bowel sounds are diminished or absent with necrotizing enterocolitis.

Palpate the Abdomen for Tenderness

Peritonitis may cause diarrhea as a result of inflammation and local enteric irritation. Signs of peritoneal irritation include a rigid abdomen, rebound tenderness (Blumberg's sign), and positive signs from the following tests: iliopsoas muscle test, obturator muscle test, and heel jar test (Markle's sign) (see Abdominal Pain, pp. 158 and 159). Tenderness is uncommon in self-limiting diarrhea. Localized right lower quadrant tenderness in a "sick" patient with acute diarrhea may indicate appendicitis, Crohn's disease, right-sided diverticulitis, or carcinoma. Localized left lower quadrant tenderness suggests diverticulitis, fecal impaction, colon cancer, and various causes of proctocolitis. Localized pain in chronic diarrhea can also occur with IBS.

Perform a Digital Rectal Examination

Look for fissures, lacerations, and feel for impacted stool. Impacted stool may be felt as a puttylike mass that fills the rectum and extends upward. Also obtain a stool sample for occult blood testing and for laboratory studies. Observe stool on finger for color and presence of blood.

Palpate Lymph Nodes

Evidence of systemic disease should be assessed. Chronic diarrhea in patients who have lymphadenopathy is associated with lymphoma and AIDS.

LABORATORY AND DIAGNOSTIC STUDIES

Laboratory or diagnostic studies are not necessary if the patient appears to have a viral or toxigenic bacterial infection because the disease is usually mild and self-limiting. Reserve stool cultures and examine for ova and parasites in patients who appear relatively ill, with signs of invasive diarrhea, persistent diarrhea, or have a history of suspected parasite infection.

Fecal Leukocytes

Fecal leukocyte detection is an easy and inexpensive test that is 75% specific for bacterial diarrhea. Leukocytes are found in inflammatory diarrheal disease and are present in bacterial infections that invade the intestinal wall (*E. coli, Shigella,* and *Salmonella* species). Leukocytes are also present in diarrhea from ulcerative colitis and Crohn's disease as well as antibiotic-related diarrhea. They are not seen in viral gastroenteritis, parasitic diarrhea, *Salmonella* carrier states, or enterotoxigenic bacterial diarrheas. Obtain a small fleck of mucus or stool. Do not allow the specimen to dry. Place the specimen on a slide, with two drops of Loffler's methylene blue stain and wait 2 minutes. Microscopic white blood cells and red blood cells indicate the presence of *Shigella,* enterohemorrhagic *E. coli,* enteropathogenic *E. coli, Campylobacter, C. difficile,* or other inflammatory or invasive diarrhea.

Fecal Occult Blood Testing (FOBT)

FOBT is used to test for occult blood in the stool. A stool sample is placed on a filter paper, and an activating solution is applied. A positive test is indicated by the appearance of a color (usually blue or green). A positive result indicates the presence of occult blood. RBCs occur more often in diarrhea caused by enteropathic bacteria or protozoa. A 3-day series of stool samples is used to screen for colon cancer and is recommended annually in adults age 50 years and older.

Fecal Fat

A 72-hour fecal fat analysis is done by instructing the patient to have a daily dietary intake of 100 g of fat for 3 days before and during a 72-hour period of stool collection. In children, a fat retention coefficient is determined. An abnormal result is greater than 6 g/day in the stool on a 80- to 100-g diet of fat and indicates a malabsorption syndrome.

D-Xylose Absorption Test

D-xylose absorption test is used to determine if diarrhea is caused by malabsorption or maldigestion. Blood is taken before the patient ingests the D-xylose. The patient is then asked to drink a fluid containing 25 g of D-xylose. Repeat venipuncture to obtain blood is done in exactly 2 hours for adults and 1 hour for children. Urine is collected approximately 5 hours after ingestion of fluid. Blood and urine levels are subsequently evaluated. An abnormal result is found if less than 4.5 g of the D-xylose is excreted in a 5-hour urine collection, and blood levels are less than 25 to 40 mg/dl in adults (30 mg/dl in children). The abnormal result means the diarrhea is caused by malabsorption.

Stool pH

The pH of the stool specimen is determined by using litmus strips. A pH of 5.5 indicates lactose or other carbohydrate malabsorption. A normal stool pH is neutral or weakly alkaline.

Wet Mount

Wet mounts are useful for trophozoites, cysts, ova, and certain helminth larvae. Obtain a sample of feces on a wooden applicator stick, mix with a drop of saline, and add iodine contrast to view and examine under a microscope. *V. cholera* can be identified by using darkfield microscopy. The characteristic darting motility of vibrios can be recognized in fresh wet preparations.

C. Difficile Toxin Assay

This assay detects *C. difficile* toxin in the stool, which is diagnostic of clostridial enterocolitis. The clostridia bacterium releases a toxin that causes necrosis of the colonic epithelium.

Stool Culture

Stool culture is used to detect common bacteria, such as Enterococcus, *E. coli,* *Proteus, Pseudomonas, Staphylococcus aureus, Candida albicans, Bacteroides,* and *Clostridia.* Special enriching techniques or media are necessary to look for some agents. Pathogenic bacteria are *Salmonella, Shigella, Campylobacter, Yersinia,* pathogenic *E. coli, Staphylococcus,* and *C. difficile.*

Stool for Ova and Parasites (O & P)

Stool can be tested for the presence of parasites. Fresh stool is required to preserve the trophozoites of some parasites. Common parasites are *Ascaris* (hookworm), *Strongyloides* (tapeworm), and *Giardia* (protozoans).

Indirect Hemagglutinin Assay (IHA)

The IHA detects antibodies to *E. histolytica.* A positive titer is >1:128.

CBC with Differential

A CBC with differential should be obtained in severely ill or dehydrated patients to screen for infection. Infection is indicated with increased leukocytes. Microcytic hypochromic anemia (MCHC <30 g/dL; MCV <85 fL) may indicate the presence of chronic disease. Most bloody diarrhea produces an elevated platelet count as an acute phase reactant in an inflammatory process. In hemolytic uremic syndrome, the platelet count may be normal or low.

Peripheral Blood Smear

Peripheral blood smear is an examination of the cellular contents of the blood under a microscope using a variety of stains. Hemoglobin can be roughly estimated by the depth of staining present. This quantitative analysis assists in characterizing a number of conditions, including hemolytic anemia associated with hemolytic uremic syndrome. In hemolytic uremic syndrome the peripheral smear shows characteristic schistocytes.

Blood Urea Nitrogen (BUN), Creatinine

BUN and creatinine tests are indicated in severely ill or dehydrated patients to ascertain adequate kidney functioning. Dehydration is a cause of pre-renal failure. Hemolytic uremic syndrome will cause impaired renal function.

Endoscopic Studies

Further endoscopic diagnostic studies such as flexible sigmoidoscopy should be considered when the cause of diarrhea is not determined or when the diarrhea lasts for longer than a week.

DIFFERENTIAL DIAGNOSIS

ACUTE DIARRHEA

Viral Gastroenteritis

Viral gastroenteritis presents with explosive onset of diarrhea, vomiting, low-grade fever, anorexia, and myalgia. Symptoms last for a week or less. Norwalk virus is a major agent and is usually seen in school-aged children and adults. Rotavirus is the most common cause of diarrhea in children 6 to 24 months and is usually seen in the winter.

Shigella

Shigella presents with acute diarrhea that contains mucus and blood. The patient has up to 7 days of watery diarrhea, then toxins are produced that result in ulceration, mucosal irritability, and frequent bowel movements. Stools are yellow or green with undigested food, mucus, and blood. Leukocytes and red blood cells are seen in the stools. It is the second most common cause of diarrhea in children 6 to 10 years old and is common in day care settings. Upper respiratory infection symptoms may also be present.

Food Poisoning With *Staphylococcus* or *Bacillus aureus*

Staphylococcal or *Bacillus aureus* food poisoning causes explosive diarrhea 2 to 6 hours after eating. High attack rates are seen among persons eating contaminated food (improperly stored meats or custard-filled pastries). Cramping and vomiting in addition to diarrhea are present. There usually is no fever. The diarrhea lasts 18 to 24 hours, and the person recovers quickly. However, the condition could be life threatening in the elderly and in persons with other serious illness.

Food Poisoning With *C. perfringens*

C. perfringens causes severe diarrhea 8 to 20 hours after eating. The patient complains of crampy abdominal pain and diarrhea. The stool is watery and non-bloody. Nausea, vomiting, and fever may be present but are less common. The diarrhea usually lasts for less than 3 days.

Salmonella

Salmonella causes severe diarrhea with fever. *Salmonella* is seen 20 times more commonly in patients with AIDS, sickle cell disease, or reticuloendothelial dysfunction. The incubation period is 3 to 40 days with insidious or abrupt onset. The patient has fever, anorexia, and weight loss. GI symptoms are first, then a fever, abdominal cramps, and vomiting appear. Stools are green, loose, slimy, and have the odor of spoiled eggs. Rarely is blood present.

Campylobacter

Campylobacter infection causes fever, headache, myalgia for 12 to 24 hours, then diarrhea develops. Two thirds of patients have watery diarrhea and a third have bloody dysentery. Incubation period is 2 to 5 days. The patient has abdominal cramping, pain, and fever, and the diarrhea contains mucus and blood. The condition may mimic appendicitis because of mesenteric lymphadenitis. Toxic megacolon and colonic hemorrhages can occur, especially if antimotility agents have been used.

Vibrio cholera

Vibrio cholera causes severe watery diarrhea without a preceding illness. It usually occurs in epidemics. The onset is acute, usually 8 to 18 hours after ingestion of contaminated seafood, water, or food prepared in contaminated water. Diarrhea resolves in 3 to 5 days. The essential element in cholera is the speed at which fluid is lost. This quick loss of fluid and dehydration can lead to death within hours. Red and white blood cells are not seen on stool examination.

Enterotoxic *E. coli*

E. coli causes moderate amounts of non-bloody diarrhea. This develops acutely 8 to 18 hours after ingestion of contaminated food/water and lasts for typically 24 to 48 hours. The patient experiences cramping and abdominal pain with the diarrhea. The organism (Gram-negative rod) is transmitted by the fecal-oral route. It is spread through contaminated water or incompletely cooked food that was cleaned in contaminated water or through incompletely cooked beef, especially ground hamburger meat, Diagnosis can be confirmed by fecal leukocytes or stool culture.

Entamoeba histolytica

Diarrhea caused by this parasite presents with large amounts of bloody diarrhea and abdominal cramping and vomiting that develop acutely 12 to 24 hours after ingestion of contaminated food or water. The diagnosis is confirmed through indirect hemagglutinin assay (IHA). Antibodies to *E. histolytica* are formed; a positive titer is >1:128.

Antibiotic-Induced

This condition produces a mild, watery diarrhea and is caused by taking antibiotics, especially ampicillin, tetracycline, lincomycin, clindamycin, and chloramphenicol. The patient often complains of crampy abdominal pain. Diagnosis is through history and clinical findings.

Pseudomembranous Colitis

Pseudomembranous colitis is most often produced by *Clostridium difficile*. This diarrhea is induced by antibiotics, most commonly ampicillin, clindamycin, or cephalosporins. An acute inflammatory bowel disorder occurs with symptoms that range from transient mild diarrhea to active colitis with bloody diarrhea, abdominal pain, fever, and leukocytosis. Symptoms usually begin during a course of antibiotic therapy but may begin 1 to 10 days after treatment is completed. Diagnosis is established by sigmoidoscopy or colonoscopy. The diagnosis is confirmed by *C. difficile* toxin assay or stool culture.

Hemolytic Uremic Syndrome (HUS)

HUS is seen in children and is usually preceded by a gastrointestinal illness. The number one bacterial cause of HUS in the United States is now *E. coli* 0157:H7 The patient presents with a history of bloody diarrhea, fever, and irritability. Initially, laboratory blood values are essentially normal except that the platelet count is normal or low. The stool culture is negative. A peripheral blood smear reveals schistocytes, confirming the diagnosis. Fragmented RBCs are often seen on the peripheral smear before complications of renal involvement occur. The child may have a sudden onset of acute renal failure. Renal function tests will be altered.

CHRONIC DIARRHEA

Irritable Bowel Syndrome (IBS)

IBS is characterized by alternating periods of constipation and diarrhea. Patients often experience mucus in stools. It is commonly seen in young and middle-aged women with a history of intermittent diarrhea. Patients often present with complaints of constipation rather than diarrhea. The patient complains of abdominal pain in the left lower quadrant, although it can occur anywhere. The pain seldom occurs at night, does not awaken the patient, and is commonly present in the morning. The patient may have rectal urgency and abdominal distention. There is no weight loss, the patient is afebrile, and the colon may be tender on palpation. IBS is a diagnosis of exclusion, and sigmoidoscopy or proctoscopy is used to rule out other disorders.

Ulcerative Colitis

Ulcerative colitis causes proctitis with rectal bleeding, tenesmus, and the passage of mucopus. Abdominal cramping is common but abdominal pain and tenderness is not a common finding. The greater the extent of colon involvement the more likely the patient is to suffer from diarrhea.

Crohn's Disease

Crohn's disease is an inflammatory bowel disease that presents with abdominal cramping, tenderness, rectal bleeding, and diarrhea. The disease may produce chronic, bloody diarrhea and cause failure to thrive in children. The patient may have a fever. Weight loss is common because of malabsorption or a reduced intake of food used to minimize postprandial symptoms. Diagnosis is made through colonoscopy and biopsy.

Carbohydrate Malabsorption; Lactose Intolerance

Malabsorption and/or lactose intolerance causes the patient to experience diarrhea, bloating, and increased flatus. Ingestion of specific disaccharides, such as lactose or sorbitol, exacerbates the episodes of diarrhea. A trial of elimination of of-fending foods often confirms the clinical diagnosis.

Fat Malabsorption

Fat malabsorption is seen with patients who have cystic fibrosis or who have vitamin A, D, or K deficiency. Patients with cystic fibrosis have foul, pale, bulky diarrhea that is greasy, oily, and consistent with steatorrhea. The diarrhea usually precedes lung involvement. Laboratory testing for fat malabsorption includes a 72-hour fecal fat analysis.

Toddler Diarrhea

Toddler diarrhea is described as abnormal amounts of formless stools with mucus in children 1 to 3 years of age. Symptoms rarely persist beyond 4 to 5 years old. The diarrhea is chronic and nonspecific with 3 to 4 stools per day, some containing mucus. Physical examination and growth are within normal limits for the child's age. This is a diagnosis of exclusion and other causes of chronic diarrhea must first be ruled out.

Celiac Sprue/Protein Hypersensitivity

This diarrhea causes increasing stool frequency, looseness, paleness, and bulkiness 3 to 6 months after dietary intake of wheat, rye, and other grains. Patients have a hypersensitivity reaction to the protein in wheat, rye, barley, and oats. Children appear lethargic, irritable, and anorexic.

Giardia

Giardia is the number one parasite causing chronic diarrhea in children in the United States and can be contracted through travel both in and outside of the country. Patients experience watery, foul-smelling diarrhea, abdominal pain, distention, and gas.

Cryptosporidium Species/*Isospora belli*

These are parasites that produce recurrent episodes of non-bloody diarrhea with variable amounts of water. The volume can be massive. The organisms are transmitted by the fecal-oral route and are spread through ingestion of contaminated water or direct oral-anal contact.

Post-Gastrectomy Dumping Syndrome

This syndrome occurs following GI surgery. The condition can occur whenever the pyloric mechanism is disrupted by pyloroplasty, gastroduodenostomy, or gastrojejunostomy. The diarrhea occurs after meals because of increased transit of food through the colon. Patients may experience associated symptoms, including diaphoresis and tachycardia.

Diabetic Enteropathy

Diabetic enteropathy occurs in patients with diabetes. Patients may experience nocturnal diarrhea, post-prandial vomiting, and fatty stools from malabsorption. The condition is a diagnosis of exclusion in diabetic persons.

HIV Enteropathy

HIV enteropathy has an insidious onset and is recurrent. Patients have large amounts of non-bloody diarrhea and mild-to-moderate nausea and vomiting. It is caused by direct infection of mucosa and neuronal cells in GI system. Patients will demonstrate other HIV-related symptoms and lymphadenopathy.

Medication Induced

Diarrhea can occur as a result of taking drugs. The most common ones are antacids that contain magnesium, antibiotics, methyldopa, digitalis, beta blockers, systemic anti-inflammatory agents, colchicine, quinidine, phenothiazine, high-dose salicylates, and laxatives.

Text continued on p. 195

Table 5-7

Differential Diagnosis of Common Causes of Acute Diarrhea

Condition	History	Physical Findings	Diagnostic Studies
Viral gastroenteritis (viral agent—Norwalk, rotavirus, etc.)	Abrupt onset 6-12 hours after exposure; non-bloody, watery diarrhea; lasts <1 week; nausea/vomiting, fever, abdominal pain, tenesmus	In children may see severe dehydration; hyperactive bowel sounds, diffuse pain on abdominal palpation	None

Continued

Table 5-7

Differential Diagnosis of Common Causes of Acute Diarrhea—cont'd

Condition	History	Physical Findings	Diagnostic Studies
Shigella (Gram-negative rod; fecal-oral transmission; common in day care setting; common in gay bowel syndrome)	Acute onset 12-24 hours after exposure; lasts 3-7 days; large amounts bloody diarrhea with abdominal cramping and vomiting	Lower abdominal tenderness, hyperactive bowel sounds, no peritoneal irritation	Fecal leukocytes; positive stool culture
S. aureus food poisoning (Gram-positive cocci; from improperly stored meats or custard-filled pastries)	Acute onset 2-6 hours after ingestion; lasts 18-24 hours; large amounts watery, non-bloody diarrhea; cramping and vomiting	Hyperactive bowel sounds	Fecal leukocytes; negative stool culture
Clostridium perfringens food poisoning (Gram-positive rod; from contaminated food)	Acute onset 8-20 hours after ingestion; lasts 12-24 hours; large amounts watery, non-bloody diarrhea; abdominal pain and cramping	Hyperactive bowel sounds, diffuse pain on abdominal palpation	Fecal leukocytes; negative anaerobic cultures of stool
Salmonella food poisoning (Gram-negative bacilli; ingestion of contaminated food, poultry, eggs)	Acute onset 12-24 hours after ingestion; lasts 2-5 days; moderate to large amounts non-bloody diarrhea; abdominal cramping and vomiting	Fever of 38.3-38.9° C (101-102° F) common; hyperactive bowel sounds, diffuse abdominal pain	Fecal leukocytes; positive stool culture; WBC normal
Campylobacter jejuni (Gram-negative rod; fecal-oral transmission; household pet)	Acute onset 3-5 days after exposure; last 3-7 days; moderate amounts bloody diarrhea	Fever, lower quadrant abdominal pain	Fecal leukocytes; positive stool culture

Table 5-7

Differential Diagnosis of Common Causes of Acute Diarrhea—cont'd

Condition	History	Physical Findings	Diagnostic Studies
Vibrio cholera (Gram-negative rod; fecal-oral transmission; ingestion of contaminated water, seafood, or food)	Acute onset 8-24 hours after ingestion of contaminated food; lasts 3-5 days; large amounts non-bloody, watery, painless diarrhea; can be mild or fulminate	Cyanotic, scaphoid abdomen, poor skin turgor, thready peripheral pulses, voice faint	Fecal leukocytes; negative stool culture
Enterotoxic *E. coli* (Gram-negative rod; fecal-oral transmission; ingestion of contaminated water or food)	Acute onset 8-18 hours after ingestion of contaminated food/water; lasts 24-48 hours; moderate amounts non-bloody diarrhea; pain, cramping, abdominal pain; adults in US generally do not develop illness from enterotoxic *E. coli*	No fever; dehydration is major complication	Fecal leukocytes; positive stool culture
Entamoeba histolytica parasite (cysts in food and water, from feces)	Acute onset 12-24 hours after ingestion of contaminated food or water; large amounts bloody diarrhea; abdominal cramping and vomiting	Right lower quadrant abdominal pain, in small number of cases hepatic abscess forms	Indirect hemagglutinin assay (IHA): antibodies to *E. histolytic;* positive titer is >1:128
Antibiotic-induced (begins after taking antibiotics)	Mild, watery diarrhea; crampy abdominal pain	Diffuse abdominal pain on palpation, fever absent	Usually not needed

Continued

Table 5-7

Differential Diagnosis of Common Causes of Acute Diarrhea—cont'd

Condition	History	Physical Findings	Diagnostic Studies
Pseudomembranous colitis (*Clostridium difficile* antibiotic-induced)	Induced by antibiotics, most commonly ampicillin, clindamycin, or cephalosporins; symptoms range from transient mild diarrhea to active colitis with bloody diarrhea, abdominal pain, fever	Lower quadrant tenderness, fever	CBC: leukocytosis, sigmoidoscopy/colonoscopy; *C. difficile* toxin assay or stool culture; *C. difficile* toxin
Hemolytic uremic syndrome (HUS) (primary cause of HUS in US is *E. coli* 0157:H7)	Child under age 4 with a history of gastroenteritis; history of bloody diarrhea, fever, and irritability	Fever, irritability; may have oliguria or anuria	CBC, platelet count, renal function tests, peripheral blood smear; negative stool culture

Table 5-8

Differential Diagnosis of Common Causes of Chronic Diarrhea

Condition	History	Physical Findings	Diagnostic Studies
Irritable bowel syndrome (IBS)	Intermittent diarrhea alternating with constipation; mucus with stool; seldom occurs at night or awakens patient; commonly present in morning; may have rectal urgency; episodes usually triggered by stress or ingestion of food; women <men, 3:1	Tender colon on palpation; may have abdominal distention; no weight loss; afebrile	Diagnosis of exclusion; sigmoidoscopy, proctoscopy

Table 5-8

Differential Diagnosis of Common Causes of Chronic Diarrhea—cont'd

Condition	History	Physical Findings	Diagnostic Studies
Ulcerative colitis (distal colon is most severely affected and rectum is involved)	History of severe diarrhea with gross blood in stools, no growth retardation; few complaints of pain; age of onset 2nd and 3rd decades with small peak during adolescence; positive family history	Overt rectal bleeding, no fever, weight loss, or pain on palpation of abdomen, initially; moderate colitis: weight loss, fever, abdominal tenderness	CBC shows leukocytosis or anemia, ESR elevated; stool cultures to rule out other causes of diarrhea; endoscopy
Crohn's disease (associated with uveitis, erythema nodosum)	History of chronic bloody diarrhea with abdominal cramping, tenderness, and rectal bleeding; in children a history of growth retardation, weight loss, moderate diarrhea, abdominal pain, and anorexia	Weight loss, rare gross rectal bleeding; fistulas common	Colonoscopy with biopsies
Carbohydrate malabsorption	Bloating, flatus, diarrhea exacerbated by ingestion of certain disaccharides, e.g., lactose, milk, milk products; may follow a viral gastroenteritis	Diffuse abdominal pain	Trial elimination of offending foods
Fat malabsorption	Greasy, fatty, malodorous stools; associated with Vitamin K, A, and D deficiencies; cystic fibrosis	Rectal prolapse, poor weight gain, abdominal distention	72-hour fecal fats sweat test

Continued

Table 5-8

Differential Diagnosis of Common Causes of Chronic Diarrhea—cont'd

Condition	History	Physical Findings	Diagnostic Studies
Toddler diarrhea	3-4 stools/day; some contain mucus; rare past 4-5 years of age	PE and growth normal	Clinical diagnosis
Celiac sprue/ protein hypersensitivity (reaction to the protein in wheat, rye, barley, and oats)	Increased stool frequency, looseness, paleness, and bulkiness of stool within 3-6 months of dietary onset; children are lethargic, irritable, and anorectic; peak frequency 9-18 months	Failure to thrive, abdominal distention, irritability, muscle wasting	Clinical findings; improvement on gluten-free diet; CBC: anemia, folate deficiency; x-ray, biopsy
Giardia parasite (primary cause of chronic diarrhea in children)	Watery, foul diarrhea; common in day care, among travelers and male homosexuals	Low-grade fever, weight loss, chronic form: fatigue, growth retardation, steatorrhea	Stool for O & P, need three specimens on different days
Cryptosporidium species/*Isospora belli* protozoan parasites (fecal-oral transmission; ingestion of contaminated water or direct oral-anal contact)	Recurrent episodes; variable amounts watery, non-bloody diarrhea; amounts can be massive	Weight loss, severe right upper quadrant abdominal pain with biliary tract involvement	Stool for O & P
Post-gastrectomy dumping syndrome	Following GI surgery, diarrhea occurs after	Diaphoresis and tachycardia	Upper GI

Table 5-8

Differential Diagnosis of Common Causes of Chronic Diarrhea—cont'd

Condition	History	Physical Findings	Diagnostic Studies
Post-gastrectomy dumping syn-drome—cont'd	meals; diarrhea occurs after meals because of increased transit of food through the colon		
Diabetic enter-opathy	Nocturnal diarrhea, postprandial vomiting, fatty stools from mal-absorption	Findings associated with diabetes	Diagnosis of exclu-sion in diabetic persons
HIV enteropathy (direct infection of mucosa and neuronal cells in GI system)	Insidious onset, recurrent large amounts non-bloody diarrhea, mild to moder-ate nausea/vomiting	Findings associated with HIV in-fection	Testing for HIV
Medication-induced	Mild to moderately severe non-watery, non-bloody diarrhea	No specific findings related to di-arrhea	Usually none needed

Constipation

There is lack of general agreement on the norms for stool frequency, size, or consistency, with considerable uncertainty on how much deviation is required to warrant the label of constipation. Gener-ally constipation refers to difficulty in defecating with infrequent bowel move-ments, straining, abdominal pain, and pain on defecating. It can also refer to hardness of stool or a feeling of incom-plete evacuation. Obstipation refers to intractable constipation or the regular passage of hard stools at 3- to 5-day intervals.

There are five areas in the defecation process where interference can cause clini-cal problems. They are (a) the peristaltic reflex, (b) the spinal arc, (c) relaxation of the anal sphincter, (d) contraction of the voluntary muscle associated with defeca-tion, and (e) the autonomic and cortical control of defecation.

Acute constipation refers to a definite change for that individual, suggesting an organic cause such as mechanical obstruc-tion, adynamic ileus or traumatic interrup-tion of the nervous system, or from medi-cations or following anesthesia. Persistent constipation occurs when the condition lasts for weeks or occurs intermittently with increasing frequency or severity. Partial obstruction or local anorectal conditions may be the cause. Chronic constipation occurs as the result of disruption of the storage, transport, and evacuation mechanisms of the colon. Functional causes are the most common and include poor bowel habits; inadequate dietary fiber, bulk, and fluids; or colonic motility disorders such as irritable bowel syndrome or psychogenic causes. Genetic predisposition to constipation seems to exist.

DIAGNOSTIC REASONING: FOCUSED HISTORY

Is this really constipation?

Key Questions
- How many stools are there per day?
- What is the consistency of the stool?

Frequency of stool. Stool frequency is the easiest parameter to quantify. In the general adult population, the "normal" frequency of bowel movements ranges from 3 to 12 per week. Less than three bowel movements per week is considered to be constipation.

Infants and children have a decreasing frequency with age, from more than four stools per day during the first week of life to 1.2 per day at age 4. Infants who have fewer number of stools than average seem to constitute a disproportionate percentage of those who develop frank constipation.

Alternating episodes of constipation and diarrhea are characteristic of irritable bowel syndrome. Patients may describe their constipation stools as hard round balls.

Stool consistency. Stools that are hard and dry are an additional parameter to consider in assessing constipation. Stools that are marginally frequent but are soft and moist may not indicate constipation,

whereas that same number that are hard and dry would indicate constipation.

Is the constipation acute or chronic?

Key Questions
- When did the constipation start?
- How long has it been going on? Is this an individual episode or is it chronic?
- At what age did the constipation first begin?

Onset and duration. Recent onset usually reflects changes in lifestyle or physical health such as dietary changes, activity changes, new medications, partially obstructing lesions, or recent illness. Chronic constipation or constipation of long duration is usually associated with either functional causes such as lack of dietary fiber and bulk or with concurrent systemic disorders such as diabetes mellitus (DM) or hypothyroidism.

Age of onset. New-onset constipation in adults over age 40 is suspicious for colon lesions. The newborn is likely to have an anatomical cause. In infants, the cause is likely inadequate fluid and fiber in the diet. In children, the cause is likely to be diet as well as developmental and psychological factors. In adults, the cause is usually related to dietary and bowel habits.

If the constipation is acute, what conditions should I consider?

Key Questions
- Have you been ill recently? Fever?
- Do you have any chronic health problems?

Recent illness. Dehydration and fever cause hardening of the stools by diminishing intestinal secretions and increasing water absorption from the colon. A transient period of constipation is common during an acute febrile illness. Also, reflex ileus is sometimes seen with pneumonia.

Chronic illness. Hardened stools are found in renal acidosis and diabetes insipidus. Infants and children with hypotonia of the abdominal and intestinal musculature from neurological conditions may be predisposed to constipation.

Medical disease can cause constipation because of neurological gut dysfunction, myopathies, endocrine disorders, and electrolyte abnormalities. Constipation in infants may be an early symptom of congenital hypothyroidism.

If the constipation is chronic or recurrent, what should I consider?

Key Questions
- What do you usually eat in a day?
- How many glasses of liquid do you drink each day?
- What are your usual bowel habits?
- How active are you?
- What medications are you taking?
- Do you use laxatives? How often? For how long?

Dietary pattern. A 3-day dietary history is more accurate than a 24-hour recall although a 24-hour recall can provide a reasonable picture of the patient's dietary habits. Diets that lack roughage result in lack of fecal bulk, causing an inadequate stimulus for peristaltic movement. Diets that are high in protein result in complete digestion of the protein, leaving little residue to stimulate movement. Diets high in calcium content lead to the formation of calcium caseinate in the stools, which does not stimulate peristalsis. Inadequate fluid intake (less than six 8-ounce glasses per day) contributes to dry, hard, and infrequent stools.

Bowel habits. Putting off a bowel movement because of time constraints or other reasons suppresses the normal gastrocolic reflex and can produce constipation.

Activity level. Constipation is a common problem in individuals with a very sedentary lifestyle. The lack of physical activity reduces the peristaltic reflex.

Medications. Medications that commonly cause or contribute to constipation include narcotics, imipramine, diuretics, calcium channel blockers, anticholinergics, psychotropic agents, antacids, decongestants, anticonvulsants, iron, bismuth, and lead.

Use of enemas, laxatives, and suppositories. Use of stimulants to empty the colon removes the peristalsis stimulus for 2 to 3 days. Diarrhea is usually followed by infrequent stools for several days. Chronic use of stimulants can produce chronic atonic constipation.

How can I further narrow the causes?

Key Questions
- What does your stool look like? Is the stool size large or small? What is the general shape? (small, round, ribbon-like)
- Is the stool formed or liquid?
- Have you had any involuntary loss of stool?
- Does the constipation alternate with periods of diarrhea?

Size or caliber of stool. Infrequent passage of small hard stools may indicate congenital aganglionic megacolon. Very large stools may indicate functional constipation, with the size of the stools a function of the size of the colon. Ribbon-like stools suggest a motility disorder such as irritable bowel syndrome (IBS). They can also be caused by narrowing of the distal or sigmoid colon from an organic lesion. A progressive decrease in the caliber of stool suggests an organic lesion.

Stools with a toothpaste-like caliber suggest fecal impaction. Constipation can also be the result of dietary habits and may be seen in teens who drink several quarts of milk per day.

Consistency of stool. Dry hard stools suggest lack of sufficient dietary fluids or fiber. Liquid stool and fecal incontinence, particularly in the elderly, may represent stool impaction and overflow.

Alternating constipation and diarrhea. Alternating episodes are characteristic of IBS. Patients often describe the stool during the constipation episodes as hard and pellet-like.

What else do I need to consider?

Key Questions
- Do you have the urge to defecate?
- Do you have any urinary symptoms?
- Do you have any nausea or vomiting?
- Is there any pain with defecation?
- Is there any bleeding with defecation? How much?
- What color are your stools? Are the stools very dark colored or black?

Urge to defecate. Children with Hirschsprung's disease (aganglionic megacolon) do not have an urge to defecate because the stool accumulates proximal to the lower portion of the rectum where the proprioceptors for defecation are located. Evidence of stiffening, squeezing, and crying indicate stool is being propelled to the rectum. Adults who overuse laxatives or other stimulants may not experience the urge to defecate.

Associated urinary problems. Voiding problems may indicate an abdominal mass. Day and night enuresis is seen in some children with encopresis (fecal soiling). Rarely does a neurological lesion produce fecal incontinence without a disturbance in bladder control.

Vomiting. Bilious vomiting may indicate intestinal obstruction in the newborn. Vomiting associated with pain in adults may indicate obstruction.

Pain. Chronic recurrent abdominal pain is commonly present in constipation. Pain is intermittent and may be localized to the periumbilical region. Crampy lower abdominal pain is usually caused by bowel distention, which can result from irritable bowel syndrome (IBS), intermittent obstruction, or adhesions. Non-crampy dull pain in the left abdomen is associated with diverticulosis. Pain on defecation may indicate an anal or rectal lesion such as hemorrhoids or anal fissures.

Bleeding. Bright red blood in the stool indicates hemorrhoids, fissure, or possible rectal mass. Black stools may indicate bleeding from a site high up in the colon because blood mixed with gastric acid makes the stools appear black. Brisk bleeding is uncommon with hemorrhoids and requires immediate thorough investigation.

Color. Red stools may be the result of using laxatives of vegetable origin. A black or very dark brown color may be caused by drugs such as iron and bismuth, both of which contribute to constipation.

If this is a child, is there anything else I need to consider?

Key Questions
- Is there fecal soiling of underpants?
- Is there crying with defecation?
- In infant: is there history of delayed passage of meconium stool?

Crying with defecation. Small children with constipation will cry with movement when a fissure is present. Also with large hard stools, the child will not want to defecate because of the pain and will do stool-holding mannerisms such as sitting, standing still.

Fecal soiling of underpants. Repeated fecal soiling from involuntary passage of small amounts of feces into the underpants of children over age 4 is consistent with encopresis from functional megacolon secondary to chronic constipation. The constipation is usually secondary to painful defecation, with a resultant anal fissure. Coercive bowel training, fear of the toilet, or reactive voluntary withholding of bowel movements can also cause this condition.

History of delayed passage of meconium stool. Such a history may indicate congenital aganglionic megacolon (Hirschsprung's disease).

Is there a family history or genetic predisposition?

Key Question

- Is there a family history of constipation or irritable bowel syndrome?

Genetic predisposition to constipation seems to exist. It is common for more than one family member to have a history of chronic constipation or IBS.

DIAGNOSTIC REASONING: FOCUSED PHYSICAL EXAMINATION

Plot Growth Curve in Children

Slow to grow may indicate congenital aganglionic megacolon. Also incorrect formula mixing, underfeeding, starvation, and anorexia nervosa may first be recognized by a complaint of constipation.

Perform Abdominal Examination

Observe abdominal contour, looking for distention. Abdominal distention is frequently not marked in patients with functional constipation but may be present with other causes. Auscultate for bowel sounds. Silent or abnormal bowel sounds may also indicate an organic cause such as obstruction. On palpation, stool may be felt as mobile, nontender masses in the left lower quadrant. Firm, rubbery masses of stool palpable in the right lower quadrant in newborns may indicate meconium ileus. Palpable abdominal masses or organomegaly point to an organic cause. Note tenderness, which may indicate an organic cause, although a tender bowel may be palpable in IBS.

Perform Digital Rectal Examination

On perianal inspection, look for skin excoriation, skin tags, fissures, strictures, tears, or hemorrhoids, any of which may cause painful defecation. Early fissures have the appearance of superficial erosions. More advanced lesions are linear or elliptic breaks in the skin. Longstanding fissures are deep and indurated. Internal fissures are seen when the anal sphincter relaxes as the examining finger is withdrawn. To examine for a fissure in a child, place the infant/child in the knee-chest position and spread the buttocks to reveal the mucocutaneous junction of the anus.

Look for rectal prolapse and feel for a rectocele, which might interfere with defecation. A normal anal sphincter with an empty rectal ampulla may indicate Hirschsprung's disease. In functional constipation, expect to find a large dilated rectum full of stool. Sphincter tone is increased in functional problems and strictures but is decreased in neurological diseases. The presence of a mass in the rectum indicates an impaction or obstructive lesion. A pilonidal dimple is seen with spinal bifida occulta.

Perform a Focused Neurological Examination

Test relevant deep tendon and superficial reflexes. Interruption of T12-S3 nerves causes loss of voluntary control of defecation (Table 5-9).

Table 5-9

Superficial and Deep Tendon Reflexes and Spinal Level Tested

REFLEX	SPINAL LEVEL TESTED
Superficial	
Upper abdominal	T7, T8, T9
Lower abdominal	T10, T11
Cremasteric	T12, L1, L2
Deep	
Biceps	C5, C6
Brachioradial	C5, C6
Triceps	C6, C7, C8
Patellar	L2, L3, L4
Achilles	S1, S2

LABORATORY AND DIAGNOSTIC STUDIES

Fecal Occult Blood Testing (FOBT)

A positive FOBT indicates blood in the stool that may be the result of ulcerative or malignant lesions. The sensitivity of this test in detecting colorectal cancers and adenomas ranges from 50% to 90%. It is an inexpensive and noninvasive method to screen for bleeding lesions. A stool sample is placed on a filter paper, and an activating solution is applied. A positive test is indicated by the appearance of a color (usually blue or green). Serial testing (3 days) is done using stool cards at home that are returned by mail for analysis. FOBT is recommended annually beginning at age 50.

Complete Blood Count (CBC)

Obtain a CBC when you suspect bleeding. Hematocrit and hemoglobin will be below the expected reference range with a bleeding lesion.

Serum Electrolytes

Severely ill patients may develop hypokalemia and hypercalcemia, which are causes of constipation. Patients on thiazide diuretics may develop hypokalemia and subsequent constipation.

Serum Thyroid-Stimulating Hormone (TSH)

An elevated TSH may suggest hypothyroidism, which can be a cause of constipation. Screen for elevated TSH in persons with other symptoms suggestive of hypothyroidism such as sparse, coarse, dry hair; hirsutism; dry skin; or hoarse speech.

Anoscopy

Anoscopy is indicated if digital rectal examination detects hemorrhoids, fissures, strictures, or masses in the anus or rectum. It enables a view of the immediate internal anal canal that is not possible on manual digital rectal examination. A hand-held anoscope is warmed and lubricated and eased slowly in while the patient bears down to relax the external sphincter. A light source is necessary; a head lamp is preferable. Anoscopy may not be possible initially with a fissure or abscess because of the pain. However, it should be performed on follow-up visit to detect inflammatory bowel disorder or rectal cancer.

Flexible Sigmoidoscopy, Colonoscopy

These tests are indicated when conservative treatment fails, for those over age 50 or with new-onset constipation, and for persons with anemia or fecal occult blood.

Barium Enema

This contrast technique can be used to detect diverticula, polyps, and masses. It is also used to determine the extent of dilated bowel in megacolon.

DIFFERENTIAL DIAGNOSIS

Despite the high incidence of constipation, only a small number of adults or children with constipation have a significant abnormality. In otherwise healthy individuals, first consider functional causes, particularly dietary, fluid, bowel, and laxative habits. In adults, depression may be associated with constipation.

Simple Constipation

Typically individuals with simple constipation report a diet low in fiber and bulk and/or inadequate fluid intake. A sedentary lifestyle is common. They also often report pain before and with bowel movements because of the hard, dry nature of the stools. Patients may also complain of loss of appetite. The physical examination of the abdomen and rectum is normal. You may feel fecal masses in the colon and rectum. No diagnostic workup is needed unless the patient does not respond to therapy.

Functional Constipation

Functional constipation is seen in children who have large, hard stools that become difficult or painful to pass. The resulting fecal retention sets up a cycle in which the sensitivity of the defecation reflex and effectiveness of persistalsis lessens. Watery stool from the proximal colon soils the underwear. On physical examination, stool is present in the LLQ and the rectum is dilated and filled with packed stool. The external sphincter is intact.

Irritable Bowel Syndrome (IBS)

IBS is common in adults, with onset usually as young adults. The presenting complaint may be either diarrhea or constipation. Alternating episodes of each is characteristic of IBS. Mucus in the stools is common. Abdominal pain often occurs, usually in the left lower quadrant, and the bowel may be tender to palpation. A tender bowel may be palpable (see also IBS in Diarrhea section, pp. 187 and 188).

Fecal Impaction

Fecal impaction is common in older adults and in those who are confined to bed. The passage of hard stools at 3- to 5-day intervals may occur. Some persons with impaction have continuous diarrhea-like passage of stools and may experience incontinence. Stools may be of small caliber, sometimes described as toothpaste-like. On rectal examination, large quantities of hard feces will be palpable in the rectal ampulla. On abdominal examination, feces-filled bowel may be palpable.

Idiopathic Slow Transit

This condition is most common in older persons, especially those who are less active and have inadequate dietary fiber and fluid intake. These patients experience decreased stool frequency; stools are typically dry and hard.

Hirschsprung's Disease (Aganglionic Megacolon)

Hirschsprung's disease is present from birth and is usually detected in young children. Delayed passage of a meconium stool may indicate Hirschsprung's disease in infants. Children with Hirschsprung's disease do not have an urge to defecate because the stools accumulate proximal to the lower portion of the rectum where the proprioceptors for defecation are located. Evidence of stiffening, squeezing, and crying indicate stool is being propelled to the rectum. On examination the rectal ampulla is empty.

Secondary Constipation From Anorectal Lesion

Because defecation is painful with an anorectal lesion, the patient suppresses it. With the eventual passage of hard stools, the patient may report blood on the surface of the stool, on the toilet paper, or in the toilet. On digital rectal examination, look for hemorrhoids, fissures, tears, or abrasions.

Drug Induced

Drug-induced constipation is consistent with a history of chronic laxative use or taking those medications that can produce constipation. It occurs most often in older persons. Abdominal and rectal examination is usually normal.

Tumors

Tumors are uncommon in children, and the frequency increases over the age of 40. Constipation occurs in less than one third of persons with colon cancer; diarrhea is more common. Onset is recent, and there may be progressive narrowing of stool caliber. Colicky abdominal pain and distention may occur in persons with bowel tumors. Persons with rectosigmoid tumors may complain of rectal discomfort, stool leakage, urgency, and tenesmus. Stool may test positive for occult blood. An abdominal mass may be palpable. Suspect right-sided lesions in elderly patients who present with constipation, anemia, anorexia, and weight loss.

Table 5-10

Differential Diagnosis Of Common Causes of Constipation

Condition	History	Physical Findings	Diagnostic Studies
Simple constipation	Low dietary fiber and bulk; inadequate fluid intake; physical inactivity; pain before and with bowel movements, anorexia	Normal abdominal and rectal examination; may feel fecal masses in colon and rectum	None if resolved; consider sigmoidoscopy if not resolved
Functional constipation	Preschool, school agers; history of abdominal pain and stool soiling	Palpable stool in LLQ; large dilated rectum with packed stool; external sphincter intact	Abdominal x-ray; unprepped barium x-ray
Irritable bowel syndrome (IBS)	Onset in young adulthood; alternating diarrhea and constipation; mucus in stools	May have tender palpable colon	Sigmoidoscopy if indicated
Obstipation/ impaction	Passage of hard stool at 3-5 day intervals; diarrhea, small caliber stools; common in those confined to bed	Hard feces in rectal ampulla; may have palpable feces-filled bowel	Sigmoidoscopy if indicated

Table 5-10

Differential Diagnosis Of Common Causes of Constipation—cont'd

Condition	History	Physical Findings	Diagnostic Studies
Slow transit	Common in older adults; physical inactivity; decreased stool frequency; stool dry and hard	Normal abdominal and rectal examination	Fecal occult blood testing to rule out tumors
Hirschsprung's disease	Delayed passage of meconium at birth; no urge to defecate	Empty rectal ampulla on examination	Colonoscopy
Anorectal lesions	Rectal pain on defecation; history of hemorrhoids; blood on stool, toilet tissue, or in toilet	On rectal examination: hemorrhoids, fissures, tears, abrasions; increased sphincter tone	Anoscopy
Drug-induced	History of chronic laxative use; history of taking those medications that produce constipation	Normal rectal and abdominal exam	None if resolved; consider sigmoidoscopy, barium enema if not resolved
Tumors	Diarrhea more common than constipation; recent onset: pain and abdominal distention; stool leakage; urgency; late: weight loss, anorexia; increased incidence over age 40; uncommon in children	May have palpable abdominal mass or organomegaly	CBC; fecal occult blood testing; sigmoidoscopy colonoscopy; barium enema

Rectal Pain and Itching

Although patients are often embarrassed by pain or problems in the anal area, anorectal problems can cause significant discomfort and anxiety. Rectal complaints include pain, irritation, discomfort, itching, or soreness in the anal area. Tenesmus is painful sphincter contraction, which may be caused by anorectal infection. Rectal pain can be caused by tears, infection, or hemorrhoids. Itching can be caused by inflammation from hemorrhoids or hypersensitivity to substances to the environment.

The anatomy of the anorectal area is important in describing the occurrence of various disorders. The anus is the most distal portion of the gastrointestinal tract and is approximately 4 cm long. It is composed of the distal end lined by stratified squamous epithelium and the proximal component lined by simple columnar epithelium. The two components are divided by the dentate line–the line where the distal end and the columns and crypts of Morgagni meet. The dentate line is also known as the anorectal junction, which also denotes the boundary between the somatic and visceral nerve supply. The columns of Morgagni are longitudinal columns of mucosa located in the proximal anus and fuse in a ring distally to form the anal papillae at the level of the dentate line. The crypts are the invaginations of the columns of Morgagni. Figure 5-2 shows the anatomy of the anus and rectum.

DIAGNOSTIC REASONING: FOCUSED HISTORY

What do the presenting symptoms tell me?

Key Questions
- Have you had any bleeding? How much? When? Describe.
- Have you had pain? When does it occur? Describe the pain.
- Specifically, do you have pain on defecation? If a child: does the child cry on defecation?
- Have you had itching? When?
- Can you feel a lump?
- Have you had any stains on your underwear? What kind? (blood, stool, pus)
- Have you had diarrhea?
- Have you been constipated?

Bleeding. Bleeding associated with defecation is characteristic of hemorrhoids and fissures. Bleeding from hemorrhoids typically occurs following defecation and is noted on the toilet paper or coating the stool. The blood is bright red and may vary from a few spots on the toilet paper to a thin stream or coating on the stool. Bleeding with fissures occurs with defecation and is accompanied by pain. Spontaneous rectal bleeding can occur with proctitis. Condyloma acuminata may grow to a size sufficient to occlude the rectal opening and will bleed on defecation.

Pain. Pain with defecation is characteristic of anal fissures. The pain may be so severe that the patient avoids defecating to avoid the pain. Children will cry with defecation. The pain may last for several hours then subside until the next bowel movement. Patients with anal fissures complain of cutting or tearing anal pain during defecation and of gnawing, throbbing discomfort after defecation.

Hemorrhoids rarely cause severe pain unless they are ulcerated or thrombosed. Thrombosed hemorrhoids cause an inflammatory reaction by activating tissue thromboplastin within the hemorrhoidal blood vessels.

Patients with a recoil abscess or fistula complain of a throbbing, continuous, progressive pain. Pain may also occur with proctitis as a result of the infectious and inflammatory processes. The pain is not limited to defecation.

Tenesmus. Tenesmus is common with anal fissures, as the tear and inflammation

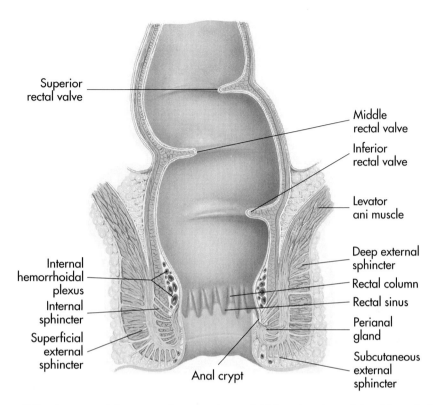

Superior
rectal valve

Middle
rectal valve

Inferior
rectal valve

Levator
ani muscle

Internal
hemorrhoidal
plexus

Internal
sphincter

Superficial
external
sphincter

Deep external
sphincter

Rectal column

Rectal sinus

Perianal
gland

Subcutaneous
external
sphincter

Anal crypt

Figure 5-2 Anatomy of the anus and rectum. (From Seidel HM et al: *Mosby's guide to physical examination,* ed 4, St. Louis, 1998, Mosby.)

involves the internal sphincter. On defecation, the sphincter may go into spasm. The patient experiences a tearing pain.

Itching. Itching is common with both hemorrhoids and fissures. Both external hemorrhoids that are covered by skin and fissures that involve breaks in the skin stimulate cutaneous sensation and lead to pain and itching.

Intense itching is a hallmark of pruritus ani, which occurs from hypersensitivity caused by irritating soap, lubricants, fragrance, or dyes present in toilet paper. Itching, particularly at night, can also be caused by pinworms.

Mass. The sensation of a mass or lump may indicate hemorrhoids or anal fissures. When the supportive tissues around the anal canal deteriorate, veins in the anorec-

tal mucosa become tortuous and dilated and then bulge and descend into the anal canal. Both external or internal hemorrhoids can protrude and then regress spontaneously or be reduced manually. The patient may feel them as a bulge or lump. With chronic anal fissures, the anal papillae hypertrophy and a skin tag ("sentinel pile") may form, which the patient may feel as a mass or lump.

Fecal soiling. Fecal soiling is common with hemorrhoids. Mucous discharge with internal hemorrhoids is less common. Fecal soiling is also common with chronic constipation in children. Some stool discharges around the feces that are in the rectum.

Diarrhea. Explosive diarrhea may be a contributing cause of anal fissures. Diarrhea can also cause irritation and excoriation, producing symptoms of itching, bleeding, and soreness.

Constipation. Constipation may be a cause or result of anal fissure. Hard dry stool can tear the rectal mucosa and produce an anal fissure. The pain associated with defecation because of a fissure may result in constipation as the patient avoids defecating.

Could this be caused by sexual practices?

Key Questions
- How many sexual partners do you have?
- Do your sexual practices include anal intercourse?
- Do you insert any objects into your rectum?

Multiple sexual partners. Multiple sexual partners place the individual at risk for developing condyloma acuminata and viral or bacterial proctitis. HIV infection is possible and places the individual at risk for the development of proctitis.

Anal intercourse. Anal intercourse predisposes individuals to anal fissure as a result of rectal trauma. The transmission of bacterial or viral organisms can result in condyloma acuminata or proctitis.

Foreign bodies. The insertion of objects into the rectum can cause anal tears and fissures.

Could this be the result of sexual abuse?

Key Questions
- Have you had unwanted sexual contact? In a child you might ask: has anyone touched your private parts?
- Do you think the child has been abused?

Sexual contact. Unwanted sexual contact that includes anal contact or intercourse may cause anal fissures as a result of

rectal trauma. The transmission of bacterial or viral organisms can result in the development of condyloma acuminata or proctitis.

A child's reporting. Children who have been abused try to tell in some way about the abuse. Subtle indications that are not proof but may indicate abuse include a preschooler's regression to earlier safer times: thumbsucking, clinging behavior, bedwetting, fear of sleeping in one's own room, and expressing feeling through art, especially drawing. Children draw what they see. Ask the child to talk about what he or she has drawn. School age children develop physical symptoms around abuse (sore throat, stomach pains). The child's play may portray intercourse and may include violence towards animals. The child's concentration may appear low, but in fact all energy is being put into keeping a secret. Some children over-compensate, getting straight As so that no one will suspect. Failure to thrive and undereating may be other behaviors that raise suspicion of abuse.

A parent's reporting. When children are sexually assaulted by a stranger, most parents bring the child into an emergency facility or clinic for immediate investigation. Abuse by a friend or family member is less overt and is often detected only when a primary care provider is alert to a suspicious history or physical findings. In some cases, a parent may voice concerns about the possibility of abuse or report that the child has told them of the incident.

A child who has been sexually abused must be referred to Children's Protective Services and to a health care provider who is an expert in the area of child abuse.

Do risk factors point to a likely condition?

Key Questions
- Do you strain to have a bowel movement?
- How often do you move your bowels? How often do you experience constipation? Are your stools hard and dry?

- What kind of work do you do? Does it require sitting for long periods?
- Describe your personal hygiene practices.
- For women: number of pregnancies, childbirth history.
- Do you have HIV/AIDS or are you on chemotherapy?
- Do you have diabetes?
- Note patient's gender.

Straining at stool. Straining during bowel movements predisposes individuals to the development of hemorrhoids and anal fissures, especially in the presence of chronic constipation. Hemorrhoids develop secondary to the pressure. Fissures develop as a result of traumatic laceration from a hard or large stool.

Chronic constipation. Chronic constipation predisposes an individual to hemorrhoids and anal fissures as a result of straining.

Prolonged sitting. Occupations that require prolonged periods of sitting predispose to the development of hemorrhoids, pruritus ani, and pilonidal cysts.

Poor hygiene. Inadequate hygiene practices are a risk factor for the development of pruritus ani and pinworms. Improper cleaning can result in excessive moisture around the canal, which causes breakdown of the epidermal layer of skin. Organisms and parasites can invade the damaged skin.

Excessive hygiene. Another risk factor in the development of pruritus ani is overzealous cleansing. Pruritus ani can result from excessive use of chemical irritants such as soap or from excessive rubbing.

Pregnancy and childbirth. The increased pressure and trauma from pregnancy and childbirth predisposes women to the development of hemorrhoids.

Diabetes mellitus (DM). DM places the individual at risk for development of pruritus ani with secondary yeast infections.

Gender. Many more males than females experience pruritus ani. The reason for this is not clear.

Might this condition require hospitalization or referral?

Key Questions

- Are you on anticoagulation therapy? Have you had bleeding?
- Do you have a bleeding disorder?
- Do you have HIV/AIDS?
- Are you on chemotherapy?
- Is there purulent discharge?

Coagulopathy with bleeding. Bleeding in anorectal problems is usually self-limiting and, if not a problem, resolves spontaneously or with local pressure. However, a bleeding internal hemorrhoid in a patient with a coagulopathy indicates the need for hospitalization.

Immunocompromised with an infection. Because of the acute infectious process, a perirectal abscess may require hospitalization, especially in a person who is immunocompromised because the infection is more likely to spread systematically. Individuals who are immunocompromised are at risk for the development of proctitis, especially by herpes simplex.

DIAGNOSTIC REASONING: FOCUSED PHYSICAL EXAMINATION

Inspect the Perirectal Area

Look for scars, warts, petechiae, bruising, and skin tags. Midline skin tags immediately anterior to the anus that have been present from birth are seen in some children. Skin tags may also develop when tears or hemorrhoidal bleeding resolves. Hemorrhoids are very uncommon in children and their presence should heighten suspicion of sexual abuse. Perirectal erythema is common with streptococcal cellulitis, and you may occasionally see vesicles surrounding the anus.

Perform a Digital Rectal Examination

A thorough gentle digital rectal examination is essential. Look for skin excoriation, skin tags, fissures, strictures, tears, or hemorrhoids, any of which may cause painful defecation. The knee-chest position affords the best visualization in both adults and children. A side-lying position can also be used. Spread the buttocks to reveal the mucocutaneous junction of the anus and carefully inspect the rectum first in the resting position and then as the patient bears down. As the patient bears down, an additional 1 to 2 cm of anorectal tissue is palpable.

Look for inflammation, swelling, and erythema that characterize inflammation or infection. These signs may be present with a fissure, fistula, abscess, or proctitis.

Note any lesions or discharge. Condyloma acuminata present as warty growths that are pink or white with a papilliform surface. In anal regions, they tend to grow in radial rows around the anal orifice, forming a confluent mass that can obscure the anal opening. Examination of the entire genital region, including the anal canal, is important because they can extend 1 or 2 cm above the dentate line. Purulent discharge may be present with proctitis or an infected fissure or fistula.

Look carefully around the periphery to see small longitudinal ulcers or tears that characterize anal fissures. Early fissures have the appearance of superficial erosions. More advanced lesions are linear or elliptic breaks in the skin. Long-standing fissures are deep and indurated. Internal fissures are seen when the anal sphincter relaxes as the examining finger is withdrawn. A sentinel tag may be visible.

External hemorrhoids, if present, will be visible as bluish swellings. Internal hemorrhoids may or may not become present as the patient bears down.

Palpate for tenderness. Hemorrhoids are generally not tender. Pain from an abscess, fissure, or fistula may preclude digital examination.

Feel for foreign bodies, which might be present as the result of insertion of objects. Foreign bodies can also be present as a result of ingestion, such as with chicken bones or small objects in children.

Perform Anoscopy

Anoscopy is essential in the evaluation of all patients with rectal pain. It enables a view of the immediate internal anal canal that is not possible on manual digital rectal examination. A hand-held anoscope warmed and lubricated is eased slowly in while the patient bears down to relax the external sphincter. A light source is necessary; a head lamp is preferable. Anoscopy may not be possible initially with a fissure or abscess because of the pain. However, it should be performed on a follow-up visit to detect inflammatory bowel disorder or rectal cancer.

LABORATORY AND DIAGNOSTIC STUDIES

Fecal Occult Blood Test (FOBT)

FOBT should be done on all patients with rectal pain. A positive test indicates blood in the stool that may be the result of ulcerative or malignant lesions. A stool sample is placed on a filter paper, and an activating solution is applied. A positive test is indicated by the appearance of a color (usually blue or green). The sensitivity of this test in detecting colorectal cancers and adenomas ranges from 50% to 90%. It is an inexpensive and noninvasive method to screen for bleeding lesions. Serial testing (3 days) can be performed through the use of stool cards at home that are returned by mail for analysis.

Flexible Sigmoidoscopy

Flexible sigmoidoscopy should be performed when you suspect inflammatory bowel disease, polyps, or carcinoma. It is particularly important for patients over 50 years of age and for those with a history of familial polyposis.

Gram Stain Rectal Discharge

Place a smear of rectal discharge on a glass slide for Gram staining. Gram-positive organisms stain purple, whereas Gram-negative organisms stain red. *N. gonorrhea,* a common cause of rectal discharge in proctitis, is a Gram-negative organism.

Cultures for Infectious Organisms

When discharge or lesions are present, collect a specimen to culture for *N. gonorrhea* or herpes. Collect the specimen on a sterile swab and place in the media provided. Bacterial culture confirms the identity of the causative organism and its sensitivity to antibiotics. A swab specimen of the perianal cellulitis usually yields a heavy growth of group A streptococcus. Viral culture is also used for the diagnosis of herpes. Results may take from 1 to 7 days, with maximum sensitivity achieved at 5 to 7 days. The herpes culture will probably not be able to identify the causative agent if the specimen is taken from a lesion that is 5 or more days old.

DNA Probe for *Chlamydia, Neisseria gonorrhea,* or *Herpes*

DNA probe testing involves the construction of nucleic acid sequence (called a probe) that will match to a sequence in the DNA or RNA of the target tissue. The results are rapid and sensitive and provide an alternative to culture for *N. gonorrhea* and *Herpes.* Obtain a sample of rectal discharge with a sterile swab and place it in the medium provided. To collect a DNA probe for herpes testing, the best specimens are those obtained from beneath the roof of a vesicle at the base and ulcer border.

VDRL, RPR, FTA-ABS

These tests are serological tests used for the screening and diagnoses of syphilis and are recommended if other STDs are found or suspected.

Microscopic Examination of Stool

Stool examination should be considered in patients with symptoms of enterocolitis to rule out infection from common causes. Fecal leukocyte detection is an easy and inexpensive test that is 75% specific for bacterial diarrhea. Leukocytes are found in inflammatory diarrheal disease and are present in bacterial infections that invade the intestinal wall (*E. coli, Shigella,* and *Salmonella* species). Microscopic white blood cells and red blood cells indicate the presence of *Shigella,* enterohemorrhagic *E. coli,* enteropathogenic *E. coli, Campylobacter, C. difficile,* or other inflammatory or invasive diarrhea. Leukocytes are also present in diarrhea from ulcerative colitis and Crohn's disease, as well as antibiotic-related diarrhea. They are not seen in viral gastroenteritis, parasitic diarrhea, *Salmonella* carrier states, or enterotoxigenic bacterial diarrheas. Obtain a small fleck of mucus or stool. Do not allow the specimen to dry. Place the specimen on a slide with two drops of Loffler's methylene blue stain and wait 2 minutes before viewing under the microscope.

Stool for Ova and Parasites (O & P)

Stool examination for O & P should also be considered in patients with symptoms of enterocolitis. Stool can be tested for the presence of parasites. Fresh stool is required to preserve the trophozoites of some parasites. Use in patients with symptoms of diarrhea to rule out infection from *Campylobacter, Shigella, Giardia,* and *Cryptosporidium.* Usually three serial samples are obtained.

Scotch Tape Test

Use this test when you suspect pinworms, which occur most commonly in children. Instruct the adult to apply adhesive cellophane tape to the perianal region early in the morning on awakening. The tape is then brought in. Place it on a glass slide and examine under a microscope for the presence of eggs. Parents may also be able to see the worms in the external anus of the child at night with a flashlight. The female worm is about 10 mm long.

DIFFERENTIAL DIAGNOSIS

Hemorrhoids

Hemorrhoids are dilated veins located beneath the lining of the anal canal. Internal hemorrhoids are located in the upper anal canal proximal to the dentate line and are covered by rectal mucosa and supported by longitudinal muscle fibers. External hemorrhoids are located in the lower anal canal, distal to the dentate line, are covered by skin, and lack muscle support.

Internal hemorrhoids are graded by size (Table 5-11) and most often present with painless rectal bleeding, which is bright red and varies in quantity from a few drops coating the stool to a spattering at the end of defecation. Patients also report a dull aching and itching with prolapse. Itching occurs only with chronic prolapse.

External hemorrhoids can also cause itching but produce pain only when they become thrombosed. With thrombosis, patients report an acute onset of constant burning and throbbing pain and a new rectal lump.

External hemorrhoids are visible on examination as bluish skin-covered lumps at the anal verge. Internal hemorrhoids may become visible when the patient bears down.

Risk factors for the development of hemorrhoids include pregnancy, childbirth, straining during defecation, and occupations requiring prolonged sitting.

Anal Fissure

Anal fissures are longitudinal ulcers that extend from just below the dentate line to the anal verge. They occur most often in the posterior midline. Acute fissures are cracks in the epithelium, but chronic fissures may result in the formation of a skin tag at the outermost edge that is visible on examination. In the chronic stage, fissures can suppurate and extend into the surrounding tissue, causing perirectal abscess.

Patients with anal fissures complain of cutting or tearing anal pain during defecation and of gnawing, throbbing discomfort after defecation. Digital and visual examination reveal presence of the fissure. Early fissures have the appearance of superficial erosions. More advanced lesions are linear or elliptic breaks in the skin. Long-standing fissures are deep and indurated. Internal fissures are seen when the anal sphincter relaxes as

---

Table 5-11

Classification of Internal Hemorrhoids

GRADE	DESCRIPTION	SYMPTOMS
1	Do not prolapse	Minimal bleeding or discomfort
2	Prolapse with straining reduce spontaneously	Bleeding, aching, pruritus when prolapsed
3	Prolapse with straining, require manual reduction	Bleeding, aching, pruritus when prolapsed
4	Cannot be reduced or require manual reduction	Bleeding, aching, pruritus when prolapsed

Modified from: Metcalf A: Anorectal disorders, *Postgrad Med* 98(5):81-94, 1995.

the examining finger is withdrawn. A sentinel tag may be visible at the anal verge.

Risk factors for the development of fissure include straining at stool, chronic constipation, and anal intercourse. Anal fissures are the most common cause of constipation or rectal bleeding in children up to 2 years old.

Perirectal Abscess/Fistula

The most common source of infection are the anal glands, located at the base of the anal crypts at the level of the dentate line. Infection may also result from fissure, Crohn's disease, trauma, or anal surgery.

Acute infection presents as an abscess and chronic infection results in a fistula. The patient complains of swelling, throbbing, and continuous progressive pain. On examination, erythema and swelling in the perirectal region of ischiorectal fossa are found. Pain may preclude examination.

Pruritus Ani

Pruritus ani is a symptom complex consisting of discomfort and itching. It is more common in men than women and is most often idiopathic. Discomfort is exacerbated by friction or a warm, moist, perineal environment. Poor anal hygiene, or conversely, over-cleansing is often a contributing factor.

Examination may reveal mild erythema and excoriation of the perirectal skin. In later stages, the skin may be red, raw, oozing, or pale and lichenified with exaggerated skin markings.

Condyloma Acuminata

Genital warts are a common STD caused by the human papilloma virus (HPV). Patients with small lesions usually have few symptoms. When the lesions become large, patients experience bleeding, discharge, itching, and pain. On examination, warts are pink or white with a papilliform surface. They may obscure the anal opening. Examination of the entire genital region, including the anal canal, is important because they can extend 1 or 2 cm above the dentate line.

Proctitis/Proctocolitis

Anorectal infection is common in individuals who engage in anal intercourse, both heterosexuals and homosexuals. Most causes of proctitis are sexually transmitted through the anal sphincter by direct invasion of the infectious agent through the mucous membrane.

Proctitis is characterized by anorectal pain, mucopurulent or bloody discharge, tenesmus, and constipation. Proctitis that is caused by a STD may be associated with intense pain. On examination, inflamed mucopurulent mucosa is present. The most common pathogens are *N. gonorrhea*, *Chlamydia*, *Treponema pallidum*, and *Herpes* virus. Herpes simplex infection can occur above or below the anal sphincter. Herpes simplex infection is common in immunocompromised individuals. Proctitis can also occur with ulcerative colitis and Crohn's disease or with patients who have an intact rectum with a colostomy or ileostomy in place. Immunocompromised patients are at greater risk for proctitis.

Proctocolitis implies involvement beyond the rectum to include the sigmoid colon. The causes may include those of proctitis but are usually due to *Shigella*, *Campylobacter*, or *Giardia*. Symptoms of proctocolitis include those of proctitis but may also include diarrhea, fever, and abdominal cramping. On examination, an inflamed mucopurulent rectal mucosa is visible. Gram stain, serology to rule out syphilis, cultures, and DNA probe assist in diagnosis.

Pinworms

Pinworms are nematodes that infect the intestine and causes perianal irritation.

The pinworm eggs are ingested and migrate to the duodenum where they hatch and mature and then travel to the cecum. The adult females emerge at night through the anus, deposit eggs in the perianal region, and die. The eggs stick to the skin and cause perianal pruritus and scratching. The worms may be visible at night, and the ova may be visible under the microscope.

Pilonidal Cyst

These dermoid cysts of involuted epithelium are caused by prolonged repetitious irritation of the sacral area. Pilonidal cysts are seen in individuals with sedentary occupations. Patients complain of pain in the sacrum superior to the rectum. There is usually erythema over the sacrum and the lesion is often fluctuant.

Perianal Streptococcal Cellulitis

Separation of the buttocks reveals erythema and occasionally vesicles surrounding the anus. The patient usually has a history of group A beta-hemolytic streptococcal (GABHS) infection. Pain, erythema, proctitis, and blood-streaked stools are common.

Sexual Abuse

Poor sphincter tone, abrasion or bruises of the perineal or perianal area, pain or itching in the genital area, warts, and large, irregular or multiple anal fissures must alert you to the possibility of sexual abuse. The presence of the following STDs suggests the likelihood of sexual abuse in children, which must be ruled out in all instances:

- Certain: gonorrhea and syphilis (if not perinatally acquired)
- Probable: chlamydia, condyloma acuminatum, *T. vaginalis,* herpes II
- Possible: herpes I (genital area)

Table 5-12

Differential Diagnosis of Common Causes of Rectal Pain and Itching

Condition	History	Physical Findings	Diagnostic Studies
Hemorrhoids	Bright red rectal bleeding with defecation or blood on stool; burning or itching; straining at stool, prolonged sitting; pregnancy and childbirth	External hemorrhoids-bluish skin-covered lumps; internal hemorrhoids—may be visible when patient bears down	FOBT

Table 5-12

Differential Diagnosis of Common Causes of Rectal Pain and Itching—cont'd

Condition	History	Physical Findings	Diagnostic Studies
Anal fissure	Cutting or tearing pain during defecation and gnawing, throbbing discomfort afterward	Early fissures appear as superficial erosions; more advanced lesions are linear or elliptic breaks in the skin; long-standing fissures are deep and indurated; internal fissures are seen when anal sphincter relaxes as the examining finger is withdrawn; sentinel tag may be visible at the anal verge	Anoscopy
Perirectal abscess	Swelling, throbbing, continuous progressive pain	Erythema and swelling in perirectal area; pain may preclude examination	Anoscopy
Pruritus ani	Discomfort and itching exacerbated by friction; history of poor anal hygiene or over-cleansing	Mild erythema and excoriation over perirectal skin; in later stages, red raw, oozing, pale lichenified perirectal skin	
Condyloma acuminata	Few symptoms with small lesions; bleeding, discharge, itching and pain with large lesions	Pink or white warty lesions with papilliform surface; may extend into anal canal	Serology to distinguish from condyloma lata caused by syphilis
Proctitis/ proctocolitis	Anorectal pain; mucopurulent discharge, tenesmus, constipation with proctitis; also diarrhea abdominal pain and fever with proctocolitis history of anal intercourse, immunocompromise	Purulent discharge, inflamed mucopurulent rectal mucosa	Cultures, DNA probe, Gram stain, serology for syphilis; stool examination, stool O & P

Continued

Table 5-12

Differential Diagnosis of Common Causes of Rectal Pain and Itching—cont'd

Condition	History	Physical Findings	Diagnostic Studies
Pinworms	Itching, especially at night	Visualize white-yellow worms 8-13 mm in length at night with a flashlight	Scotch tape test positive for eggs
Infected pilonidal cyst	Pain in sacrum, superior to rectum; history of a sedentary occupation	Erythema, swelling over sacrum, which can be fluctuant	None, resection of cyst done 4 weeks after antibiotic treatment
Perianal streptococcal cellulitis	History of GABHS, local itching, pain	Erythema, proctitis, blood streaked stools	Culture of perianal area
Sexual abuse	History of abuse; perianal pain, itching	Large irregular anal fissures, bruising, rectal tone decrease, warts, presence of semen	Serology for syphilis; culture (gonorrhea, *T. vaginalis,* herpes) DNA probe (chlamydia, gonorrhea)

Chapter 6

Common Problems of the Genitourinary System

Urinary Incontinence

Urinary incontinence is the involuntary leakage of urine. It occurs as a result of pathological, anatomical, psychological, or physiological factors that produce obstruction, bladder irritability, or interference with neurological functioning. Environmental factors such as decreased mobility or inaccessibility of toilet facilities may also produce periodic incontinence.

Urinary incontinence is a common problem, particularly in older adults. It is so common in older women that some think of it as "normal." The prevalence in U.S. women is 26% during reproductive years and 30% to 40% in post-menopausal years. In non-institutionalized elderly women, the prevalence is 15% to 30%, and, in men, it is 8% to 22%. In elderly in nursing homes, the rate rises to almost 50%.

Urinary incontinence in adults is categorized according to the underlying anatomical or physiological impairment, specifically, stress incontinence, urge incontinence, overflow incontinence, and incontinence from reversible causes.

Stress incontinence is leakage of urine during activities that increase abdominal pressure, such as coughing, sneezing, laughing, or other physical activities. It occurs most often in females and is caused by hypermotility at the base of the bladder and urethra associated with pelvic floor relaxation or intrinsic urethral weakness.

Urge incontinence is an abrupt and strong desire to void with the inability to delay urination and is caused by bladder hyperactivity, or hypersensitive bladder. Detrusor muscle over-activity occurs when pathological brain disorders interfere with central inhibitory centers and fail to prevent detrusor muscle contractions.

Overflow incontinence occurs with over-distention of the bladder caused by an underactive or acontractile detrusor muscle, sphincter-detrusor dyssynergia, which is loss of the synergistic urinary sphincter relaxation that normally occurs with bladder detrusor muscle contraction, or from bladder outlet or urethral obstruction. Sphincter weakness can occur from damage to the urethra or its innervation or from pelvic floor muscle relaxation.

Incontinence from reversible factors originates outside of the lower urinary tract and is caused by mental status impairment, immobility, or medication. Some sources term this "functional" or "transient" incontinence.

A final category of incontinence is called mixed incontinence. This occurs when the incontinence is produced as the result of several anatomical, physiological, or functional factors.

Involuntary discharge of urine in children is abnormal beyond the age of 4 years for daytime wetting and beyond the age of 6 for nighttime wetting. Daytime wetting constitutes diurnal enuresis; nighttime wetting is known as nocturnal or sleep enuresis. In children, enuresis may be organic or nonorganic. Nonorganic enuresis can be primary or secondary. Primary nonorganic enuresis occurs in 75% to 90% of children. This enuresis is defined as wetting that has continued since infancy without an established pattern of dryness. Secondary nonorganic enuresis occurs in 10% to 25% of children and is defined as recurrence of wetting after continence has been established for at least 6 months. The possibility of abnormal urinary anatomy is high in young children who present with urinary tract symptoms.

DIAGNOSTIC REASONING: FOCUSED HISTORY

ADULTS

Could this be the result of reversible factors? (Box 6-1)

Key Questions
- What medications are you taking?
- Do you have any of the following urinary symptoms: urgency, frequency, burning, pain, blood in urine, flank pain?
- Do you have vaginal dryness or itching?
- Do you have pain/discomfort with sexual activity?
- Have you had changes in bowel function? When was your last BM?
- Are you feeling depressed or blue?
- Are you aware of incontinence?
- How mobile are you?
- Are you able to get to the toilet easily?
- Do you have any chronic health problems?

Medications. Sedatives, hypnotics, diuretics, anticholinergic agents, adrenergic agents, and calcium channel blockers can cause incontinence. Alpha-adrenergic agonists and beta-adrenergic agonists increase sphincter tone and may cause retention. Anticholinergics, prostaglandin inhibitors, calcium channel blockers, and narcotic analgesics decrease detrusor tone. Diuretics can cause incontinence because of in-

---

Box 6-1	

Reversible Factors That Can Cause Urinary Incontinence In Adults

D	Delirium, dementia, depression
I	Infection
A	Atrophic vaginitis/urethritis
P	Pharmaceuticals
E	Endocrine/excess urine production
R	Restricted mobility, retention
S	Stool impaction

Modified from Resnick NM: Initial evaluation of the incontinent patient, *J Am Geriatr Soc* 38(3):311, 1990.

creased production of urine, and central nervous system depressants such as hypnotics and sedatives can interfere with functional ability.

Urinary tract infection (UTI), vaginal dryness, and dyspareunia. UTI and atrophic vaginitis can cause incontinence through local irritation and loss of muscle tone.

Bowel function. Fecal impaction can cause incontinence through mechanical obstruction of the urethra.

Mental status, mobility, chronic health problems. Excessive urine production may be a problem if mobility is restricted, health is poor, or orientation is variable. Chronic health problems, psychological factors, and restricted mobility can result in incontinence because of loss of functional ability and/or mentation.

What do the presenting symptoms tell me?

Key Questions
- What is the primary symptom? (Urgency; dribbling; lack of sensation; nocturia; abdominal discomfort; leakage with laughing, coughing, sneezing, etc.)
- How frequently do you urinate?
- How much urine is lost each time?
- Do you have difficulty starting to urinate?
- Does your urine stream start and stop while you are urinating?

Primary symptom. Urgency is the primary symptom of detrusor instability. Dribbling indicates overflow incontinence, and sphincter weakness usually increases with postural changes. Men often complain of nocturia and dribbling with overflow incontinence. Abdominal discomfort often occurs with overflow incontinence because of bladder distention. Incontinence with increase in intra-abdominal pressure is usually stress incontinence but

can also be the result of detrusor overactivity and bladder irritability.

Frequency of voiding. Increase in frequency of voiding occurs with detrusor instability or hyperactivity and may occur with some transient causes such as use of diuretics or large-volume fluid intake. Decreased frequency is common in overflow incontinence.

Amount of urine lost with each episode. Small amounts of urine loss occur with stress and overflow incontinence.

Character of stream. A small-caliber stream, intermittent stream, or difficulty in starting the stream indicates obstructive uropathy. In males, this may be secondary to an enlarged prostate gland.

Are there any other symptoms that will point me in the right direction?

Key Questions
- How much fluid do you drink in a day?
- How much caffeine and alcohol do you drink?
- What time of day do you drink fluids?
- How thirsty are you?
- Have you lost or gained weight recently?

Fluid intake. A significant increase in the amount of fluid intake or an unusually large volume may indicate diabetes mellitus. Caffeine and alcohol can act as diuretics and may be a cause of reversible incontinence. Caffeine can also be a bladder irritant and either produce or exacerbate urge incontinence. A large volume of fluid intake may produce enuresis secondary to a large urine volume, particularly if fluids are consumed in the evening before bedtime.

Thirst. Unusual thirst accompanied by an unusually large intake of fluid may indicate diabetes mellitus (DM).

Weight loss or gain. Weight loss may indicate a chronic health problem, tumor, or dementia. Weight gain may indicate congestive heart failure (CHF), diabetes mellitus, or loss of mobility.

CHILDREN

Is this primary or secondary enuresis?

Key Question

• Has the child ever had consistent dryness for at least 6 months?

   Primary enuresis occurs when a child has never achieved consistent dryness. Secondary enuresis is involuntary voiding of urine in a child who has had a period of dryness greater than 6 months. Secondary enuresis is often indicative of some other form of voiding dysfunction or significant underlying pathology. In children, daytime urinary incontinence beyond the age of 4 years may indicate congenital abnormalities in the urinary tract or nervous system.

Is this organic enuresis?

Key Questions

• Does the child have pain on urination?
• Does the child have intermittent daytime wetness?
• Does the child seem very thirsty and urinate a lot?
• Has the child had any nervous system trauma?
• Does the child have constipation or encopresis?
• Does the child have constant wetness or dribbling throughout the day?
• Does the child have an abnormal stream, such as dribbling or hesitancy?
• Has the child had a change in gait?
• Has the child had a lumbar puncture recently?
• Does the child snore or have apnea at night?
• Does the child complain of rectal itching at night?

   Organic explanations of enuresis focus primarily on the genitourinary and nervous systems.

Genitourinary system. Fifteen percent of children with a urinary tract infection (UTI) present with enuresis. It is uncertain whether UTI causes the enuresis or vice versa. A wet perineum predisposes to ascending infection, and prompt treatment of the infection cures the enuresis in about one third of the cases. Asymptomatic bacteremia in school children is associated with enuresis.

   Fecal retention that is chronic or intermittent is responsible for production of "functional" bladder neck obstruction. Displacement of the bladder and posterior urethra by the full rectum in the fixed and limited space of the bony pelvis causes detrusor perineal dyssynergism, which is thought to be the mechanism responsible for urinary stasis and interference with micturition produced by constipation.

   Abnormal daytime voiding suggests urological abnormality. Dribbling suggests the presence of an ectopic ureter. Chronic leakage of urine in females may indicate an ectopic ureter that terminates in the vagina. Partial distal urethral obstruction can cause straining to urinate.

   Polyuria from a glucose-induced osmotic diuresis can be seen in diabetes mellitus. Renal tubules lose their ability to concentrate urine, resulting in polyuria of large volumes of very dilute urine.

Nervous system. Lumbosacral disorders affect bladder innervation and may cause enuresis. Head injury or brain tumor can cause polyuria and polydipsia. The kidneys are unable to concentrate urine, related to a deficiency in the hypothalamic production of ADH, producing central diabetes insipidus (DI) or related to renal unresponsiveness to ADH (nephrogenic DI).

   Interference with the nerve supply to the bladder causes a neurogenic bladder and obstruction. This can be functional, resulting from an imbalance between the detrusor muscle contraction and urethral sphincter relaxation. It can also be congenital or acquired, such as with meningomyelocele or spinal cord injury.

Sleep apnea interferes with the child's ability to wake appropriately in response to stimuli to void.

Other. Pinworms *(Enterobius vermicularis)* primarily inhabit the cecum and lower bowel and are the most common cause of rectal itching in children. Pinworms have been implicated in incontinence in children, although the reason is not clear.

What risk factors does this child have for nonorganic enuresis?

Key Questions
- Is the child a boy or girl?
- Is there a history of bedwetting in the family?
- Is the child a twin?
- Has the child been institutionalized?
- What is the child's birth order?
- Does the child have sickle cell disease?
- What is the child's daily fluid intake?

Gender. Boys are more likely to have nocturnal enuresis. Girls are more likely to have diurnal enuresis related to UTI.

Family history. Children with nonorganic enuresis often have a very strong family history of fathers who had nocturnal enuresis as a child.

Twin/birth order. Nocturnal enuresis is most common in the firstborn and in twins.

Institutionalization. Institutionalized children have a greater tendency to enuresis because of developmental delay.

Sickle cell disease. Children with sickle cell anemia may have a concentrating defect and excrete low specific gravity urine in large volumes, which may make the child wet the bed.

Fluid intake. A large volume of fluid intake may produce enuresis secondary to a large urine volume, particularly if the fluids are consumed in the evening before bedtime.

DIAGNOSTIC REASONING: FOCUSED PHYSICAL EXAMINATION

Perform Mental Status Examination

Assess orientation and cognitive function. In adults, incontinence can occur as the result of disorientation, delirium, or dementia.

In children, secondary enuresis can be caused by the presence of stress factors during the developmental period from 2 to 4 years of age. Separation from family, death of a parent, birth of a sibling, a move, marital conflict, and other stress-related causes may produce transient and intermittent enuresis.

Observe Gait

The urinary bladder receives extensive autonomic as well as somatic innervation. Lesions at all levels of the neuraxis from the cortex to peripheral nerves produce abnormalities of micturition.

Take Vital Signs

Blood pressure readings in children are important to rule out nephrotic causes of enuresis. When chronic renal failure is the result of an inadequate amount of normally functioning renal tissue, the clinical presentation may be enuresis. Fever in infants without any other signs is likely caused by UTI.

Examine the Abdomen

Palpate for masses, suprapubic tenderness, or fullness. Palpate the bladder. Abdominal distention or palpable bladder is suggestive of urinary retention and overflow incontinence.

Examine Genitalia in Males

Look for abnormalities of the foreskin, glans, meatus, penis, and perineal skin that might contribute to or produce incontinence.

Perform Pelvic Examination in Females

Note signs of pelvic prolapse (cystocele, rectocele). Palpate for pelvic mass and perivaginal muscle tone. Note condition of the vaginal mucosa and look for atrophic vaginitis. Vaginitis can cause urinary incontinence in children and adults, whereas atrophic vaginitis will produce incontinence only in adults.

Observe for evidence of sexual abuse such as abrasions, tears, or bruising. Urethral irritation, especially if discharge is present, may suggest sexual abuse in children.

Perform Provocative Stress Testing

During the pelvic examination, ask the patient to relax then cough vigorously (or perform a Valsalva maneuver) and watch for urine loss from urethra. A positive test indicates stress incontinence.

Perform Digital Rectal Examination

Assess for perineal sensation, resting and active sphincter tone, rectal mass, fecal impaction, and fissures. A lax sphincter suggests spinal cord involvement.

In men, assess consistency and contour of the prostate. Prostate enlargement or masses suggests the possibility of overflow incontinence from obstruction.

Conduct a Neurological Examination

Assess the intactness of the neurological system. Note focal deficits and test reflexes. Assess nerve roots S2-4. Test perineal sensation and deep tendon reflexes. Test for muscle tone and strength. Deficits may point to a neurological cause for the incontinence.

Examine/Palpate the Spine in Children

Look for an undetected birth defect that may be causing a neurological disturbance. A spinal dimple or hair tuft may alert you to a potential problem.

Perform Musculoskeletal Examination

Assess mobility, strength, and functional ability. In many older adults, the inability to get to a toilet causes incontinence.

An easy assessment of mobility is the timed get-up-and-go test. Time the patient getting up from a chair, walking 10 feet, and sitting back down. Although the time required to perform this test will vary, a mobile, independent, older adult can perform this activity in about 10 seconds.

Additional Procedures

Postvoid Residual (PVR)

Have the patient void without straining, then catheterize. A residual volume greater than 100 ml suggests either bladder weakness (stress incontinence) or outlet obstruction (overflow incontinence).

Observe Voiding

Note hesitancy, dribbling, interrupted stream, decreased force, and caliber of stream. These symptoms suggest outlet obstruction and overflow incontinence.

LABORATORY AND DIAGNOSTIC STUDIES

Urinalysis (U/A)

Dipstick U/A can rule out or point to infection or systemic disease as a cause of the incontinence. Note hematuria, pyuria, bacturia, or the presence of leukocytes esterase or nitrites as indicators of urinary tract infection. Glycosuria or proteinuria suggests DM or renal disease.

Urine Culture

A culture can be used to determine the organism(s) producing a UTI and can confirm diagnosis.

Blood Urea Nitrogen (BUN)/Creatinine

Use these indicators of renal function if you suspect obstruction or urinary retention.

Urine Cytology

Urine for cytology is indicated if microscopic or gross painless hematuria is present in the absence of infection.

Specific Gravity

A specific gravity of >1.015 rules out diabetes insipidus as the cause of incontinence.

Gram Stain, Potassium Hydroxide (KOH), or Vaginal Culture

These tests can confirm vaginal infection. See Chapter 7, Vaginal Discharge and Itching, on the procedures for these tests, pp. 270 and 271.

Office Cystometrography

Have the patient void and empty the bladder. Have men lie supine and place women in the dorsal lithotomy position. Insert a sterile 12-14 French (nonballooned) catheter and empty the bladder. (Measure the postvoid residual and collect urine for U/A at that time). Insert a 50-ml syringe with plunger removed into the end of catheter and position it about 15 cm above the urethra. Fill the syringe by pouring sterile water into it in 25- to 50-ml amounts. Record cumulative total fluid instillation in the bladder and note the volume at which the patient first reports the urge to void. Continue adding fluid slowly until the fluid level in the syringe rises, indicating a rise in intrabladder pressure and contraction of the detrusor muscle. The rise may be gradual or sudden. Detrusor contraction at less than 300 to 350 ml of bladder volume indicates detrusor instability (urge incontinence). Have the patient void at the end of the procedure. The amount instilled minus the amount voided will also provide a measure of postvoid residual.

Complete Urodynamic Testing

Complete urodynamic testing includes full cystometrography, perineal electromyelography, and voiding cystourethrography. It is indicated when a presumptive diagnosis cannot be made and when surgical repair of stress incontinence is a consideration.

Cystoscopy and Contrast Radiography

These procedures are indicated for detection of neoplasms or stones.

Ultrasound

Ultrasonography may be useful in determining the presence of an obstruction.

DIFFERENTIAL DIAGNOSIS

INCONTINENCE FROM ANATOMICAL CAUSES

Stress Incontinence

Stress incontinence is associated with activities that increase intra-abdominal pressure, such as coughing, sneezing, running, or laughing. The amount of urine lost with each episode is small. The patient usually has a history of childbirth. On examination, pelvic floor relaxation may be evident with presence of a cystocele and/or rectocele. The urethral sphincter may appear lax, and there is loss of urine with provocative testing. Atrophic vaginitis is a common finding in post-menopausal women.

U/A and culture may be performed to rule out infections or urinary tract problems. Postvoid residual is normal.

Urge Incontinence

Urge incontinence is characterized by an uncontrolled urge to void, secondary to detrusor muscle irritability or hyperactivity or a hypersensitive bladder. The urine volume lost is large. Physical examination is usually normal. Postvoid residual is normal. Diagnostic testing includes U/A and culture to rule out infection, and BUN and creatinine to rule out nephropathy. On office cystometrography, the urine volume is <300 to 350 ml before the urge to void occurs. Complete urodynamic testing can confirm the diagnosis.

Overflow Incontinence

Overflow incontinence occurs in the presence of obstruction or interruption in the nervous system. It is a result of overdistention of the bladder from an underactive or acontractile detrusor, sphincter-detrusor dyssynergia (loss of the synergistic urinary sphincter relaxation that normally occurs with bladder detrusor muscle contraction), or from bladder outlet or urethral obstruction. Sphincter weakness can occur from damage to the urethra or its innervation or from pelvic floor muscle relaxation.

Overflow incontinence is small-volume incontinence, with symptoms of dribbling and hesitancy. In men, symptoms of an enlarged prostate may be present (i.e., nocturia, dribbling, hesitancy, and deceased force and caliber of stream). On examination, look for distended bladder, prostate hypertrophy, evidence of spinal cord disease, or diabetic neuropathy. Postvoid residual is >100 ml. Diagnostic testing includes U/A and urine culture as well as BUN and creatinine levels.

Interference with the nerve supply to the bladder can result in neurogenic bladder, obstruction, and consequent overflow incontinence, caused by an imbalance between the detrusor muscle contraction and urethral sphincter relaxation. Functional incontinence can also be congenital or acquired, such as with meningomyelocele or spinal cord injury, or as a surgical complication from radical prostatectomy. On examination, the anal sphincter may be lax. Neurological testing may reveal deficits.

INCONTINENCE FROM REVERSIBLE FACTORS

Medications

Sedatives, hypnotics, diuretics, anticholinergic agents, alpha-adrenergic agents, and calcium channel blockers can cause incontinence. Alpha-adrenergic agonists and beta-adrenergic agonists increase sphincter tone and may cause retention and can cause urge incontinence. Anticholinergics, prostaglandin inhibitors, calcium channel blockers, narcotic analgesics decrease detrusor tone and can produce incontinence. Diuretics can cause incontinence because of increased production of urine, and central nervous system depressants such as hypnotics and sedatives can interfere with functional ability.

Urinary Tract Infection (UTI)

The patient with UTI has symptoms of lower or upper tract infection, such as burning, dysuria, frequency, urgency, flank pain, fever. The urine may have a foul odor. The patient may exhibit suprapubic or CVA tenderness. In infants, a fever with no localizing signs frequently indicates UTI. Urine analysis and culture can confirm diagnosis of a lower urinary tract infection.

Vaginitis

Vaginitis produces incontinence as a result of local irritation. Atrophic vaginitis indicates a loss of estrogen and a concomitant loss of the vesicourethral angle, which predisposes women to stress incontinence. Provocative stress testing can demonstrate stress incontinence. Gram stain, KOH, or culture can confirm vaginal infection.

Constipation, Fecal Impaction

Constipation or fecal impaction can produce an obstructive overflow incontinence by mechanical pressure on the urethra. The patient may experience abdominal pain and fecal soiling. On examination, stool may be felt in the colon and/or ampulla.

Change in Mental or Functional Status

Depression, dementia, or confusion can all produce incontinence (see Chapter 11, p. 401). Restricted mobility can result in incontinence because of loss of functional ability.

Diabetes Insipidus

In diabetes insipidus (DI), the kidneys are unable to concentrate urine because of a deficiency in the hypothalamic production of ADH (central DI) or a renal unresponsiveness to ADH (nephrogenic DI). The result is polyuria, which may cause incontinence. The patient also exhibits polydipsia.

Diabetes Mellitus

Diabetes mellitus (DM) often presents with excessive fluid intake and urination. The excess fluid volume can result in incontinence, particularly in older adults with chronic health problems, restricted mobility, or compromise in mental or functional health.

ENURESIS FROM ORGANIC CAUSES

Genitourinary Causes

Genitourinary disorders that can produce enuresis include UTI, ectopic ureter, or urethral obstruction. Physical examination is usually normal. Fever and abdominal tenderness may be present with a UTI. Anatomical genitourinary abnormalities may signal an ectopic ureter. Diagnostic testing includes urinalysis, urine culture, and specific gravity to rule out infection and DM. Referral for further evaluation may be necessary.

Neurological Causes

Nervous system involvement can also produce enuresis. Lumbosacral disorders affect bladder innervation and may cause enuresis. Head injury or brain tumor can cause polyuria and polydipsia. Interference with the nerve supply to the bladder causes neurogenic bladder and obstruction, which can result in enuresis. Interference in innervation can occur from congenital or acquired causes. Sleep apnea interferes with the child's ability to wake appropriately in response to stimuli to void. Diagnostic testing includes urinalysis, urine culture, and specific gravity to rule out infection and DM. Referral for further evaluation may be necessary.

ENURESIS FROM NON-ORGANIC CAUSES

Primary Enuresis

Primary enuresis occurs when a child has never achieved consistent dryness. The normal developmental patterns of micturition follow a characteristic pattern in children but at an individual rate. The usual progression depends on the maturation of the central nervous system. Generally the following stages are seen:

- Birth to 6 months—Bladder emptying is an uninhibited reflex action.
- 6-12 months—Bladder emptying is less frequent because of CNS inhibition of reflex action.
- 1-2 years—Child consciously perceives bladder fullness; CNS inhibition increases.
- 3-5 years—At age 5 years most children are aware of bladder fullness;

they develop the ability to inhibit the need to void both voluntarily and unconsciously.

Primary enuresis may represent a developmental delay or maturational lag. Often there is a family history of enuresis. The enuresis usually is nocturnal only. The incidence is higher in boys than girls and usually resolves as the child matures. Physical examination is normal. Diagnostic testing includes urinalysis, urine culture, and specific gravity to rule out other causes.

Developmental (Secondary) Enuresis

Developmental enuresis, which is secondary, may be related to changes or stresses in a child's life. It can also occur as the result of genital trauma, infection, distended colon, or fecal impaction. The enuresis occurs in a child who has had a period of dryness greater than 6 months. Diagnostic testing includes urinalysis, urine culture, and specific gravity to rule out other causes.

Small Bladder

An anatomically small bladder can also produce enuresis. The child voids frequently but not in excessive volume. Physical examination is normal. Diagnostic testing includes urinalysis, urine culture, and specific gravity to rule out other causes.

Sickle Cell Anemia

Children with sickle cell anemia have a concentrating defect and may experience enuresis because of volume excess. Physical examination findings are consistent with the sickle cell disorder. Diagnostic testing includes urinalysis, urine culture, and specific gravity.

Table 6-1

Differential Diagnosis of Common Causes of Urinary Incontinence

Condition	History	Physical Findings	Diagnostic Studies
Incontinence from Anatomical Causes			
Stress incontinence	Small-volume incontinence with coughing, sneezing, laughing, running; history of prior pelvic surgery	Pelvic floor relaxation; cystocele, rectocele; lax urethral sphincter; loss of urine with provocative testing; atrophic vaginitis	U/A and culture; PVR normal
Urge incontinence	Uncontrolled urge to void; large-volume incontinence; history of central nervous system disorders, such as stroke, multiple sclerosis, parkinsonism	Normal exam	U/A and culture; PVR normal; office cystometrography: <300-350 volume; BUN, creatinine, urodynamic testing

Table 6-1

Differential Diagnosis of Common Causes of Urinary Incontinence—cont'd

Condition	History	Physical Findings	Diagnostic Studies
Incontinence from Anatomical Causes—cont'd			
Overflow incontinence	Small-volume incontinence, dribbling; hesitancy; in men symptoms of enlarged prostate: nocturia, dribbling, hesitancy, decreased force and caliber of stream; in neurogenic bladder: history of bowel problems, spinal cord injury, or multiple sclerosis	Distended bladder; prostate hypertrophy, stool in rectum; fecal impaction; in neurogenic bladder, evidence of spinal cord disease or diabetic neuropathy; lax sphincter; gait disturbance	U/A and culture; PVR >100 ml; BUN, creatinine; in neurogenic bladder, refer for testing
Incontinence from Reversible Factors			
Medications	Hypnotics, diuretics, anticholinergic agents, alpha-adrenergic agents, calcium channel blockers	Normal except for findings related to other physical conditions	U/A to rule out tract problems; blood chemistry to rule out systemic problem
Urinary tract infection (UTI)	Dysuria, urgency, daytime accidents	Frequency, odor, fever	U/A and culture
Vaginitis	Itching, odor	Discharge; atrophic vaginitis; evidence of sexual abuse	Gram stain, KOH, culture
Constipation/fecal impaction	Abdominal pain	Soiling, stool felt in colon and/or ampulla	None
Change in mental or functional status	Change in mental status; impaired mobility; new environment	Impaired mental status; impaired mobility	U/A and culture; blood chemistry
Diabetes insipidus (DI)	History of trauma to head; thirst, frequency	Weight loss	U/A specific gravity >1.015
Diabetes mellitus (DM)	Thirsty, increased frequency	Weight loss	U/A; serum glucose

Continued

Table 6-1

Differential Diagnosis of Common Causes of Urinary Incontinence—cont'd

Condition	History	Physical Findings	Diagnostic Studies
Enuresis from Organic Causes			
Genitourinary causes	UTI history; dribbling; urine leakage	Fever, abdominal tenderness; anatomical abnormalities (ectopic ureter); exam may be normal	U/A and culture; specific gravity; referral for testing
Neurological causes	Head injury; spinal cord injury; polydipsia, polyuria; sleep apnea	Lax sphincter, spinal tuft, neurological deficits; altered gait; exam may be normal	U/A and culture; specific gravity; referral for evaluation
Enuresis from Non-Organic Causes			
Primary enuresis	Child has never been dry; may have family history	Normal exam; developmental delay	U/A and culture; specific gravity to rule out other causes
Developmental (secondary) enuresis	Child has been dry for 6 months in a row; changes or stresses in child's life	Examine for genital trauma or abuse, infection, distended colon, fecal impaction	U/A and culture; specific gravity to rule out other causes, screen for glycosuria
Small bladder	Void frequently, not in excessive volume	None	Bladder capacity = child's age +2 up to 11 yr
Sickle cell anemia	Family history	Findings related to sickle cell disease	U/A and culture, specific gravity

Urinary Problems in Females and Children

Common urinary complaints from females include changes in usual urination patterns (frequency, urgency, nocturia, incontinence), changes in urine appearance (color, cloudiness), and pain (dysuria, flank pain, or suprapubic pain).

Urinary problems in females may be caused by infection, inflammation, calculi (stones), congenital malformation, or trauma. The majority of urinary tract infections (UTIs) are caused by Gram-negative bacteria, predominantly *Escherichia coli*. The sexually transmitted pathogens *Chlamydia trachomatis*, *Neisseria gonorrhea*, and *Herpes simplex* are common causes of urethritis. Vaginitis also causes urinary symptoms in women. Urinary stones may occur anywhere in the urinary tract and are common causes of pain, bleeding, obstruction, and secondary infection.

Urinary tract infection in children is the second most common clinical disease of childhood, next to respiratory tract disorder. The symptoms of urinary tract disorder may be vague or absent, making the diagnosis easily overlooked. The infection may be present without symptoms, with symptoms that are obviously related to the urinary system, or with symptoms that may divert attention to another organ system problem. Abdominal masses in the newborn are most frequently caused by renal enlargement, specifically dysplastic kidney and/or congenital hydronephrosis. Vesicoureteral reflux is the major structural abnormality associated with UTI and renal damage.

Trauma to the urinary tract may be caused by penetrating, blunt, or crushing injuries or by surgery or instrumentation. Hematuria, oliguria, and pain are the most common symptoms.

DIAGNOSTIC REASONING: FOCUSED HISTORY

Are there systemic or upper urinary tract symptoms present?

Key Questions
- Have you had a fever or chills?
- Have you had nausea or vomiting?
- Have you had acute pain in the abdomen or back?
- Are you HIV positive or on chemotherapy?
- Infant: Has the infant been irritable or had anorexia or lethargy?

Fever and chills. The presence of fever and chills suggests a systemic inflammatory response and indicates an acute condition that should be aggressively treated.

Suspect pyelonephritis or lithiasis of the upper urinary system. Urinary tract infection is the most common bacterial infection found in febrile infants and children who present without an obvious source of infection.

Nausea and vomiting. Nausea and vomiting often accompany upper urinary tract infection, pyelonephritis, or lithiasis. Like fever and chills, these suggest a systemic inflammatory response and indicate that the patient may be acutely ill. In newborns and infants, non-specific symptoms, such as vomiting, diarrhea, and feeding difficulties, may indicate UTI.

Acute pain. Acute pain in the back or abdomen suggests upper urinary tract infection and pyelonephritis. Flank pain occurs with stretching of the renal capsule, associated with parenchymal swelling, and may indicate infection, obstruction, or primary renal disease.

Urinary tract stones may produce localized back pain or excruciating pain that radiates to the thigh.

Immunocompromised patients. Immunocompromised patients are susceptible to overwhelming infections by both common and atypical organisms, and aggressive investigation is warranted.

Irritable infant. Urinary tract infection in neonates and infants is manifested in subtle ways, such as irritability, anorexia, and weight loss. Some infants with urinary tract infection present with bacteremia.

Is there hematuria?

Key Questions
- Have you had blood in your urine? When in the stream does it occur?
- Do you have pain with urination?
- Do you have bleeding without urination?
- Have you done any strenuous exercise recently?

Hematuria. Red-to-brown discoloration is commonly caused by infection, trauma, or urinary tract stones. It can also be caused by parenchymal renal disease, systemic disease, medications, or coagulopathies.

Pyelonephritis or urinary tract stones are common causes of gross (macroscopic) hematuria. Neoplasm, trauma, and some medications can also produce gross hematuria. Gross hematuria occurs in 60% to 90% of bladder tumors. Both bladder and renal neoplasms are less common in women than men. Hematuria can be produced by local irritation in cystitis. Qualitative and quantitative platelet disorders as well as hemophilia can cause both gross and microscopic bleeding. Urinary frequency or urgency, dysuria, or suprapubic pain suggest that the origin of hematuria is confined to the lower urinary tract.

Initial hematuria (at the beginning of urination) suggests the urethra is the source, while terminal hematuria (at the end of urination) suggests posterior urethra or bladder base involvement. Total hematuria means red blood cells are dispersed throughout the urinary stream, characterizing origination in the kidney, ureter, or bladder.

Pain. Hematuria without pain is usually caused by renal disease or tumor of the bladder or kidney. Other causes of painless hematuria include stones, polycystic kidney disease, renal cysts, sickle cell disease, and hydronephrosis. When discomfort such as renal colic accompanies hematuria, suspect a ureteral stone. Hematuria with dysuria suggests bladder infection or lithiasis.

Bleeding without urination. Bladder lesions may produce bleeding independent of micturition.

Strenuous exercise. Transient hematuria is frequent after strenuous exercise proportional to the amount of exercise and trauma to the urinary tract. Exercise-related hematuria is caused by direct trauma to the kidney and bladder, as well as by ischemic injury. It is caused by the shifting of blood flow from the renal circulation to the heart, lung, and skeletal muscles during periods of high demand.

Can the symptoms be localized to the lower urinary tract?

Key Questions
- What are your primary symptoms? (pain, frequency, urgency, small amounts of urine, nausea, nocturia, itching)
- Have you had any suprapubic pain?
- Do you have involuntary urination?

Primary symptoms. Dysuria suggests irritation or inflammation in the bladder neck or urethra, usually caused by bacterial infection or irritation. These cause injury to the bladder mucosa, leading to inflammatory changes, infiltration, and edema. These changes can result in urgency and frequency, from mild stretching of the bladder to a loss of bladder elasticity.

Dysuria is the cardinal symptom of acute bacterial cystitis. In children, it may also be the first indication of an anatomical lesion such as obstruction of the urinary tract or vesicoureteral reflux (VUR). Other common symptoms include frequency, mild nausea, nocturia, urgency, and voiding small amounts. Fever is notably absent. Infants may have strong-smelling urine and continuously damp diapers.

Dysuria also suggests urethritis, especially if accompanied by vaginal discharge. External dysuria, a burning sensation as the urine passes inflamed labia, suggests vulvovaginitis. Patients with vulvovaginitis may also complain of discharge, odor, or itching. Women who have active herpes lesions may also experience external dysuria. Young children with pinworms (*Enterobius vermicularis*) may have dysuria and vaginitis because of the abrasions that result from periurethral and perivaginal itching and scratching.

Interstitial cystitis produces diminished bladder capacity along with symptoms of frequent painful urination. Hematuria may be present. Frequency can also occur as a result of stones or tumor.

Suprapubic discomfort and urinary incontinence. Discomfort in the suprapubic area is indicative of bladder involvement and urinary incontinence and is characteristic of bladder neck irritability caused by inflammation. Local causes of incontinence can also include pelvic relaxation and impaired bladder muscle activity. Preschool children with UTIs frequently have enuresis. See Urinary Incontinence, p. 218.

Could this be the result of trauma?

Key Questions
- Have you had any recent injury?
- Have you been hit recently?
- Have you noticed the child putting foreign objects in her genital tract?

Recent injury. Injury or a blow to the flank area can produce hematuria, originating from the kidney. Straddle injury may result in abrasions and local inflammation causing pain on urination.

About 5% of childhood trauma involves the kidney, making it a relatively uncommon event. About 10% of the kidneys injured have underlying abnormalities, such as hydronephrosis or a horseshoe shape, making them more vulnerable to injury.

Trauma. Domestic violence may present with blood in urine because of trauma. Trauma may or may not be associated with pain. Active children may not remember trauma to the area.

Foreign objects. Children have a propensity to put foreign objects in any orifice. Placing foreign objects in the vagina may cause dysuria and pyuria.

Could this be genitourinary in origin?

Key Questions
- Are you sexually active? How frequently?
- Have you had a new sexual partner recently?
- How many sexual partners do you have?
- Does your sexual partner have any symptoms?
- Do you use a diaphragm?
- Do you have any vaginal discharge?
- Post-menopausal women: are you on hormone replacement therapy?

Sexual activity. Factors that contribute to the development of acute bacterial cystitis include frequent sexual intercourse, use of a diaphragm, and use of spermicidal gel for contraception. Urethritis is associated with a history of a new sexual partner, a partner with urethritis, and multiple sexual partners. Masturbation may also cause dysuria in girls, as a result of either local irritation or the introduction of organisms that produce a lower UTI.

Organisms from sexually transmitted diseases can cause urethritis when they are present in large numbers in the urethra. A local inflammatory response results. *Chlamydia trachomatis* is the most common pathogen, although *Neisseria gonorrhea, Trichomonas vaginalis,* and *Herpes simplex* may also cause urethritis. Active herpes lesions can also produce dysuria as the urine passes across the inflamed external mucosa.

Diaphragm use. Some women who use a diaphragm experience mechanical compression of the urethra, with subsequent urine retention that predisposes them to the development of cystitis.

Vaginal discharge, hormone replacement therapy. Vaginal infections are a common cause of dysuria, particularly in college-aged women. Atrophic vaginitis can also cause dysuria. Post-menopausal women who are not on hormone replacement therapy are more likely to have atrophic vaginitis.

Are there any specific risk factors to point me in the right direction?

Key Questions

- Have you had this or similar problems before? If yes, when and how many times?
- Have you had recent catheterization or urinary tract procedures performed?
- Is there a family history of kidney or urinary problems?
- Do you have diabetes?
- How much spicy foods, caffeinated beverages/food, carbonated beverages, or alcohol do you consume?
- How much water do you drink?
- Do you suppress the urge to urinate? (postpone urination)
- Do you use bubble bath, shampoos, feminine hygiene products, powders, and soaps?
- Do you have constipation?

History of previous similar problems. Patients with previous urinary problems are at risk for chronic relapsing conditions, such as unresolved infections, resistant strains of organisms, or reinfection.

Recent instrumentation. Recent instrumentation of the urinary tract places the patient at risk for infections.

Family history of urinary problems. A family history of renal or kidney problems puts the patient at increased risk for urinary problems. A family history of deafness or renal insufficiency suggests hereditary nephritis or Alport's syndrome.

History of diabetes mellitus. Diabetes mellitus is associated with recurrent bacterial cystitis.

Types of food consumed. Dysuria without pyuria can be caused by chemical irritants such as spicy foods, caffeine, carbonation, and alcohol.

Decreased fluid intake. Decreased fluid intake with concentrated urine produces an irritant effect on bladder mucosa and may be a cause of dysuria without pyuria. It can also predispose to the development of bacterial cystitis.

Urge to urinate. Women who ignore the urge to urinate or who postpone urination are predisposed to the development of bacterial cystitis. Urine in the bladder for a prolonged period promotes bacterial growth.

Girls who have a history of squatting or leg crossing to stop urination may have a UTI. Uncontrolled bladder contractions against a closed bladder sphincter cause the behavior. These children may develop vesicoureteral reflux and infection.

Bubble bath and hygiene products. Common chemical irritants can cause dysuria without infection. The most common irritant, particularly in children, is bubble bath.

Constipation. Mechanical factors related to compression of the bladder and bladder neck by a hard mass of stool from constipation may cause UTI. There is also a relationship between constipation and dysfunctional voiding accompanied by incomplete bladder emptying.

What else could this be?

Key Questions

- Have you had recent treatment for a sexually transmitted disease?
- Have you been diagnosed with, but not treated for, a sexually transmitted disease?
- Have you had excessive urination?
- Have you had a sore throat or been treated for strep throat recently?

Sexually transmitted disease. Because vaginitis may cause urinary symptoms in females, a sexually transmitted vaginitis may be producing symptoms. Recent treatment for a sexually transmitted disease may indicate treatment failure, a coinfection that was not covered by the prescribed drug, or a reinfection (see Chapter 7, Vaginal Discharge and Itching, p. 263).

Excessive urination. The presence of polyuria suggests diabetes mellitus or diabetes insipidus. Women with diabetes mellitus are also prone to UTI.

Recent streptococcal infection. Poststreptococcal glomerulonephritis may develop after a 1- to 3-week latent period following pharyngeal or skin infections with certain strains of group A beta-hemolytic streptococci. The peak incidence is at age 7.

DIAGNOSTIC REASONING: FOCUSED PHYSICAL EXAMINATION

Note General Appearance

A patient who appears ill or who is pacing in pain is likely to have an upper urinary tract problem such as pyelonephritis or urolithiasis. Patients with lower urinary tract problems usually do not present with signs of systemic involvement, are free of fever, and generally appear well. Neonates present with malaise, irritability, and difficulty feeding. Toddlers and preschoolers appear ill with nausea, vomiting, and diarrhea.

Obtain Vital Signs, Height, and Weight

Failure to thrive is a common presenting sign of urinary tract disease in neonates or young children. Hypertension is seen in patients with nephritis.

Examine the Skin

Neonates with UTI may present with jaundice.

Palpate and Percuss for Flank Pain and at the Costovertebral Angle Bilaterally

Pain that is reproducible is indicative of renal capsule distention and characterizes acute pyelonephritis or acute ureteral obstruction.

Palpate and Percuss the Abdomen

Polycystic kidneys may produce abdominal distention. A flank mass may indicate a hydronephrotic kidney. Pain in the lower quadrant indicates lower ureter involvement. Suprapubic tenderness is characteristic of lower urinary tract infection. Perform deep palpation to identify kidneys or other abdominal masses. Normal kidneys are usually not easily palpated. A distended bladder rises above the symphysis pubis and is characteristic of residual urine resulting from incomplete bladder emptying. Palpating an enlarged bladder may cause pain. In hypertensive patients, auscultate at the subcostal anterior abdomen for bruits that could indicate a renovascular cause of hypertension.

Inspect the Perirectal Area

Inspect the skin and hair for inflammation or lesions, parasites, or dermatitis. Note inflammation, presence of lesions, or vaginal discharge. Observe for the presence of labial adhesions that might predispose the child to perineal bacterial colonization. Note personal hygiene. External excoriation could be the cause of burning or pain on urination. Note if there are any abrasions, tears, or bruising present, which might indicate trauma and/or sexual abuse.

Perform a Pelvic Examination if Indicated

A pelvic examination is essential if you suspect vaginitis or vulvovaginitis as a cause of the urinary symptom(s). On internal examination, note vaginal color, moistness, rugation, and characteristics of discharge. Pale, dry mucosa with lack of rugation characterizes atrophic vaginitis in a mature woman. Vaginal discharge not characteristic of physiological discharge suggests a vaginal infection. For discussion of vulvovaginitis, see Chapter 7, Vaginal Discharge and Itching, p. 272. Determine rectal tone. An atonic anal sphincter suggests a neurogenic bladder. Rectal examination for fecal impaction is indicated if the history suggests significant constipation or encopresis.

LABORATORY AND DIAGNOSTIC STUDIES

The extent of diagnostic investigation is determined by the history and the findings of the examination. The symptoms reported by the patient are taken into account when ordering diagnostic tests in order to corroborate or verify the diagnosis. General screening tests can be used to provide additional data for patients with urinary tract problems.

Urine should be freshly voided and usually midstream. If not examined immediately, the specimen should be refrigerated because cells begin to disintegrate after 1 to 2 hours.

Urine Dipstick

Reagent strips can be used to screen urine in the clinical setting.

Specific Gravity

Urine specific gravity depends on the patient's hydration. The urine pH also depends on the level of hydration as well as acid base status, time of urine collection, diet, and drugs that may affect the urine pH.

Leukocyte Esterase

The leukocyte esterase strip is calibrated to turn purple in 60 seconds, indicating 5 or more white blood cells in the urine. A positive test is indicative of urethritis (75% to 90% sensitivity, 95% specificity). Urine that tests positive for leukocyte esterase should be cultured for bacteria. Vaginal infection with *Trichomonas* can produce false positives; diets high in vitamin C can produce false negatives.

Nitrite

The nitrite strip is calibrated to turn pink within 30 seconds and signifies nitrite produced by $>10^5$ or more organisms/ml. Urine that tests positive for nitrites should be cultured for bacteria. However, note that some organisms that cause UTIs do not convert nitrate to nitrites (e.g., *Staphylococcus* or *Streptococcus*).

Protein

The normally small amount of protein excreted by a healthy adult is usually not detectable by dipstick analysis until the patient excretes 150 to 300 mg/day. At this level the patient will show trace amounts. In healthy persons, urine contains no protein or only trace amounts of proteins, which consists of albumin and globulins from the plasma. Glomerules usually prevent passage of protein from the blood to the glomerular filtrate. Therefore the persistent presence of protein in urine is a strong indication of renal disease. If more than a trace of protein is found, then a quantitative 24-hour evaluation is necessary. False positives can occur with alkaline urine.

If the patient has trace levels of proteinuria, then use of 20% sulfosalicylic acid testing for protein is appropriate. Add 8 drops of 20% sulfosalicylic acid to a sample of fresh, concentrated urine. Protein concentration is directly proportional to the degree of white turbidity produced. The absence of white turbidity indicates a false positive by dipstick analysis.

A typical scale to indicate progressively increasing amounts of protein is 1+ (30 mg/dL), 2+ (100 mg/dL), 3+ (300 mg/dL), and 4+ (500 to 1000 mg/dL). Peripheral edema and ascites may be present in an adult who has 3+ or 4+ proteinuria and is typically excreting 3 g or more of protein/day. Proteinuria reported for a single urinalysis is not an absolute guide in a differential diagnosis because proteinuria may be glomerular or tubular.

Glucose

Glucose in the urine is indicative of an elevated serum glucose of >200 mg/dL. If serum glucose levels are normal while urine glucose is elevated, then proximal renal tubular damage should be suspected.

Ketones

Ketones are detected earlier in the urine than in the blood and may indicate starvation or diabetic ketoacidosis.

Blood

Reagent strips are calibrated to detect red cells present. The strip detects heme at 0.05 to 0.3 mg hemoglobin/dL (see Red Blood Cells section following).

Urinalysis with Microscopic Examination

Color

The urine should be clear to yellow, depending on the concentration. The precipitation of calcium phosphate or urates can turn the urine milky, especially when stored in the refrigerator. Warming the urine to body temperature causes these precipitated salts to return to solution, removing the milky appearance. Methylene blue and indigo blue can make the urine blue. Vegetable dyes and paint from toys ingested by young children can turn their urine various colors. Brown urine is often observed in glomerulonephritis. Turbidity with a foul odor indicates infection. Color changes of the urine may result from various sources: hemoglobin from systemic red blood cell lysis; myoglobin from damaged muscle cell or rhabdomyolysis; vegetable pigment from food, such as red beets; and pigment from drugs, such as rifampin and phenazopyridine, or porphyrins from porphyria.

Discoloration of the urine should be investigated with microscopic examination to determine if red blood cells (RBCs) or any foreign substances are present. Pyuria results from white blood cell (WBC) debris and leukocytes in the urine, but cloudy urine can also result from other causes.

Sediment

Sediment for casts, blood cells, and bacteria can be detected by microscopic examination. Casts indicate hemorrhage or various conditions of the nephron. Red blood cells (RBC) indicate acute inflammatory or vascular disorders of the glomerulus. More than 1 to 2 RBC/high power field (HPF) is abnormal and can indicate renal or systemic disease or trauma to the kidney. Sediment is labeled as active when an abnormal number of cells, tubular casts, crystals, or infectious organisms are found.

A healthy person's urinalysis usually contains no cells, although an occasional cell/HPF is seen. More than 1 tubular epithelial and transitional epithelial cell/HPF suggests damage to the tubules or bladder wall. More than 1 RBC or WBC/HPF is considered abnormal. The more cells/HPF, the more active the renal disease may be.

Microscopic examination of the urine, resulting in 20 or more organisms/HPF, indicates urinary tract infection. Less than 20 organisms/HPF merits further study such as culture and sensitivity.

Red Blood Cells

Hematuria is >3 RBC/HPF. Distorted, irregularly shaped cells suggest a glomerular problem. The major causes of hematuria include acute and chronic prostatitis or urethritis, hemorrhagic cystitis, renal stones, or tumors of the kidney, renal pelvis, ureter, bladder, and urethra. Hematuria with proteinuria usually suggests a renal origin. Isolated hematuria is usually produced by sites outside the kidneys.

White Blood Cells

Pyuria (>5 WBC/HPF) is highly sensitive for the presence of a UTI. However, it may occur with dehydration, renal stones, appendicitis, or other extrinsic ureteral irritation in the absence of demonstrable microbial infection.

Casts

Tubular casts are formed in the distal portion of the nephron. A hyaline cast is a wispy, translucent, cylindrical replica of the tubular lumen. Red cell casts are characteristic of glomerular origins. The presence of abnormal cells, protein, hemoglobin, myoglobin, or other debris with a cast helps identify the type of renal disease.

Urine Culture and Sensitivity

Culture is indicated in children if you are uncertain of a diagnosis of acute bacterial cystitis based on clinical findings and urinalysis, or if the patient has signs and symptoms of an upper UTI or complicated UTI.

Potassium Hydroxide (KOH)/Wet Mount

Perform these procedures if you suspect vulvovaginitis as a cause of the urinary symptoms. See Chapter 7, Vaginal Discharge and Itching, p. 270, for explanation and discussion of these procedures.

Vaginal Culture/DNA Probe

Use these testing procedures to diagnose or confirm vaginal infection (see Chapter 7, Vaginal Discharge and Itching, p. 271).

Ultrasonography

Ultrasonography is a noninvasive technique than can provide information about kidneys, ureters, bladder, and vascular structures. Renal ultrasound is a good first test to determine kidney size, contour, and the presence of calculi. Urinary bladder sonogram is used to identify tumors of the bladder, thickening of the bladder wall, posterior masses behind the bladder, or obstruction of the lower urinary tract showing residual urine.

X-Ray

A flat plate of the abdomen can be used to identify structures of the kidney, ureters, and bladder. Urinary calculi are usually visible on x-ray.

DIFFERENTIAL DIAGNOSIS

Bacterial Cystitis

Acute bacterial cystitis accounts for 25% to 33% of lower urinary tract infections. Patients present with dysuria and may have urinary frequency, mild nausea, nocturia, urgency, and voiding of small amounts. Fever is notably absent in adults but may be present in pediatric patients. Neonates may present with prolonged jaundice and failure to thrive.

The adult patient appears well and on physical examination has no CVA tenderness. Suprapubic tenderness may be present. Clinical diagnosis is supported by urine dipstick findings, which may include the presence of blood, leukocyte esterase, and nitrites. Microscopic analysis may show the presence of RBCs and WBCs. No casts will be present. Urine culture and sensitivity will confirm the diagnosis.

Urethritis

Dysuria suggests urethritis, especially if accompanied by vaginal discharge. The history often includes a new sex partner, frequent sex, a partner with urethritis, or multiple sex partners. As with bacterial cystitis, the patient appears well, and on physical examination has no CVA tenderness or fever. On urinalysis using a dipstick, findings may include the presence of blood, leukocyte esterase, and nitrites, although the patient may have urethritis in the absence of these findings. Urine culture or DNA probe confirms the presence of the offending pathogens, usually *Chlamydia*, *N. gonorrhea*, *Trichomonas*, and *Herpes*.

Vulvovaginitis

Vulvovaginitis is a common cause of dysuria. The patient often describes the dysuria as "external"—a burning sensation as the urine passes inflamed labia. The patient often has a history of vaginal discharge, odor, and/or itching. On physical examination, discharge is usually present in the vagina or from the cervix. Wet prep, KOH, and vaginal culture or DNA probe can confirm diagnosis (see Chapter 7, Vaginal Discharge and Itching, p. 272).

In older women, atrophic vaginitis may produce urinary symptoms. These women may be peri- or post-menopausal. Women with atrophic vaginitis may complain of vaginal dryness or discomfort during sexual intercourse. On physical examination, the vaginal mucosa is thin, pale, dry, with less rugation. Diagnosis is made on the basis of clinical findings.

Interstitial Cystitis

Interstitial cystitis produces diminished bladder capacity along with symptoms of frequent, painful urination. Hematuria may be present. The cause is unknown but may be related to collagen disease, may be an autoimmune disorder, an allergic manifestation, or secondary to an unidentified infectious agent. The bladder wall becomes inflamed, with mucosal ulceration and scarring that produces contraction of the smooth muscle and causes the symptoms. Middle-aged women are most often affected. Typically, the patient appears well and has no physical findings. Suprapubic tenderness may be present. Urinalysis is usually negative. This is a diagnosis of ex-

clusion, and the patient is often frustrated because no cause has been previously found for her long-standing and persistent symptoms. The patient has no evidence of urological disease on x-ray and cystometric studies. Cystoscopic evidence of interstitial disease includes focal ulceration, edema, and perivascular infiltrates.

Pyelonephritis

The patient presents with fever, chills, appears toxic, and complains of back pain. Nausea and vomiting may be present. Some patients also complain of lower urinary tract symptoms, including frequency and dysuria. The patient feels and looks ill. On physical examination, CVA tenderness is usually present. The abdomen may also be tender. On microscopic examination, WBCs are usually present. White cell casts suggest pyelonephritis. Bacterial casts, although rare, are pathognomonic of pyelonephritis. Urine culture and sensitivity confirm diagnosis and identify the pathogen, usually *E. coli*, *Klebsiella* sp., *Proteus mirabilis*, and *Enterobacter* sp.

Urolithiasis

Urinary stones can occur anywhere in the urinary tract and may produce symptoms of acute pain, hematuria, and secondary infection. Many calculi are "silent" and may cause only hematuria, microscopic or gross. Renal calculi may occur when a stone obstructs the urinary tract. Typical symptoms of renal colic include severe flank pain that radiates along the pathway of the ureter to the inner thigh. Chills, fever, and urinary frequency are common. The patient may have nausea, vomiting, and abdominal distention.

The clinical diagnosis is supported by urinalysis and imaging findings. The urine may be normal; however, gross or microscopic hematuria is common. Pyuria (WBCs) with or without bacteria may be present. Crystalline structures may be present. Most stones are visible on x-ray or by ultrasound.

Poststreptococcal Glomerulonephritis

This condition is an immune-mediated nephritis. It occurs most commonly in elementary school children. There is a history of recent streptococcal skin or pharyngeal infection within the past 1 to 3 weeks. Anorexia, vomiting, fever, abdominal pain, headache, and lethargy are reported. On physical examination, periorbital edema is usually present as is hypertension. Orthopnea, dyspnea, cough, and rales may be present. Hematuria and proteinuria are present. A positive serum ASO titer confirms recent infection. A depressed serum concentration of C3 is found in the first few days of the disease.

Chemical Irritation

There is a history of use of bubble bath, body lotions, soaps, and sprays. The patient experiences frequency, burning, and urgency with small volumes of voided urine. Children will frequently suppress voiding because of pain. Physical examination may reveal erythema of the labia and urethral outlet. Laboratory examination may reveal pyuria and bacteriuria as a result of local infection and denudation.

Table 6-2

Differential Diagnosis of Common Causes of Urinary Problems in Females and Children

Condition	History	Physical Findings	Diagnostic Studies
Bacterial cystitis	Dysuria, frequency, mild nausea, nocturia, urgency, and voiding small amounts; neonates and young infants present with anorexia, irritability, fever	No fever; appears well; no CVA tenderness; may have suprapubic tenderness; NOTE: neonates and young infants may present with failure to thrive, bacteremia	Urine dipstick: + blood, + leukocyte esterase, + nitrites; microscopic analysis: RBCs, WBCs, no casts; urine C & S; in children, a voiding cystourethrogram and renal ultrasound are recommended
Urethritis	Dysuria; vaginal discharge; history of new sex partner, frequent sex, partner with urethritis, multiple sex partners	Appears well, has no CVA tenderness or fever	Urine dipstick: may have + blood, + leukocyte esterase, + nitrites; urine culture or DNA probe: Chlamydia, N. gonorrhea, Trichomonas
Vulvovaginitis	History of vaginal itching, discharge, burning, dryness; postmenopausal	Inflamed or atophic labia; vaginal or cervical discharge	Microscopic exam, vaginal cultures, DNA probe

Table 6-2

Differential Diagnosis of Common Causes of Urinary Problems in Females and Children—cont'd

Condition	History	Physical Findings	Diagnostic Studies
Interstitial cystitis	Frequent painful urination; hematuria; most often middle-aged women; often frustrated because no cause has been previously found for long-standing and persistent symptoms	Appears well and has no physical findings; suprapubic tenderness may be present	Urinalysis usually negative; x-ray and cystometric studies to rule out other urological disease; cystoscopy
Pyelonephritis	Fever, chills, back pain, nausea and vomiting, toxic appearance; some patients also have frequency and dysuria	Feels and looks ill; fever; CVA tenderness; abdomen may be tender	Microscopic examination: WBCs may have white cell casts or bacterial casts; urine C & S: *E. coli, Klebsiella* sp, *Proteus mirabilis, Enterobacter* sp; blood cultures
Urolithiasis	Pain, hematuria, may have symptoms of secondary infection; renal colic: pain that radiates to the inner thigh; nausea, vomiting	May have CVA tenderness; looks ill during periods of acute pain; may have abdominal distention	Urinalysis: gross or microscopic hematuria; WBCs with or without bacteria; crystalline structures may be present; x-ray or ultrasound
Poststreptococcal glomerulonephritis	History of skin or throat infection 1-3 weeks prior; lethargy, anorexia, vomiting, abdominal pain	Hypertension, periorbital edema, CVA tenderness; may have dyspnea, cough, pallor	U/A+, + proteinuria, hematuria, + ASO titer, serum C3 low early in disease
Chemical irritation	History of bubble bath, soaps, lotions, sprays; urgency, dysuria	No fever; erythematous labia, urethral opening	Hematuria common, gross hematuria unusual and casts never seen

Genitourinary Problems In Males

Urinary tract problems in males represent a range of conditions from infections, inflammation, and urine outlet obstruction to congenital malformation, trauma, or neoplasm. Any part of the renal/urological/reproductive tract can be involved, and symptoms may often be localized to a single site. Symptoms may also be vague, can reflect the involved area, or be referred from the actual site of involvement.

Dysuria in males is most commonly caused by urethritis, prostatitis, cystitis, and mechanical irritation of the urethra. Inflammation, although infrequent in young males, increases with age until elderly males are affected as frequently as elderly females.

Cystitis in men results from ascending infection of the urethra or prostate or occurs secondary to urethral instrumentation. The most common cause of recurrent cystitis in men is chronic bacterial prostatitis. *Escherichia coli* is the usual Gram-negative pathogen. *Chlamydia trachomatis* is the major cause of prostatitis and nongonococcal urethritis in men under age 40 and is sexually transmitted. Recurrent urinary tract infections may involve resistant Gram-negative *Klebsiella* sp., *Enterobacter* sp., *Pseudomonas, Proteus mirabilis,* or Gram-positive *Enterococcus* and *Staphylococcus aureus*. Infection may involve the kidneys and cause pyelonephritis. Secondary infection can occur as the result of urinary stones.

The male patient with urinary problems may also present with symptoms involving urinary flow. Urine flow may be altered by compression of the urethra as it passes through an enlarged prostate, obstructing the flow of urine and producing hesitancy, slowing of the urinary stream, dribbling, and nocturia. Benign prostatic hyperplasia (BPH) is common in men over age 50 and progresses with age until 80% of men over 80 are affected. Patients with BPH are more prone to urinary tract infections and incontinence. Urinary stones may occur anywhere in the urinary tract and are common causes of obstructive symptoms, bleeding, and pain.

Trauma to the urinary tract may be caused by penetrating, straddle, blunt, or crushing injuries or by surgery or instrumentation. Hematuria, oliguria, and pain are the most common symptoms.

Neoplasms occur more often in males than females. Kidney, prostate, and bladder neoplasms are more common in elderly men. Kidney and bladder neoplasms often produce painless hematuria. Prostate cancer produces symptoms of outlet obstruction.

Kidney problems can range from asymptomatic blood chemical changes to life-threatening abnormal renal function that could manifest in fluid-electrolyte imbalance and acid-base imbalance. Patients with renal insufficiency may present with nonspecific complaints such as fatigue, anorexia, or weakness. However, a discussion of renal insufficiency and renal failure is beyond the scope of this chapter.

DIAGNOSTIC REASONING: FOCUSED HISTORY

Are there systemic or serious symptoms present?

Key Questions
- Have you had fever or chills, nausea or vomiting?
- Are you HIV positive or on chemotherapy?
- Are you having acute pain?
- Have you been able to pass any urine?

Fever and chills. The presence of fever and/or chills suggests a systemic inflammatory response and indicates that the patient may be acutely ill and should be aggressively treated. Specifically, suspect pyelonephritis or lithiasis of the upper urinary system or prostatitis, orchitis, or epididymitis of the lower urinary tract.

Immunocompromised patients. Immunocompromised patients are susceptible to overwhelming infections by both common and atypical organisms, and aggressive investigation is warranted.

Acute pain. Acute pain in the abdomen or flank is characteristic of bladder, ureter, and kidney involvement. Acute pain in the scrotum or testicles may indicate infection or pathology of the scrotal contents or be referred from other sites in the urinary tract. Pain in the scrotum or testicles is characteristic of inflammation of the testicles, epididymitis, or torsion of a testicle (see Penile Discharge, p. 259).

Anuria. A sudden decrease in urinary output may result from compromised renal blood supply (prerenal); damaged interstitia, glomeruli, or tubules (intrarenal); or obstructed urine flow (postrenal). Patients with prerenal failure usually have a history of volume depletion or a reduction in arterial blood volume such as in low cardiac output states. Patients with intrarenal failure may present with history of renal damage from nephrotoxic agents. Postrenal failure is the least likely cause of anuria, but it should be ruled out first, because when failure results from obstructive causes, mechanical intervention may reestablish kidney function before permanent nephron damage occurs. Patients at greatest risk for acute renal failure are the elderly, diabetic patients, and those with a history of renal, heart, or liver disease.

Anuria may represent obstruction or renal failure.

Is there hematuria?

Key Questions

• Have you noticed blood in your urine?
• Is there blood every time you urinate or just sometimes?
• Does the blood start with the beginning of urination, continue through-

out urination, or occur only at the end of urination? Is there blood without urinating?
• Do you have pain with the blood?

Hematuria. Blood can enter the urinary tract at any site. The most common source of isolated hematuria is extrarenal. A lesion of the bladder or lower urinary tract is demonstrated in over 60% of patients. The most common causes of gross hematuria from the kidney are nephropathy and polycystic kidney disease. No cause for hematuria can be found in 10% to 15% of patients.

Timing. Initial hematuria becomes clear during voiding and is indicative of anterior urethral lesions such as urethritis, stricture, or meatal stenosis. Terminal hematuria begins with clear urine, then becomes bloody and is suggestive of prostatic lesions or lesions in the prostatic urethra. Total hematuria is usually characteristic of lesions in the kidneys and ureters. Bladder lesions may produce bleeding independent of micturition. Recent trauma to the kidneys can also produce hematuria. Gross hematuria is often transient but may continue microscopically.

Pain. Hematuria with pain usually indicates the passage of a stone or sloughed renal papilla, often with concurrent infection. Painless gross hematuria is consistent with upper or lower tract tumor, systemic coagulopathy, or excessive anticoagulant effect. Less common causes include acute necrosis or sloughing of a papilla. In elderly males, painless hematuria may be a late presenting sign of renal cancer.

Can the symptoms be localized to a part of the urinary tract?

Key Questions

• Do you have trouble starting to urinate? (slow/weakened urinary stream, dribbling of urine)

- Do you have low back, flank, or abdominal pain?
- Do you have aching in the perineal area?
- Do you have suprapubic discomfort?
- Have you had involuntary urination?
- Do you have frequency, urgency, dysuria, or penile discharge?
- Do you have to urinate at night?
- Do you have an excessive volume of urine?

Hesitancy, slow urinary stream, and dribbling of urine. In men over age 50, the presence of hesitancy, slow urinary stream, and dribbling of urine with a gradual onset over time indicates obstructive problems from benign prostatic hypertrophy. Have the patient complete the American Urological Association (AUA) Symptom Index (Table 6-3). Using the Index, classify symptoms as mild (0-7), moderate (8-19), or severe (20-35).

Low back, flank, or abdominal pain. Patient reports of low back, flank, or abdominal pain are often indicative of ureteral and kidney involvement. Renal tract pain may present with a constant dull ache in the costovertebral angle area. Dislodged kidney stones will produce an acute ureteral pain that is colicky and cyclic in nature. Gross blood in the urine and infection may accompany the ureteral pain. The pain can radiate to the abdomen, testes, and penis. However, renal disorders do not frequently cause pain. True renal pain can originate from the calyces or renal pelvis. Pain can result from stretching of the kidney capsule, interstitial edema, or inflammation of the capsule.

Aching in the perineal area. Prostate pain is often interpreted by the patient as a vague ache in the perineal area. The usual cause of perineal aching is infection. Another cause may be prostatic stones with infection.

Suprapubic discomfort and urinary incontinence. Discomfort in the suprapubic area is indicative of bladder involvement, whereas urinary incontinence is characteristic of bladder neck irritability caused by inflammation. Bladder pain is most often caused by infection; however, it can also be produced by obstruction and bladder distention as the result of tumor or stones.

Penile discharge with frequency, urgency, and dysuria. Penile discharge with frequency, urgency, and dysuria are characteristic of anterior urethral irritation in males and of exposure to a sexually transmitted disease (see Penile Discharge, p. 258).

Nocturia. Primary bladder disease from infection, stones, or tumors can produce nocturia. Prostate enlargement characteristically produces nocturia. Most adults do not need to void during the night, but some may get up once during the night depending on the amount and timing of fluid ingestion.

Usually patients who complain of daytime frequency without nocturia are free of organic disease.

Polyuria. Polyuria is defined as a volume greater than 3 L of urine/day and depends on fluid intake and the patient's state of hydration. Polyuria may be an early indication of renal disease progression because of the kidneys' inability to concentrate urine. Taking a history of fluid intake is important to identify possible causes of polyuria. Pseudo-polyuria results from increased fluid ingestion that may present with certain personality disorders. With the current emphasis on water ingestion, a large intake can also produce a pseudo-polyuria. Alcohol ingestion inhibits antidiuretic hormone; glycosuria promotes excess solute excretion. Diabetes insipidus may also be implicated. Nocturia can occur with the mobilization of fluid during sleep, secondary to congestive heart failure.

Table 6-3

The American Urological Association Symptom Index

Patients rate their answers to each question on a scale of 0 to 5.

QUESTIONS	AUA SYMPTOM SCORE (CIRCLE ONE NUMBER ON EACH LINE)					
	NOT AT ALL	LESS THAN 1 TIME IN 5	LESS THAN HALF THE TIME	ABOUT HALF THE TIME	MORE THAN HALF THE TIME	ALMOST ALWAYS
1. Over the past month, how often have you had a sensation of not emptying your bladder completely after you finished voiding?	0	1	2	3	4	5
2. Over the past month, how often have you had to urinate again less than 2 hours after you finished urinating?	0	1	2	3	4	5
3. Over the past month, how often have you found you stopped and started again several times when you urinated?	0	1	2	3	4	5
4. Over the past month, how often have you found it difficult to postpone urination?	0	1	2	3	4	5
5. Over the past month, how often have you had a weak urinary stream?	0	1	2	3	4	5
6. Over the past month, how often have you had to push or strain to begin urination?	0	1	2	3	4	5
7. Over the past month, how many times did you most typically get up to urinate from the time you went to bed at night until the time you got up in the morning?	0	1	2	3	4	5

AUA Symptom Score = sum of above 7 circled numbers: _____.

Symptoms are classified as: mild (0-7), moderate (8-19), severe (20-35).

From Barry JB et al and The Measurement Committee of the American Urological Association: The American Urological Association Symptom Index for Benign Prostatic Hyperplasia, *J Urol* 148:1549-1557, 1992.

Are there any specific risk factors to point me in the right direction?

Key Questions
- Have you had this or similar problems before? If yes, when and how many times?
- Do you have a family history of renal or kidney problems, prostatitis, or prostate cancer?
- How old are you? (What is the patient's age?)
- Have you been confined to bed? (especially if elderly)
- Are you sexually active? How many partners?

History of previous similar problems. Patients with previous urinary problems are at risk for chronic relapsing conditions, such as unresolved infections, resistant strains of organisms, or reinfection. Recurrent infections, pyelonephritis, or complications warrant urological referral for workup and evaluation.

Family history of urinary problems. A family history of renal or kidney problems or prostatitis puts the patient at increased risk for urinary problems. Familial disorders that may be implicated in kidney disease include diabetes mellitus, hypertension, collagen vascular disease, nephrolithiasis, and polycystic kidney disease.

Age. Urinary tract infection in males increases with age. Slow development of prostatic obstruction is common in men over age 50 and is usually painless. Patients have difficulty in starting the urine stream, and there is a decreased force of stream and dribbling after voiding. *Chlamydia* is the major cause of prostatitis, epididymitis, and nongonococcal urethritis in males under 40 years of age. Adolescents who are sexually active are at particular risk for sexually transmitted diseases.

Confined to bed. Elderly patients confined to bed are at an increased risk of infection. Likely mechanisms include urinary stasis and reflux.

Sexually active. Sexually active males, especially those who engage in unprotected sex, are at risk for sexually transmitted diseases, which can produce urethritis. The risk increases with multiple partners.

What else could this be?

Key Questions
- Have you had recent instrumentation of the urethra or urinary tract?
- Have you had recent treatment for a sexually transmitted disease?
- Have you been recently diagnosed with but not treated for a sexually transmitted disease?
- What drugs have you taken? (prescription, over the counter, or illicit)
- What do you do for a living? As hobbies? (toxic exposure)

Recent instrumentation. Recent instrumentation of the urinary tract places the patient at risk for infections. Patients with indwelling catheters are also at risk for infection.

Recent sexually transmitted disease. Sexually transmitted diseases can produce urethritis and urinary symptoms. Recent treatment for a sexually transmitted disease may indicate treatment failure, a coinfection that was not covered by the prescribed drug, or a reinfection.

Drug review or history. The most prevalent nephrotoxic drugs include aminoglycosides, nonsteroidal anti-inflammatory drugs, iodinated radiocontrast media, and angiotensin-converting enzyme inhibitors. Less prevalent are antibiotics such as amphotericin B, chemotherapeutic agents, cocaine, H2 receptor antagonists, phenytoin, sulfonamide diuretics, and volatile hydrocarbons.

Toxic exposures. Occupational hazards that may cause kidney problems include exposure to volatile hydrocarbons, benzene, aniline, xylene, heavy metals, and ionizing radiation.

DIAGNOSTIC REASONING: FOCUSED PHYSICAL EXAMINATION

Note General Appearance

A patient who appears ill or who is in pain is likely to have an upper urinary tract problem such as pyelonephritis or urolithiasis. Patients with lower urinary tract problems usually do not present with signs of systemic involvement, are free of fever, and generally appear well.

Obtain Vital Signs

Hypertension is seen in patients with nephritis.

Inspect Skin and Mucous Membranes

A pale skin color may suggest anemia caused by poor nutrition or chronic renal failure. A yellow- to brown-colored skin without scleral icterus may indicate severe chronic uremia. Other skin changes seen with renal problems may range from rash to purpura.

Hypertension and edema are two findings that usually indicate renal problems; however, a physical examination may not provide much data because few physical signs found on examination indicate the presence of kidney disease.

Palpate and Percuss for Flank Pain at the Costovertebral Angle

Pain that is reproducible is indicative of renal capsule distention and characterizes acute pyelonephritis or acute ureteral obstruction. Perinephric abscess may cause flank swelling and redness.

Palpate and Percuss the Abdomen

Abdominal distention suggests ascites or fluid collection in the bowel. Pain in the lower quadrant indicates lower ureter involvement. Perform deep palpation to identify kidneys or other abdominal masses. Normal kidneys are usually not easily palpated. A distended bladder rises above the symphysis pubis and is characteristic of residual urine from incomplete bladder emptying. Palpating an enlarged bladder may cause pain. Chronic bladder distention is usually painless and cannot always be determined by manual palpation alone.

If the patient is hypertensive, auscultate at the subcostal anterior abdomen for bruit that could indicate a renovascular cause of hypertension.

Inspect and Palpate the External Genitalia

Inspect the skin and hair for inflammation or lesions, parasites, or dermatitis. Note hair pattern distribution and level of development of structures for age group. Palpate the shaft of the penis for strictures. Observe for phimosis if uncircumcised and retract the foreskin. Note inflammation or presence of smegma. Inspect glans, coronal, and frenulum areas for lesions. Note personal hygiene, phimosis in uncircumcised males, and presence of urine, discharge, and fecal stains on undergarments. Check position of urethral meatus. Strip or milk the penis from the base towards the glans or head of the penis. Note any discharge for color, consistency, and amount.

Check scrotum skin surfaces and testicles for tenderness and masses; also check epididymis, spermatic cords, and inguinal canals. The left scrotal sac usually hangs lower than the right. Elevation of an affected testicle may relieve discomfort and is characteristic of epididymitis. A painful scrotal mass is usually associated with inflammation or testicular torsion.

Perform scrotal transillumination in a darkened room. Do not use a halogen light source as it may burn the patient. A solid mass prevents the passage of light and requires further examination. A hydrocele is a nontender firm mass that results from fluid accumulation. It will transilluminate but may make testicular palpation impossible. A spermatocele (a cystic swelling on the epididymis) is not as large as a hydrocele but does not transilluminate. Dilated veins in the scrotal sac, or varicocele, is the most common scrotal mass, usually occurring on the left side. It is often more prominent when the patient is standing and regresses with the patient in the prone position. It is classically described as a "bag of worms."

Observe Voiding

Observing the patient urinating may be useful to check for hesitancy in initiating the urine stream, force of stream, and dribbling at end of micturition. Observe the abdominal force used during urination. Patients will use abdominal muscles to increase the intraabdominal pressure to force urine from the bladder while holding their breath.

Perform Digital Rectal Prostate Examination

Digital rectal examination of the prostate is done to identify irregularities of the prostate that are suggestive of cancer and to note any tenderness or inflammation. The size and consistency should be noted. The median sulcus and lateral margins should be palpated. Induration or firmness is characteristic of early prostate disease; a hard stony gland suggests advanced prostatic carcinoma. The gland may feel soft because of inflammation or infection. If hypertrophied, the prostate gland will extend into the rectal canal, and the median sulcus may be obliterated. Do not massage the prostate if acute prostatitis is suspected because of the possibility of spreading the infection. Document the amount of prostate extension into the rectum using an acceptable clinical scale:

- Grade I: protrudes <1 cm into the rectum
- Grade II: protrudes 1 to 2 cm into the rectum
- Grade III: protrudes 2 to 3 cm into the rectum
- Grade IV: protrudes >3 cm into the rectum

LABORATORY AND DIAGNOSTIC STUDIES

The history and the findings of the physical examination determine the extent of diagnostic investigation. The symptoms reported by the patient are taken into account when ordering diagnostic tests in order to corroborate or verify the diagnosis. General screening tests can be used to provide additional data for patients with urinary tract problems.

Specific tests for kidney function include urinalysis, screening blood chemistry tests such as urea nitrogen and serum creatinine, and hematological studies. Abnormal blood tests include elevated creatinine, blood urea nitrogen, hyperkalemia, and hypocalcemia.

Urine collected for urinalysis should be freshly voided and usually midstream. If not examined immediately, the specimen should be refrigerated because cells begin to disintegrate after 1 to 2 hours.

Urine Dipstick

Reagent strips can be used to screen urine in the clinical setting.

Specific Gravity

Urine specific gravity depends on the patient's hydration. The urine pH also depends on the level of hydration as well as acid-base status, time of urine collection, diet, and drugs that may affect the urine pH.

Leukocyte Esterase

The leukocyte esterase strip is calibrated to turn purple in 60 seconds, indicating 5 or more white blood cells in the urine. A positive test is indicative of urethritis (75% to 90% sensitivity, 95% specificity). Urine that tests positive for leukocyte esterase should be cultured for bacteria. Diets high in vitamin C can produce false negatives.

Nitrite

The nitrite strip is calibrated to turn pink within 30 seconds and signifies nitrite produced by $>10^5$ or more organisms/ml. Urine that tests positive for nitrites should be cultured for bacteria. However, note that some organisms that cause UTIs do not convert nitrate to nitrites (e.g., *Staphylococcus* or *Streptococcus*).

Protein

Protein portions of the dipstick do not detect light chain proteins. If the patient has trace levels of proteinuria, then use of 20% sulfosalicylic acid testing for protein is appropriate to determine false positives (see p. 232 for explanation of this procedure). The normally small amount of protein excreted by a healthy adult is usually not detectable by dipstick analysis until the patient excretes 150 to 300 mg/day. At this level, the patient will show trace amounts. A typical scale to indicate a progressively increasing amount of protein is 1+ (30 mg/dL), 2+ (100 mg/dL), 3+ (300 mg/dL), and 4+ (500 to 1000 mg/dL). Peripheral edema and ascites may be present in an adult who has 3+ or 4+ proteinuria and is typically excreting 3 g or more of protein/day. Proteinuria reported for a single urinalysis is not an absolute guide in a differential diagnosis because proteinuria may be glomerular or tubular.

Glucose

Glucose in the urine is indicative of an elevated serum glucose >200 mg/dL. If serum glucose levels are normal while urine glucose is elevated, then proximal renal tubular damage should be suspected.

Ketones

Ketones are detected earlier in the urine than in the blood and may indicate starvation or diabetic ketoacidosis.

Blood

Reagent strips are calibrated to detect if red cells are present. The strip detects heme at 0.05 to 0.3 mg hemoglobin/dL (see Red Blood Cells section following).

Urinalysis with Microscopic Examination

Color

The urine should be clear to yellow, depending on the concentration. Turbidity with a foul odor indicates infection. Color changes of the urine may result from various sources: hemoglobin from systemic red blood cell lysis; myoglobin from damaged muscle cell or rhabdomyolysis; vegetable pigment from food, such as red beets; and pigment from drugs such as rifampin and phenazopyridine and porphyrins from porphyria.

Discoloration of the urine should be investigated with microscopic examination to determine if red blood cells (RBCs) or any foreign substances are present. Pyuria results from pus cells and white blood cells (WBCs) in the urine, but cloudy urine can also result from other causes.

Sediment

Sediment for casts, blood cells, and bacteria can be detected by microscopic examination. Casts indicate hemorrhage or conditions of the nephron. RBCs indicate acute inflammatory or vascular disorders of the glomerulus. More than 1 to 2 RBCs/high-powered field (HPF) is abnormal and can indicate renal or systemic disease or trauma to the kidney. Sediment is labeled as active when an abnormal number of cells, tubular casts, crystals, or infectious organisms are found.

A healthy person's urinalysis usually contains no cells, although an occasional cell/HPF may be found. However, more than 1 tubular epithelial and transitional epithelial cell/HPF suggests damage to the tubules or bladder wall. More than 1 RBC or WBC/HPF is considered abnormal. The more cells/HPF, the more active the renal disease may be.

Microscopic examination of the urine, resulting in 20 or more organisms/HPF indicates urinary tract infection. Less than 20 organisms/HPF merits further study such as culture and sensitivity.

Red Blood Cells

Hematuria is >3 RBCs/HPF. If the red blood cells are distorted, irregularly shaped, or membranous, then a glomerular problem is suggested. The major causes of hematuria include acute and chronic prostatitis or urethritis, hemorrhagic cystitis, renal stones, or tumors of the kidney, renal pelvis, ureter, bladder, prostate, and urethra. Hematuria with proteinuria usually suggests a renal origin. Isolated hematuria is usually produced by sites outside the kidneys.

If urinalysis fails to reveal evidence of infection with hematuria, then a calcium to creatinine ratio is obtained. A ratio greater than 0.18 may indicate hypercalciuria. A 24-hour urine test for calcium level is then done. The normal result should be less than 4 mg/kg/day.

White Blood Cells

Pyuria is greater than 5 WBCs/HPF and is highly suggestive for the presence of a UTI.

Casts

Tubular casts are formed in the distal portion of the nephron. A hyaline cast is a wispy, translucent, cylindrical replica of the tubular lumen. Red cell casts are characteristic of glomerular origins. The presence of abnormal cells, protein, hemoglobin, myoglobin, or other debris with a cast helps identify the type of renal disease. Significant proteinuria results from glomerulopathies, whereas tubular disorders cause little proteinuria. Therefore the sediment findings are helpful to correlate with the degree of proteinuria.

Segmented Urine Collection for Gram Stain and Culture and Sensitivity

Segmented urine collection is used to identify the site along the urinary tract where the colonization of organisms is occurring:

- Voided specimen #1: 5 to 10 ml of first voided urine collected
- Voided specimen #2: Sterile midstream urine collected
- Specimen #3: Prostatic massage performed; prostatic secretion collected from meatal opening
- Voided specimen #4: Complete emptying of bladder; urine specimen collected

Label each of the specimens and perform culture and sensitivity or Gram staining.

Urine Flow Studies (Uroflowmetry)

Urine flow studies can be used as a screening tool to determine diminished force of urination and obstruction. Flow rate is defined as the volume of fluid expelled from the urethra/ unit time and is expressed in ml/second. The patient must have a full bladder because urine flow rate depends on voided volume. The patient urinates into an insert in the toilet, which measures the flow rate of the urine. The normal flow pattern exhibits a rapid increase to maximal flow rate, within one third of the ultimate voiding time. After achieving maximal rate, flow decreases more slowly; average flow rate should be approximately 50% of the maximal urine flow rate.

Gram Stain

Gram stain of urethral exudate or spun urine should be performed to determine inflammation (WBCs) and the presence of either Gram-negative or Gram-positive bacteria. Gram-negative bacteria stain pink-red. Gram-positive bacteria stain dark blue to purple. The nuclei of polymorpho-nuclear (PMN) leukocytes stain pink-red. A Gram stain with more than 4 PMNs/HPF is indicative of urethritis because urethritis is defined by the presence of 5 to 10 PMNs/HPF. Practically, however, any number of WBCs is suggestive of urethritis. A symptomatic patient with risk factors but no positive laboratory results should be retested using the first voided urine of the day.

If the stain is positive for PMN leukocytes, then the smear is examined for Gram-negative intracellular diplococci (GNICDC). If found, the smear is considered positive for gonococcal urethritis. A smear that is equivocal or atypical indicates a mixed gonococcal and nongonococcal urethritis. If there are no GNICDC, then a nongonococcal urethritis is indicated. The Gram stain has 95% specificity in gonococcal urethritis, with nearly 100% sensitivity in urethritis.

Culture and Sensitivity

Culture and sensitivity should be performed on specimens to identify the causative organism and its sensitivity to antibiotics. This is especially important in populations at increased risk for resistant organisms.

Creatinine/Blood Urea Nitrogen (BUN)

Serum creatinine and BUN are used to indicate kidney function.

Prostatic Specific Antigen (PSA)

Tumor markers such as prostatic specific antigen (PSA) may be used to detect or monitor prostatic cancer. PSA results should be correlated with the digital rectal examination. Currently the use of PSA testing to screen men is under debate. Some authorities recommend screening males over age 50 and those at risk (i.e.,

patients with a family history or black males). Others do not recommend routine screening based on lack of empirical evidence of the benefit. In either case, the patient should be told of the potential benefits, known harms, and treatment options available and should be assisted in making an individual decision about testing.

For normal-risk males, levels of 1 to 4 ng/mL are considered within reference range while 4 to 10 ng/ml are elevated levels that fall into a gray zone and may require other tests such as transrectal ultrasound (TRUS) and prostate biopsy. PSA levels 10 or above are abnormal and indicate malignant activity of the prostate. Conditions such as BPH also correlate with high PSA levels. The threshold level for black males who are at risk may be lower than for other groups of males. A test measuring the free or unbound amount of PSA is currently being developed and validated. It is thought that this free PSA test will be able to specifically identify prostate cancers more readily than is possible with the current test.

X-Ray

If microscopic hematuria is present and the patient is under 50 years of age, obtain a flat plate of the abdomen to identify structures of the kidney, ureters, and bladder (KUB). Urinary calculi are usually visible on x-ray.

Ultrasonography

Ultrasonography is noninvasive and provides information on kidneys, ureters, bladder, vascular structures, prostate, and testicles. Renal ultrasound is a good first test to determine kidney size, contour, and the presence of calculi. Urinary bladder sonogram is used to identify tumors of the bladder, thickening of the bladder wall, posterior masses behind the bladder, and obstruction of the lower urinary tract evidenced by residual urine. Scrotal sonogram is used to evaluate chronic scrotal swelling. It can be used to identify abscess, infected testes, tumor, hydrocele, spermatocele, adherent scrotal hernia, and chronic epididymitis. However, because it does not assess perfusion, it is less helpful in the initial examination of an acute scrotum where a Doppler blood flow is more appropriate. Transrectal prostate sonogram or ultrasound (TRUS) can be used to evaluate the prostate for tumors or nodules as well as to determine the volume of the prostate. It is also useful in diagnosing prostatitis, benign prostatic hypertrophy, and cancer of the prostate.

Doppler Flow Studies

Doppler blood flow studies are used to measure blood flow to the scrotal structures. Color Doppler provides a color image, depicting the direction of the flow and the velocity in shades of blue and red. It is useful in the differential diagnosis of torsion testicle and epididymitis. A torsion testicle demonstrates reduced or absent blood flow, while epididymitis will show blood flow.

Biopsy

Biopsy of the prostate is necessary for definitive diagnosis of cancer. Guided biopsy is performed using transrectal ultrasound.

DIFFERENTIAL DIAGNOSIS

Cystitis/Urethritis

Males can have inflammation limited to the penile segment of the urethra. The history would include meatal burning and discharge. Classic symptoms are frequency, urgency, and dysuria. Nocturia with suprapubic or low back pain are common.

Screening can be done in most settings with urine dip strips. A positive leukocyte esterase and nitrate indicates infection. Urine culture and sensitivity confirms diagnosis and identifies the causative organism(s). Urinalysis with microscopic exami-

nation can determine if 20 or more organisms/HPF are present, which is indicative of UTI. Less than 20 organisms/HPF merits further study such as culture and sensitivity. Colonization has taken place if 10^3 or more organisms/ml are present in the culture.

Pyelonephritis

The patient with pyelonephritis presents with fever, chills, appears toxic, and complains of back pain. Nausea and vomiting may be present. Some patients also complain of lower urinary tract symptoms, including frequency and dysuria. The patient feels and looks ill. On physical examination, CVA tenderness is usually present. The abdomen may also be tender. On microscopic examination, WBCs are usually present. White cell casts suggest pyelonephritis. Bacterial casts, although rare, are pathognomonic of pyelonephritis. Urine culture and sensitivity confirm diagnosis and identify the pathogen, usually *E. coli, Klebsiella* sp., *Proteus mirabilis,* and *Enterobacter* sp.

Urolithiasis

Urinary stones can occur anywhere in the urinary tract and may produce symptoms of pain, hematuria, and secondary infection. Many calculi are "silent" and may cause only hematuria, microscopic or gross. Renal calculi may occur when a stone obstructs the urinary tract. Typical symptoms of renal colic include severe flank pain that radiates along the pathway of the ureter to the scrotum or inner thigh. Chills, fever, and urinary frequency are common. The patient may have nausea, vomiting, and abdominal distention. There may be a history of hematuria. Painful hematuria is characteristic of a stone, and the pain is described as colicky. Evaluate if the hematuria occurs at the time of urine initiation, at termination of micturition, or throughout micturition. This may be helpful in localizing the stone.

The clinical diagnosis is supported by urinalysis and imaging findings. The urine may be normal; gross or microscopic hematuria is common. Pyuria (WBCs) with or without bacteria may be present. Crystalline structures may be present. Most stones are visible on x-ray or by ultrasound.

Acute Prostatitis

The patient with acute prostatitis is obviously ill and presents with chills, high fever, urinary frequency and urgency, perineal pain, and low back pain. The patient may exhibit varying degrees of obstructive symptoms, dysuria or burning, nocturia, hematuria, arthralgia, and myalgia. On examination, the prostate gland is tender, swollen, indurated, and warm. Do not massage the gland, because bacteremia can result from expression of microorganisms. Urine or prostate secretion culture can confirm the diagnosis.

Chronic Prostatitis

Chronic prostatitis is a common cause of recurrent cystitis in men. It is caused by the same pathogens seen in acute prostatitis. Patients may be asymptomatic. Common symptoms, if evident, include low back pain and perineal discomfort, urinary frequency, and painful urination. Infection can involve the scrotal contents, producing epididymitis. Palpation of the prostate may reveal no specific findings. It may be moderately tender and irregularly indurated or boggy. Copious secretion may be present. Diagnosis is made on the basis of clinical symptoms and by culture of prostatic secretion.

Epididymitis/Orchitis

The patient with epididymitis/orchitis is usually a sexually active young male, and pain is the likely presenting symptom. The patient may be febrile. The history usually indicates a slow onset of discomfort over hours or days as compared to torsion testicle, which has a rapid onset of symptoms. Elevation of the affected testicle may reduce the discomfort. Swelling of the scrotum and testicle may be present. Doppler flow studies with color can locate hot spots and identify intact blood flow.

Testicular Torsion

The patient with testicular torsion is usually a pubescent male, with previous episodes of testicular pain. The history indicates a rapid onset of acute pain. Nausea and vomiting may have occurred or be present. Doppler blood flow studies may support the diagnosis by identifying lack of blood flow to the affected testicle. This is an emergent condition, and intervention must take place within the first 4 to 6 hours in order to salvage the testicle from infarction.

Benign Prostatic Hyperplasia (BPH)

Prostatic hypertrophy is common in men over age 50. Presenting symptoms include hesitancy, slow urine stream, and dribbling. Digital rectal examination reveals an enlarged prostate with a reduced or obliterated median sulcus. Induration or firmness is characteristic of early prostate disease, and a hard stony gland suggests advanced prostatic carcinoma. The gland may feel soft because of inflammation or infection. The American Urological Association (AUA) Symptom Index (Table 6-3) is useful in determining treatment options based on severity of symptoms, ranging from mild to severe. Digital rectal examinations combined with PSA tests are done annually by many clinicians for men over age 50 and for men at risk, including black males starting at age 40, to differentiate between BPH and prostate cancer.

Prostate Cancer

Patients with prostate cancer often present with the same obstructive symptoms as with BPH but may also be asymptomatic. Males presenting with complaints of lower abdominal pain probably represent extension of the cancer with metastasis. On examination, the prostate is stony hard and protrudes into the colon. PSA levels may be elevated and transrectal ultrasound indicates enlargement or nodules. PSA levels between 4 and 10 ng/mL may necessitate a biopsy to determine or rule out prostate cancer. A refined PSA test is currently being readied that determines the amount of free or unbound PSA and will be able to identify more accurately those with prostate cancer.

Bladder or Kidney Tumor

Silent hematuria in elderly patients is often a late presenting indication of cancer. It is more common in men than women. Patients often have a history of smoking or alcohol abuse.

Table 6-4

Differential Diagnosis of Common Causes of Genitourinary Problems in Males

Condition	History	Physical Findings	Diagnostic Studies
Cystitis/ urethritis	Frequency, urgency, and dysuria; nocturia with low back pain	Discharge may be present; may have suprapubic tenderness	Urine dipstick: positive leukocyte esterase; hematuria; urinalysis with microscopic exam; segmented urine collection; Gram stain; C & S
Pyelonephritis	Fever, chills, back pain, nausea and vomiting, toxic appearance; some patients also have frequency and dysuria	Feels and looks ill; fever >101° F; CVA tenderness; abdomen may be tender	Microscopic examination: WBCs may have white cell casts or bacterial casts; urine C & S; blood cultures
Urolithiasis	Pain, hematuria, may have symptoms of secondary infection; renal colic: pain that radiates to the inner thigh; nausea, vomiting	May have CVA tenderness; looks ill during periods of acute pain; may have abdominal distention	Urinalysis: gross or microscopic hematuria; WBCs with or without bacteria; crystalline structures may be present; x-ray or ultrasound
Acute prostatitis	Chills, high fever, urinary frequency, urgency; perineal pain and low back pain; varying degrees of obstructive symptoms, dysuria or burning, nocturia, hematuria, arthralgia, and myalgia	Fever >101° F; prostate gland tender, swollen indurated, warm; do not massage as can cause bacteremia	Urinalysis, urine culture, prostate secretion culture

Table 6-4

Differential Diagnosis of Common Causes of Genitourinary Problems in Males—cont'd

Condition	History	Physical Findings	Diagnostic Studies
Chronic prostatitis	Common cause of recurrent cystitis in men; same pathogen as in prostate secretion; may be asymptomatic; commonly have low back pain and perineal pain, urinary frequency, and painful urination	Infection can involve the scrotal contents, producing epididymitis; palpation of prostate reveals no specific findings; may be moderately tender and irregularly indurated or boggy; may have copious secretion	Culture prostatic secretion
Epididymitis/ orchititis	Abrupt onset over several hours, febrile, pain in scrotum and/or testicles	Tender swollen epididymitis and/or testicles; elevation of affected testicle may lessen the discomfort; may have fever	Doppler flow studies with color
Testicular torsion	Sudden onset of testicular pain, which radiates to groin; may also have lower abdominal pain	Exquisitely tender testicle; testicle may ride high because of shortened spermatic cord; cremasteric reflex absent	Scrotal ultrasonography; however, this is a surgical emergency
Benign prostatic hyperplasia (BPH)	Hesitancy, slow urine stream, dribbling, nocturia	Prostate protrusion into rectum; median sulcus reduced; prostate boggy	TRUS; PSA 1-4 ng/mL
Prostate cancer	Hesitancy, slow urine stream, dribbling, nocturia; low back pain	Prostate protrusion into rectum; prostate hard	TRUS; PSA elevated; biopsy
Bladder or kidney tumor	More common in men than women; patients often have a history of smoking or alcohol abuse	Usually no symptoms other than silent hematuria	U/A: hematuria

Penile Discharge

Penile discharge results from an infectious or inflammatory process secondary to exposure or contact with secretions containing causative organisms that enter and ascend the urethra. Males infected with *Chlamydia* may be asymptomatic 25% of the time, and symptoms may be absent in a few men with *gonorrhea* infections. Co-infections with both *Neisseria gonorrhea* and *Chlamydia* organisms may be present in up to 25% of heterosexual males.

Urethritis in males, usually related to a sexually transmitted disease (STD) that is acquired during unprotected sexual contact, is classified as either gonococcal or nongonococcal urethritis (NGU). It is not possible to accurately determine the causative organism based on symptoms or from physical examination alone. Although patients may be tentatively classified clinically, laboratory tests are used to direct diagnosis and treatment. Nongonococcal infections may result from several causative organisms, but the most frequently identified organism (40% of the time) is *Chlamydia trachomatis*. Other organisms identified in NGU include *Ureaplasma urealyticum* and, less frequently, *Trichomonas*.

DIAGNOSTIC REASONING: FOCUSED HISTORY

Is this an upper urinary tract problem?

Key Questions
- Have you had a fever or chills?
- Have you noticed any blood in your urine?
- Are you having any acute pain? Where?

Fever. The presence of fever indicates an ascending infection of the upper urinary tract (pyelonephritis) or a descending infection of the lower urinary tract (prostatitis, epididymitis). A fever over 101° F (39° C) should be cause for concern and aggressive treatment.

Hematuria. Blood in the urine signifies renal involvement, specifically pyelonephritis or lithiasis. Painless hematuria in the elderly is characteristic of bladder tumor or is a late symptom of carcinoma of the kidney.

Acute pain. Abdominal, flank, and costovertebral angle pain are characteristic of bladder, ureter, and kidney involvement. Urinary tract pain is usually perceived locally in the area where sensory fibers of nerves are located. However, pain can be referred to a site distant from the area that is affected because sensory nerves of the lower body are concentrated in the same segments of the spinal cord. Most pain in the urinary tract is referred pain and may not actually be perceived by the patient in the site where the problem actually occurs. A dull ache may be felt at the costovertebral angle or flank. Pain may be elicited by putting tension on the renal capsule, pelvis, or ureter. Ureter pain may be perceived in the bladder, penis, scrotum, or perineum. Testicular pain may be a result of renal calculi. Pain may vary in intensity from a dull ache to a sharp, stabbing, colicky pain that is unbearable.

Is this a lower urinary tract problem?

Key Questions
- Are you having acute pain in the scrotum that came on suddenly?
- Are you having acute pain in the scrotum that developed over a period of hours or days?

Acute pain. Acute pain in the scrotum with sudden onset is the first symptom of testicular torsion. The twisting of the spermatic cord results in vascular ischemia and decreased enervation. The pain may increase in severity, and one third of patients report previous episodes of testicular pain. Nausea and vomiting are common.

Scrotal area pain. Scrotal area pain developing over a period of hours or days is characteristic of epididymitis. Fever and chills can develop with severe infection.

Is this likely a sexually transmitted disease (STD)?

Key Questions
- When did you last have sex?
- How many sexual partners do you have?
- Do you have any new partners?
- How many days from exposure to onset of symptoms?
- What color is the discharge?
- How much discharge are you having?
- What is the consistency of the discharge?

Sexual history. A history of multiple sexual partners signifies a risk for exposure to sexually transmitted diseases. The incidence of *Ureaplasma urealyticum* increases with the number of sexual partners. A new partner also is a risk factor as is a sexual partner who has other sexual partners.

Number of days between exposure and symptom onset. For patients with a single exposure, a shorter incubation period is characteristic of *N. gonorrhea* (2 to 6 days) and a longer period of 8 to 21 days for *C. trachomatis*. For patients with multiple or unknown exposures, the time interval may not be useful.

Color, consistency, and amount of discharge. The presence of copious amounts of spontaneous yellow-greenish drainage is indicative of a gonococcal infection. A scant mucoid discharge is characteristic of a nongonococcal infection.

Is this a local infection or process?

Key Questions
- Is the end of your penis red and inflamed?
- Tell me how you clean yourself.

Red, inflamed glans penis. A beefy-red, inflamed glans penis is indicative of a yeast infection or a fixed drug reaction often caused by tetracycline. Lubricated condoms or spermicidical gel can cause contact dermatitis.

Hygienic practices. Poor hygiene or aggressive hygiene with inappropriate or harsh cleansers can cause local irritation and result in inflammation.

Are there any risk factors that point me in the right direction?

Key Questions
- When is the last time you used street or illicit drugs?
- When is the last time you had sex that was risky, such as unprotected sex, a same sex partner, or oral or anal sex?
- Is this a sexually active adolescent?

History of drug or substance abuse. Substance or drug abuse is a risk factor for unprotected and indiscriminate sexual relations. Substance or drug abuse may produce a scant, whitish penile discharge.

Risky sexual preferences and practices. Unprotected sex increases the chances of sexually transmitted diseases. A same sex partner provides information about risk as does unprotected sex. Oral and anal sexual practices increase the possibility of sexually transmitted disease at these sites.

Sexually active adolescent. Sexually active adolescents, about 40% of persons between 14 and 18 years, are at risk for sexually transmitted diseases (STDs) because of their lack of barrier protection use, impetuous sexual activities, and use of alcohol or drugs. STDs are a serious health problem, occurring in about 25% of sexually active adolescents.

Is this complicated urethritis?

Key Questions

- Are you having frequency, urgency, nocturia or perirectal, testicular, or low back pain?
- Do you have any joints or tendons that hurt, eye infections, sloughing of skin on your penis, or red spots and sores on your hands, arms, legs, or feet?

Symptoms that may indicate complicated urethritis. Symptoms or urinary frequency, urgency, and nocturia may indicate complications of a urethral infection caused by spreading of the infection to other urinary tract structures such as the prostate (see Genitourinary Problems in Males, p. 249). Further involvement may include symptoms of perirectal, testicular, or low back pain, indicating involvement of the vas deferens and the epididymis, which can lead to acute epididymitis and/or the involvement of the testicle and the development of orchitis.

Symptoms that may indicate Reiter's syndrome. Reiter's syndrome is a complication of nongonococcal urethritis (NGU) that follows urogenital infection and classically includes arthritis, conjunctivitis, oral mucosal ulcers, and dermatitis. More common is the joint and tendon involvement following *C. trachomatis* infection. This complication has also been reported in HIV-positive patients. It is less common in non-white populations, and the incubation period is usually 1 to 4 weeks after the onset of urethritis.

Disseminated systemic urethral infection. A disseminated gonococcal infection can produce papules or petechiae that progress to pustules on the skin surfaces of the hands, arms, and legs.

What else could this be?

Key Questions

- Have you had recent instrumentation of the urethra? (e.g., catheterization)

- Have you been treated recently for a sexually transmitted disease?
- Are you or your partner an immigrant, alien, or have you recently engaged in foreign travel?

Recent treatment or instrumentation. Recent treatment or instrumentation of the urethra produces a risk for infection. Elderly males are especially at risk because they often undergo urinary tract treatment or instrumentation secondary to benign prostatic hypertrophy.

Recent treatment for an STD. Recent treatment for an STD may indicate treatment failure, a coinfection that was not covered by the prescribed drug, or recent exposure. The appropriate laboratory test may have not been done or was not available, or treatment may have been empirically based on presenting symptoms. Infection with more than one organism or a coinfection may take place. Urethritis can also develop from a nongonococcal organism that has a longer incubation period and was not sensitive to the drug prescribed. The urethritis episode may also represent a recent exposure after treatment. Another possibility could be lack of patient compliance with treatment. The patient does not take the medication as directed or stops taking the medication when the symptoms disappear but before the causative organism is eliminated from the urethra.

Immigrant or alien patient or partner or recent foreign travel. Immigrants, aliens, or partners of foreigners or patients with a history of foreign travel may have exposure to other STDs that are not seen as frequently in the United States but which have a higher incidence and prevalence in foreign countries. Resistant strains of common organisms are also prevalent in foreign countries. Referral or infectious disease consultation may be necessary from urologists, infectious disease departments, or public health departments in order to identify and treat patients with unusual STDs.

DIAGNOSTIC REASONING: FOCUSED PHYSICAL EXAMINATION

Note General Appearance

If the patient appears systematically ill, a more aggressive and immediate approach should be taken and an expanded examination becomes appropriate. An ascending infection is usually limited to the anterior portion of the male urethra and is most likely to cause local signs and symptoms in the male patient. The patient who appears to be in acute pain from sites other than the urethra warrants more than a focused physical examination.

Examine skin surfaces, exposed orifices, and eyes as well as mucous membranes and bordering areas around sites that may have been exposed during sexual activity.

Note eyes for discharge or infection. Check around nares and lips for signs of infection or lesions. Inspect the chest, back, palms, and bottoms of the feet for rashes or lesions. Secondary syphilis produces typical rashes and lesions in these areas, as does Reiter's syndrome. Spontaneous greenish-yellow discharge from the eyes is indicative of gonococcal infections.

Inspect the skin of the abdomen, inguinal areas, and thighs for lesions or rashes. Disseminated gonococcal infections may produce papules, petechiae, and pustules on the hands, arms, and feet. *Chlamydia* may produce hyperkeratotic lesions on skin surfaces and a rash on the penis in the uncircumcised male.

Palpate Lymph Nodes

Palpate the cervical, axillary, inguinal, and femoral lymph nodes for adenopathy. Although a nonspecific indicator of infection, lymph nodes may enlarge in response to exposure from several organisms. Virus exposure may cause lymph node enlargement, or there may be extension of bacterial organisms into adjacent lymph chains, indicating regional infections. It is impor-

tant to ascertain how long the nodes have been enlarged and what symptoms have appeared during the course of enlargement. Assess the state of the nodes, such as any redness, swelling, heat, or pain, or if they are firm, mobile, or boggy. Sexually active males may have some inguinal lymph node enlargement, and the patient may or may not be aware of the enlargement. Lymph node enlargement should be documented and described.

Examine Body Hair

Examine hair on the head and in the pubic area and inspect underlying skin areas. Hair shafts can be infected with lice and nits. Hair follicles can be irritated from scratching and from secondary infection by other organisms.

Examine the Penis and Urethral Meatus

Inspect penile skin surfaces for lesions, especially the underside of the head of the penis around the area of the frenulum where viral lesions may be found. Palpate the shaft of the penis for tenderness or for strictures of the urethra. Retract the foreskin if present and inspect the glans penis, corona, and frenulum for lesions. Inspect the meatus for redness, discharge, patency, or growths. If there is discharge, note if it is spontaneous or produced by milking or stripping the penis. Document a tender urethra and describe the character of any discharge. Note whether the discharge is a profuse yellow green, which indicates gonococcal infection, or scant and mucoid-like, which is characteristic of *C. trachomatis* and nongonococcal infection.

Examine Scrotum and Testicles

Inspect and palpate the scrotum for lesions. Palpate the testicles and epididymitis for tenderness and any signs of inflammation. Elevating a tender testicle may alleviate pain and reduce discomfort in epididymitis. The testicle may not be able to be defined when there is an acute infection present because of examiner-produced pain with palpation. The borders of the testicle may also be obliterated from swelling and edema.

Inspect and Examine Other Sites for Lesions and Discharge

Inspect other sites such as the mouth and pharynx using a tongue depressor to visualize buccal skinfolds for any lesions. The pharyngeal area may be asymptomatic. Depending on the patient's sexual practices and preferences, other sites exposed to sexual contact such as the rectum need to be examined. Rectal bleeding, pus, and mucus may indicate proctitis and require further anoscopic examination and special cultural and laboratory consideration (see Chapter 5, Rectal Pain and Itching, p. 204). Examine any joints or tendons that are inflamed or tender or any limited range of motion.

LABORATORY AND DIAGNOSTIC STUDIES

In order to improve the probability of identifying the causative organism, the patient should be examined and specimens obtained at least an hour after the last voiding, ideally up to 4 hours after voiding. Manufacturer directions should be followed for all materials used to collect specimens, and policies and procedures should be adhered to in order to obtain valid and reliable results from laboratory and diagnostic tests.

Urine Dipstick

Urine dipstick is used as a screening test for urethritis. The leukocyte esterase strip is calibrated to turn purple in 60 seconds, indicating 5 or more white blood cells in the urine. A positive result is indicative of urethritis (75% to 90% sensitivity, 95% specificity). The nitrite strip is cali-

brated to turn pink within 30 seconds and signifies nitrites produced by $>10^5$ or more organisms/ml. Urine that tests positive for leukocyte esterase and nitrites should be cultured for bacteria. However, note that some organisms that cause UTIs do not convert nitrate to nitrites (e.g., *Staphylococcus* or *Streptococcus*).

Urinalysis with Microscopic Examination

Look for proteinuria and glycosuria that suggests kidney involvement. The presence of casts, red blood cells, and bacteria is also important. Casts indicate hemorrhage or pathological conditions of the nephrons. Red blood cells indicate acute inflammatory or vascular disorders of the glomerulus. More than 1 or 2 RBCs/high-powered (HPF) field is abnormal and can indicate renal or systemic disease or kidney trauma. Microscopic examination of the urine resulting in 20 or more organisms/HPF indicates urinary tract infection. Less than 20 organisms/HPF merits further study such as culture and sensitivity.

Segmented Urine Collection for Culture and Sensitivity

Obtaining segmented urine specimens is a procedure used to identify the site along the urinary tract where the colonization of organisms is occurring and is useful in diagnosing prostatitis (see Genitourinary Problems in Males, p. 246).

Gram Stain of Specimens

The Gram stain has 95% specificity in gonococcal urethritis. Sensitivity in urethritis is nearly 100%. Gram stain of urethral discharge should be performed to determine inflammation (WBCs) and the presence of either Gram-negative or Gram-positive bacteria.

If the stain is positive for PMNs, then the smear is examined for Gram-negative intracellular diplococci (GNICDC). If found, the smear is considered positive for gonococcal urethritis. A smear that is equivocal or atypical indicates a mixed gonococcal and nongonococcal urethritis. If there are no GNICDC, then a nongonococcal urethritis is indicated.

Culture and Sensitivity

Culture and sensitivity should be performed on specimens to confirm the identity of the causative organism and its sensitivity to antibiotics. This is especially important in populations with resistant organisms.

Other Diagnostic Tests to Detect Specific Organisms

Other available diagnostic methods, depending on the practice setting, include gonococci enzymes, antigens, DNA, and liposaccharides. Recently, polymerase chain reaction tests are being used to determine minute traces of chlamydial DNA particles from urine samples. Ligase chain reaction, a similar noninvasive method for amplifying and detecting trace amounts of genetic material, can also be performed on urine samples. Although these newer tests may be used for screening purposes, they are for

specific organisms and do not provide information about other causative organisms that may also be present as coinfections. These newer diagnostic tests will become more widely used and available over time. See Table 6-5 for a summary of screening tests for STDs in males.

Doppler Blood Flow

Doppler blood flow studies can be done to support the diagnosis of torsion testicle and epididymitis. Torsion testicle results in a lack of blood flow to the testicle, while in epididymitis the blood flow is intact. Color Doppler flow studies also provide information concerning blood flow to the testicles as well as identifying hot areas of infection.

Complete Blood Count (CBC)

CBC with differential can be done to indicate a systemic response to infection.

Serology for Syphilis

Serological tests can be used to screen for syphilis. They are nontreponemal tests so are not specific for syphilis (see Treponemal Tests following). The tests include VDRL (Veneral Disease Research Labora-

---

Table 6-5

STD Screening Tests for Males

SCREENING TEST	SITE	HETEROSEXUAL PRACTICES	HOMOSEXUAL/ BISEXUAL PRACTICES
Gram stain	Urethral	X	X
	Rectal		X
Cultures for *N. gonorrhea*	Urethral	X	X
	Rectal		X
	Pharyngeal		X
DNA probe/antigen detection for	Urethral	X	X
Chlamydia	Rectal		X
Syphilis serology		X	X
HIV screening		X	X
Hepatitis B screening			X

tory), RPR (Rapid Plasma Reagin), and USR (Unheated Serum Reagin).

Treponemal Tests

Treponemal tests are used to confirm positive nontreponemal tests as mentioned previously. The tests include FTA (Fluorescent Treponemal Antibody) and MHA-TP (Microhemagglutination—*T. pallidum*).

Human Leukocyte Antigen

The human leukocyte antigen test is done to determine antigens that are present for specific diseases. Histocompatibility locus-A (HLA-B27) tissue haplotype is associated with sexually acquired reactive arthritis seen in Reiter's syndrome. This test is not specific but is used to confirm the diagnosis.

DIFFERENTIAL DIAGNOSIS

URETHRITIS

Urethritis presents with itching, burning, or pain around the urethral opening. Symptoms vary in severity. Discharge may range from copious amounts of greenish-yellow to scant mucoid-like discharge that may only be visible before the first voiding of the day. Patients commonly present with complaints of urinary frequency, urgency, and/or burning with urination as well as penile discharge. Patients may also report a known sexual partner or that the public health department has contacted them indicating that they need to be checked for a sexually transmitted disease. If you are unable to make a diagnosis based on history and physical findings, diagnostic testing is necessary for specific organism identification.

Neisseria gonorrhea and nongonococcal urethritis caused by *Chlamydia trachomatis* are the two most common infectious causes of urethritis. A coinfection with both organisms is common in up to 25% of the cases.

Gonococcal Urethritis

Gonococcal STDs are usually the easiest to diagnose because the patient often presents with complaints of a yellow-green discharge and burning on urination. Unprotected sexual relations increase the risk for contracting this STD. Gonococcal infection often becomes symptomatic in 2 to 6 days after exposure and produces the classic yellow-green profuse spontaneous drainage. On examination, the penis will be normal in appearance except for the copious discharge. Diagnosis is established by DNA probe and is confirmed by Gram stain and urethral culture.

Nongonococcal Urethritis (NGU)

NGU can produce penile discharge although, on examination, discharge may not be present. Nongonococcal urethritis typically develops over a longer incubation period of 8 to 21 days, and 75% of patients present with a clear or mucoid discharge.

Chlamydia is the most common nongonococcal causative organism. The resulting urethritis is characterized by a scant mucoid discharge visible before the first urination of the day. The patient may complain of irritation around the meatus of the urethra or have vague symptoms. On examination, stripping the penis may produce scant mucoid discharge. DNA probes are used to diagnose *Chlamydia,* and Gram stains are used to rule out and establish nongonococcal disease, of which chlamydial infection is the most frequent. Urine screening tests can be used to identify DNA chlamydial particles.

COMPLICATED URETHRITIS

The examiner should recognize common complications of urethritis. Periurethritis may progress to urethral stricture in untreated cases, causing banding of the penile urethra in the shaft of the penis. Prostatitis can develop and progress to a systemic inflammatory response, causing chills and fever. Extension of inflammation to other structures of the urinary tract may result in acute infection of the epididymis and testicles. Orchitis, a testicular inflammation, presents with a swollen and tender testicle. Disseminated systemic urethral infection produces small tender papules or petechiae on the skin surfaces of the hands, arms, and legs. They may further develop into pustules and become hemorrhagic or necrotic. Joints can become involved with tenosynovitis and arthritis with synovial effusion in Reiter's syndrome. Monarticular joint or tendon involvement should be investigated further.

Prostatitis

Patients with acute prostatitis is likely to look and feel sick and be febrile. They usually complain of dysuria, burning, frequency, and nocturia (see Genitourinary Problems in Males, p. 249). Prostatic massage is contraindicated in acute prostatitis.

Patients with chronic prostatitis do not present as acutely ill but have a history of prostate problems. A causative organism may not be identified.

Epididymitis/Orchitis

The patient with epididymitis/orchitis is usually a sexually active young male, and pain is the likely presenting symptom. The patient may be febrile. The history usually indicates a slower onset of discomfort over hours or days as compared to torsion testicle, which has a rapid onset of symptoms. Elevation of the affected testicle may reduce the discomfort. Swelling of the scrotum and testicle may be present. Doppler flow studies with color can locate hot spots and identify intact blood flow (see Genitourinary Problems in Males, p. 248).

Reiter's Syndrome

As a complication of a urethral infection, Reiter's syndrome commonly includes joint or tendon involvement, but conjunctivitis and skin lesions may also be present. History includes a urethral infection within 1 to 3 weeks. HLA-B27 antigen typing may support confirmation of the diagnosis.

TESTICULAR PROBLEMS

Testicular Torsion

The patient with testicular torsion is usually a pubescent male, with previous episodes of testicular pain. The history given by the patient indicates a rapid onset of acute pain. Nausea and vomiting may have occurred or be present. Doppler blood flow studies may support the diagnosis by identifying lack of blood flow to the affected testicle. This is an emergent condition, and intervention must take place within the first 4 to 6 hours in order to salvage the testicle from infarction.

Table 6-6

Differential Diagnosis of Common Causes of Penile Discharge

Condition	History	Physical Findings	Diagnostic Studies
Urethritis			
Gonococcal urethritis	Unprotected sexual activity; abrupt onset of symptoms 3-5 days after exposure; yellow-green discharge; classic symptoms reported by males: frequency, urgency, dysuria; dysuria may be worse at beginning of urine flow	Yellow-green discharge; spontaneous or copious amounts with stripping of penis	Collect specimens at least 1 hour, preferably 4 hours, after last voiding; Gram stain, culture, DNA probe for *Gonococcus*
Nongonococcal urethritis	Unprotected sexual activity; longer incubation period 8-21 days; meatal itching or irritation; scant mucoid-like discharge, if present, before first voiding of the day; symptoms vary and range in severity for urgency, frequency, and dysuria	Thin mucoid discharge may be absent or minimal with penile milking or stripping	Gram stain; culture; DNA probe for *Chlamydia;* urine screen for DNA; *Chlamydia* particles
Complicated Urethritis			
Prostatitis	Chills, fever; 30-50 years of age; onset of symptoms over days; pain in rectal, perianal area, low back, and abdomen	May have fever; painful prostate; do not massage	Segmental urine specimens; culture & sensitivity

Table 6-6

Differential Diagnosis of Common Causes of Penile Discharge—cont'd

Condition	History	Physical Findings	Diagnostic Studies
Epididymitis/ orchitis	Abrupt onset over several hours, febrile, pain in scrotum and/or testicles	Tender swollen epididymis and/or testicles; elevation of affected testicle may lessen the discomfort; may have fever	Doppler flow studies with color
Reiter's syndrome	Joint and tendon involvement; urethritis	Joint and tendon involvement, decreased range of motion; skin and mucous lesions; conjunctivitis	Blood, synovial fluid, HLA-B27 antigen; x-rays
Testicular Problems			
Testicular torsion	Usually a pubescent male, with previous episodes of testicular pain; rapid onset of acute pain with nausea and vomiting	Exquisitely tender swollen testicle; testicle may ride high because of shortened spermatic cord; cremasteric reflex absent	Doppler blood flow studies: lack of blood flow to the affected testicle; emergent condition: intervention must take place within the first 4-6 hours in order to salvage the testicle from infarction

Chapter 7

Common Gynecological Problems

≡ Vaginal Discharge and Itching

Vaginitis is an inflammation of the vagina that can cause a vaginal discharge. Vaginal infections are common in postpubertal women. *Trichomonas vaginalis, Candida,* and bacterial vaginosis (BV) (the epithelium is not inflamed with this syndrome) account for 95% of all vaginal infections in the United States. Often patients have more than one infection at a given time.

In women of childbearing age, the top three vaginal discharges are associated with bacterial vaginosis, *Candida,* and *Trichomonas.* Some studies suggest that pregnant women with BV have premature rupture of membranes and early delivery. The most common cervicitis infections are *Chlamydia trachomatis, Neisseria gonorrhea,* and *Herpes simplex.* Postmenopausal women often have discharge related to atrophic vaginitis, caused by the deficiency of estrogen in the vaginal tissues.

Vulvar itching, burning, and a foul odor often accompany vaginal discharge. Pubic lice, scabies, pinworms, and genital warts (condyloma acuminata) can all cause itching. Common foreign bodies found in the vagina of adults are lost or forgotten tampons that can produce a foul-smelling discharge.

Chemical vaginitis in a young girl is usually caused by a sensitivity to "bubble bath," while in the adolescent or woman it occurs because of use of scented douches, lubricants, or hygiene sprays. Vulvovaginitis is one of the most common gynecological disorders in children. The reason for this is two-fold—first, their perineal hygiene is often poor, and, second, they are hypoestrogenic. The vaginal mucosa is thin and less resistant to infectious organisms. The postmenopausal woman can experience these same symptoms from estrogen deficiency.

In childhood and adolescence, complaints of vulvar itching, soreness, or vaginal discharge occur in most girls. The lack of estrogen stimulation, neutral pH of the vaginal secretions, lack of protective thick labia and pubic hair of adult females, and daily living habits (e.g., wiping, clothing, play equipment and environment, baths, foreign bodies, and pinworms) lead to this complaint.

The most accurate method of diagnosing the patient with vulvovaginitis consists of a careful history, pelvic examination, and microscopic evaluation of the vaginal fluid. At times a culture of the vaginal fluid or cervix is also necessary.

DIAGNOSTIC REASONING: FOCUSED HISTORY

What kind of vaginitis might this be?

Key Questions
- What is the amount, color, and consistency of your discharge?
- Do you have itching, swelling, or redness?
- Is there an odor?

Characteristics of discharge. Copious amounts of greenish, offensive-smelling discharge are most consistent with *Trichomonas* vaginitis. Mucopurulent or purulent discharges are associated with *gonorrhea* and *Chlamydia*. A moderate amount of white, curd-like discharge is consistent with *Candida* vulvovaginitis. Bacterial vaginosis typically produces a discharge that is thin and either white, green, gray, or brownish in color. While characteristic symptoms associated with each type of vaginal discharge can be helpful in arriving at a diagnosis, they are not diagnostic in and of themselves. Microscopic examination of the vaginal discharge is more sensitive than the clinical picture in confirming the diagnosis (Figure 7-1).

Itching, swelling, redness. Vaginitis causes inflammation of the tissues, resulting in erythema and edema. Because of the inflammatory process, the amount of discharge will produce a concomitant amount of swelling and redness of the vulva and vagina. BV does not involve the inflammatory process and results in a discharge with little vulvovaginal erythema and edema. Itching is consistently present with candidiasis. It can lead to excoriations and satellite lesions. Itching is infrequently seen with BV.

Odor. A fishy odor caused by the release of amines from organic acids is prominent with BV. It is accentuated by the addition of potassium hydroxide (KOH) to the wet mount slide and is considered a positive "whiff" test. Odor commonly accompanies trichomonal infections; retained tampons or other foreign bodies can also cause a foul odor.

Is this likely a sexually transmitted infection?

Key Questions
- Are you sexually active? Do you have multiple partners? Do you have a new partner?
- Have you had sex against your will? In a child you might ask: has anyone touched your private parts?
- What form of protection do you use? How often?
- Have you or your partner(s) ever been tested or treated for a sexually transmitted disease (STD)?
- Do you have any rashes, blisters, sores, lumps, or bumps?

Sexual activity. Early-age onset of sexual activity, multiple partners, and nonuse of barrier contraceptives, particularly condoms, increases the risk of a vaginal infection. STDs are common in women of childbearing age (12 to 50) who have acquired a new partner. The patient who has a high rate of sexual partner changes, or who participates in risky sexual practices (e.g., rectal intercourse without a condom) is at high risk for sexually transmitted diseases.

Do not ignore the possibility of a STD in the older woman. She may be sexually active after a divorce or widowhood or because of sexual abuse. Fifty percent of all

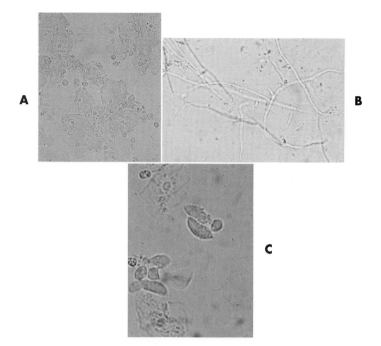

Figure 7-1   Microscopic differential diagnoses of vaginal infections. "Clue cells," epithelial cells with clumps of bacteria are evident in BV (**A**); budding, branching hyphae characterize candidiasis (**B**); motile trichmonads are seen with trichomoniasis (**C**). (From Zitelli BJ, Davis HW: *Atlas of pediatric physical diagnosis,* ed 3, St. Louis, 1997, Mosby-Wolfe.)

children with a STD have been found to be sexually abused. *Trichomonas* vaginitis is rare in children but can be transmitted to the neonate from an infected mother.

Lesions. Vesicles usually indicate herpes infection. Patients typically notice them on the external labia and complain that they itch or burn. Condylomata lata, condylomata acuminata, and molluscum contagiosum are all papular lesions found on the labia, perineum, and anal regions. Molluscum contagiosum, when occurring in the genital area, may extend to include the inner thighs. Typically, condylomata acuminata (genital warts) are rough, verrucous lesions that are usually located inferiorly from fossa navicularis to the fourchette and the perineal area. A painless ulcer suggests syphilis and classically appears as a solitary lesion. However, there can be more than one chancre, especially if the patient is immunocompromised.

Are there any risk factors for non-STD vaginitis?

Key Questions
- Have you ever been told that you have diabetes, Cushing's syndrome, or that you are HIV positive?
- Have you been ill recently?
- Are you taking antibiotics, hormones, or oral contraceptive pills?
- Have you received chemotherapy?
- Does the itching seem to be worse at night?
- Describe some of your recent activities.

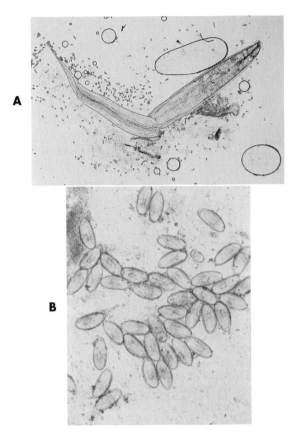

Figure 7-2 Pinworms *(Enterobius vermicularis).* On this wet mount a mature worm is shown surrounded by eggs **(A),** which are shown more clearly at higher power **(B).** (From Zitelli BJ, David HW: *Atlas of pediatric physical diagnosis,* ed 3, St. Louis, 1997, Mosby-Wolfe.)

Immunocompromised states. Refractory fungal vulvovaginitis may indicate undiagnosed diabetes or an immunocompromised state.

Recent illness. Chickenpox, scarlet fever, and measles can cause vaginitis.

Medications or chemotherapy. Birth control pills, corticosteroids, antibiotics, and chemotherapy are associated with vulvovaginitis candidiasis. Oral contraceptives may alter the vaginal pH, and antibiotics may alter the normal vaginal flora; both predispose to fungal infection. Corticosteroids and chemotherapy can produce an immunocompromised state and offer the opportunity for fungal infection.

Night itching. Pinworms are an intestinal parasite that inhabits the rectum or colon and emerges to lay eggs in the skinfolds of the anus. Perianal pruritus, especially at night, along with pain or itching of genitals is common (Figure 7-2).

Activities. Bicycle riding, using pools or hot tubs, or wearing tight-fitting pants or pantyhose can lead to heat and moisture in the genital area, causing mechanical irritation and infection such as candidiasis or BV.

Is this an acute or chronic condition?

Key Questions

- How long have you had this? Is it getting better or worse?
- Have you ever had these symptoms before?
- How many episodes have you had in the past year?
- Are the episodes related to any particular activity or time?

Chronology of symptoms. The occurrence of a vaginal discharge after having a new sex partner suggests an acute condition, such as a sexually transmitted infection. Symptoms associated with use of condoms or spermicide suggest sensitivity to the product. If the discharge occurs monthly, becoming worse after menses, suspect a chronic condition such as vulvovaginitis candidiasis. Recurrent episodes related to bathing activities point to chemical irritation.

If this is acute, could it be related to a previous infection?

Key Questions

- Have you been tested and treated for this condition recently?
- What medication was prescribed? How long ago?
- Did you take all the medication?
- What other prescriptions were you taking at that time?

Adequate diagnosis. Diagnoses made clinically by the color or appearance of a discharge may be incorrect, or a concomitant vaginal infection may have been missed. However, self-diagnosis and treatment is common, especially with the over-the-counter medicines for "yeast infection."

Adequate therapy. Most medications that are prescribed are not taken exactly as directed. Women will quit using their vaginal medications when menses begins and resume after it ends. This practice can lead to treatment failure. They may also discontinue the therapeutic agent early, as soon as relief from symptoms takes place or a drug side effect is experienced (e.g., the metallic taste of metronidazole). Drug interactions may account for inadequate therapy, or there may be the need to alter dietary regimen (e.g., abstain from alcoholic beverages).

If this is chronic, what should I suspect?

Key Questions

- Do any family members or sexual partners have vaginal or urinary infections? Any itching, rashes, sores, lumps, or bumps?
- Do you have a new or untreated partner?
- What are your sexual practices? Vaginal, oral, or anal sex?
- How many yeast infections have you had this year?

Transmission. Caregivers, parents, and siblings can spread infections like candidiasis, molluscum contagiosum, herpes, lice, and pinworms to children by poor hygiene practices. Autoinoculation is also possible, especially for herpes, genital warts, and molluscum contagiosum.

New or untreated partner. The most common cause of reinfection is intercourse with a new or untreated partner.

Sexual practices. Possible infection reservoirs are oral and anal cavities, which may need to be cultured for *Herpes* or *gonorrhea*. Additionally, materials used during intercourse may need to be disinfected (e.g., diaphragm). Less common modes of transmission include shared intimate clothing.

Chronic vulvovaginitis. If the patient has more than three separate episodes of candidal vulvovaginitis in 1 year, consider diabetes or the immunocompromised state of HIV/AIDS as the underlying etiology. Yeast grows best in areas that are dark, moist, warm, and high in glucose—areas where the normal flora has been compromised. The use of oral contraceptive pills or hormone replacement therapy, antibiotic (e.g., tetracycline for acne) or steroid therapy, diets high in carbohydrates or artificial sweeteners, and clothing that holds moisture against the vulva (e.g., pantyhose, tight jeans) are excellent potentiators for infection.

What are other possible causes for this vaginitis?

Key Questions

- What are your personal hygiene practices?
- Do you douche?
- Have you changed brands of contraceptive products?
- Could you have forgotten to remove your diaphragm or tampon?

Hygiene practices. Feminine hygiene practices may contribute to vaginitis by causing a local allergic reaction, altered vaginal flora, or contamination of the vagina from the rectum. Perfumes in douches, sprays, lubricants, and bubble baths are frequent offenders in allergic vaginitis.

Once a child is out of diapers, toileting is less closely assisted, and wiping techniques may be poor, leading to contamination of the vagina by bowel flora.

Douching. Frequent douching may change the balance of normal vaginal flora by altering the pH. This allows recolonization of the vagina with enteric bacteria, leading to pruritus and discharge. Douching can cause an allergic reaction. Colored or perfumed toilet paper can irritate the perineum, causing redness and itching. Wiping with tissue after urination or defecation in the direction from the anus toward the vagina can inoculate the vagina with rectal microbes.

Contraceptive products. Contraceptive products (e.g., spermicidal jellies, suppositories, foam, or condoms) may cause an allergic inflammation of the sensitive mucosa and produce itching, erythema, tenderness, and an increase in usual vaginal secretions.

Foreign body. A foul-smelling vaginal discharge can be caused by a lost tampon, condom, or forgotten diaphragm. A child who puts a foreign object into her vagina may have pruritus, burning, or a foul, purulent vaginal discharge. Foreign bodies in the vagina are associated with vaginal bleeding or spotting. If the object is left for some time, it can imbed and perforate the vaginal wall.

Are there any associated symptoms that point to a cause?

Key Questions

- Do you have burning or pain with urination? Frequency, hesitation, nocturia?
- Do you have painful intercourse?
- Do you have abdominal or pelvic pain?
- If an infant: Does the infant have an eye infection?
- If an infant: Does the infant have a cough?

Urinary symptoms. Atrophic vaginitis is often accompanied by dysuria, dyspareunia, and vaginal dryness. Estrogen deficiency affects the woman's entire lower genital tract and may produce symptoms that can be confused with a urinary tract infection. Low estrogen levels may exacerbate stress and urge incontinence. *Trichomonas* and *Chlamydia* may produce a coexisting urethritis that causes frequency and dysuria.

Dyspareunia and pain. Vaginal atrophy, genital warts, or vaginal infections can cause introital dyspareunia. A more likely reason for deep vaginal dyspareunia is endometriosis, pelvic inflammatory disease

(PID), or fibroids. Sexually transmitted diseases like gonorrhea and chlamydia can cause cervicitis, which, if left untreated, can progress to PID and produce abdominal and/or pelvic pain (see Chapter 5, Abdominal Pain, p. 164).

Eye infection. Eye infections in the newborn may be associated with *gonorrhea* and *Chlamydia* (see Chapter 2, Red Eye, p. 58).

Cough. Pneumonia in the newborn may be an indication of chlamydiosis (see Chapter 4, Cough., p. 138).

DIAGNOSTIC REASONING: FOCUSED PHYSICAL EXAMINATION

Note Vital Signs

The presence of a fever may alert you to a serious infection such as PID. Fever is uncommon with vaginitis.

Perform an Oral Examination

Oral thrush may accompany vulvar candidiasis, particularly in children. Look for white patches that bleed when you try to scrape them off.

Perform an External Genitalia Examination

Palpate for inguinal lymphadenopathy and tenderness, which can be present with vaginal infections. Inspect the vulva and labia, looking for erythema, excoriations, and induration. The skin is often bright red and swollen with small fissures or excoriations from candidiasis. Also, thick white curds of discharge are often noted in the labial folds. Bacterial vaginosis (BV) often produces a profuse, thin, whitish discharge that will leak out of the vagina onto the perineum. Palpate the Bartholin's and Skene's glands and milk the urethra for discharge. Palpable Bartholin glands often coexist with STDs. If purulent discharge is

seen, consider the diagnoses of *gonorrhea* or *Chlamydia* and obtain cultures.

Condylomata lata, condylomata acuminata, and molluscum contagiosum are all papular lesions found on the labia, perineum, and anal regions. Molluscum contagiosum, when occurring in the genital area, may extend to include the inner thighs. Herpes lesions are usually ulcerative in nature when seen clinically and need to be differentiated from other similar lesions (e.g., syphilitic chancre can be more than one lesion and tender if secondarily infected). Herpetic lesions are found in clusters and can extend from the labia into the vagina. Typically, condylomata acuminata (genital warts) are rough, verrucous lesions that are located inferiorly from the fossa navicularis to the fourchette and the perineal area.

In the overweight patient, vulvovaginitis candidiasis is frequently accompanied by intertriginous candidiasis (e.g., under the breasts and the abdominal apron).

Perform an Internal Vaginal Examination

Note the condition of the vaginal walls. A plastic speculum makes vaginal wall inspection easy and helps in the identification of a foreign body for removal. In children, the knee-chest position is very useful for inspecting the vagina. In children, an otoscope or nasal speculum may be used; rarely is a hysteroscope (under anesthesia) needed. Pale or mottled red splotches of the vaginal mucosa are associated with atrophic vaginitis, and the sticky discharge is a yellow or brown color. In severe cases of atrophic vaginitis, the pale, thin mucosa may have adhered to the opposing vaginal wall, and the speculum examination often causes an oozing bloody discharge.

The appearance of the cervix should be noted. A friable or "strawberry" appearance of cervical petechiae with a frothy, foul-smelling discharge is descriptive of a *Trichomonas* infection. A mucopurulent discharge from the cervical os is an indication to obtain an endocervical sample for *gonorrhea* and *Chlamydia* cultures. This discharge is yellowish green in color when collected on an endocervical swab. The character of the discharge does NOT consistently identify common infectious causes of vaginitis. Three positive characteristics for any one etiology can correctly identify the causative agent (e.g., an increased pH, the presence of "clue cells," and a thin gray discharge seen in BV) (see Table 7-1).

The wet mount is a valuable diagnostic tool, and a sample of vaginal discharge is best obtained from the lateral vaginal fornices. Cultures for BV, fungal infections, and *Trichomonas* vaginitis are not routinely recommended and are usually reserved for determining resistant organisms. Treat vaginal infections before the Papanicolaou test is obtained because BV and trichomoniasis may cause inflammatory atypia results.

Perform a Bimanual Examination

Assess the condition of the uterus, fallopian tubes, and ovaries by checking for uterine and cervical motion tenderness (CMT), ovarian size, and presence of masses. CMT or pain on palpation of the uterus and adnexa confirms the spread of vaginitis or cervicitis to the upper genital tract. This warrants immediate evaluation, treatment, or referral to prevent tubal scarring, ectopic pregnancy, and infertility.

Perform a Vaginal-Rectal Examination

Vaginal-rectal examination is an important technique in assessing the posterior uterus and condition of the cul-de-sac as well as the rectum. Make sure that the internal examination glove is changed before rectal insertion to prevent contamination of the rectum with vaginal discharge organisms. A rectal examination is used to palpate a foreign body and to check for normal pelvic anatomy in the child.

LABORATORY AND DIAGNOSTIC STUDIES

Potassium Hydroxide (KOH) and Wet Mount

Obtain a discharge sample from the lateral fornices of the vagina, using a cotton-tipped applicator. There are several acceptable techniques for preparing a KOH and wet mount. One technique is to prepare two slides with a smear of vaginal discharge. To one, add a drop of 10% KOH and put a cover slip in place. To the other, add a drop of normal saline and put a cover slip in place. The whiff test is positive when the addition of the 10% KOH produces a fishy odor, which is caused by the release of amines. The whiff test has a positive predictive value of 76% for BV. Look under the microscope at the KOH slide for the presence of branching and budding hyphae that are characteristic of yeast infection. Examine the saline wet mount microscopically for motile trichomonads that signal the presence of *Trichomonas*. Clue cells, which are epithelial cells full of bacteria that obscure the cell border, are characteristic of bacterial vaginosis (see Figure 7-1).

Test for pH

Most litmus paper reads the pH ranges from 3.0 to 9.0. This is a simple inexpensive test to aid in determining the etiology of the vaginal discharge. Normal vaginal secretions are less than 4.5 pH. A pH greater than 4.5 is consistent with BV, trichomoniasis, or atrophic vaginitis.

Fungal Culture or Sabouraud Agar Culture

Fungal culture may be needed in the diagnosis of non-*Candida albicans* species (e.g., *C. glabrata, C. tropicalis, C. kruse*) that are refractory to medication regimens.

Herpes Culture

Viral culture is the most reliable method of diagnosing herpes. Results may take from 1 to 7 days, with maximum sensitivity achieved at 5 to 7 days. The herpes culture will probably not be able to identify the causative agent if the specimen is taken from a lesion that is 5 or more days old. It is important to document positive genital herpes infections in the pregnant woman and in skin lesions of the newborn.

Tzanck Smear

Tzanck smear characteristic findings are multinucleated giant cells that are likely to be found if the specimen comes from an intact herpes lesion. Prepare the Tzanck smear by removing the roof of the vesicle and scraping the skin with a scalpel blade. Make sure that the base and the margins of the vesicle are scraped; do not use the vesicular fluid for this specimen. The cellular material is spread onto a glass slide, fixed with absolute alcohol for 1 minute, then stained with Wright's stain. Alternative staining methods are available, and guidelines can be obtained from local laboratories.

Modified Diamond's Culture

Diamond's culture is used to identify *Trichomonas*. However, it is seldom needed to make the diagnosis.

Thayer-Martin Culture

Thayer-Martin medium is a bacterial culture that identifies gonococcal infections. A culture is taken from the endocervical canal of the uterine cervix. First remove excess mucus from a portion of the cervix, using a cotton ball held in ring forceps or a large cotton-tipped procto-swab. Insert a sterile cotton-tipped applicator (Q-tip) into the endocervical canal and allow it to absorb the mucus for 10 to 30 seconds before inoculating the medium. Inoculate the medium bottle or plate in a zigzag manner, while simultaneously rolling the small cotton-tipped applicator. When opening the Thayer-Martin culture bottle, avoid holding the bottle totally upright, which will allow for the loss of the carbon dioxide from the specimen collection bottle.

DNA Probe for *Chlamydia, gonorrhea,* and *Herpes*

The DNA probe is a highly sensitive and specific test with excellent predictive values. Use a dacron swab (with plastic or wire shaft) when collecting your specimen because wooden, cotton-tipped applicators may interfere with the test results. The sample should be taken from the endocervical canal because *Neisseria gonorrhea* has a predilection for the columnar and transitional cells. The swab is rotated in the endocervical canal for 30 seconds. Care should be taken to avoid contact with the vaginal mucous membranes, which would contaminate the specimen. The DNA probe collection technique is the same for *Chlamydia* as described for *gonorrhea,* and one specimen for both tests is all that is usually collected. To collect a DNA probe for *Herpes* testing, the best specimens are those obtained from beneath the roof of a vesicle at the base and at the ulcer border.

Serology for Syphilis: VDRL, RPR, FTA-ABS

These serological tests are used for screening and diagnosing syphilis and are recommended if other STDs are found or suspected.

Urinalysis

Obtain a U/A if the patient has dysuria. However, external pain on urination may come from urine on inflamed vulvar tissue, eliminating the need for urinalysis.

Microscopy/Skin Scraping

Viewing a skin scraping under the microscope is used to assist with the differential diagnosis of scabies and pubic lice (see Chapter 3, Rashes and Skin Lesions, p. 73).

Tape Test

Microscopic identification of pinworm ova on transparent tape that has been pressed to the perianal skin is taken and affixed, adhesive side down, to a microscope slide and scanned for the presence of eggs. Positive findings are diagnostic for *Enterobius vermicularis* (pinworms) (see Figure 7-2).

Acetic Acid Test (Acetowhite)

The acetic acid test is best used to detect subclinical lesions caused by human papilloma virus (HPV) when a genital wart has been identified on the patient, sexual contact, or when the Pap test indicates dysplasia. Applying 5% acetic acid (vinegar) to the cervix, labia, or perianal area causes the lesion to turn white (acetowhite). Saturate a gauze pad with vinegar and place on the lesion for 5 to 10 minutes. After this soaking, the white wart will have a sharp circumscribed macular or papular border. The surface will appear verrucous. False-positives can occur with candidiasis, psoriasis, lichen planus, and sebaceous glands.

Follicle-Stimulating Hormone (FSH)

FSH levels that are greater than 30 mU/mL are diagnostic of perimenopause, and levels of 40 mU/mL or higher represent menopause. This test is particularly helpful in establishing the hypoestrogenic status of a young woman who is experiencing premature menopause and atrophic vaginitis.

DIFFERENTIAL DIAGNOSIS

DISCHARGES

Physiological Discharge

Normal vaginal discharge is produced by the cervical and vulvar glands. It is mucoid, clear, or white in color and has no foul odor. The amount varies from scant to profuse, depending on the amount of estrogen stimulation to the tissues. On occasion physiological discharge can lead to slight vulvar irritation and mild itching secondary to wetness. The vaginal pH is less than 4.5. Wet mount reveals up to 3 to 5 WBCs and the presence of epithelial cells and lactobacilli.

Bacterial Vaginosis (BV)

BV is the most common cause of vaginal discharge and is considered a disturbance in normal vaginal flora. It is often found after intercourse with a new partner or in conjunction with other sexually transmitted diseases. Fifty percent of women are asymptomatic; hence treatment may not be necessary except during pregnancy (increased preterm labor) or in those having vaginal surgical procedures (increased infection). Consistent symptomatology includes a thin homogeneous white, gray, green, or brownish discharge that has a foul odor; there can be pelvic tenderness or pain, but no CMT. The vaginal pH is greater than 4.5. Wet mount shows "clue" cells and a few lactobacilli; the "whiff" test is positive (see Figure 7-1).

Candida Vulvovaginitis

Ninety percent of women with *Candida* vulvovaginitis present with vulvar pruritus. In children, it may be accompanied by oral thrush. The discharge is often thick, white, and "curdy"; the labia are erythematous and edematous. A 4.0 to 4.7 vaginal pH is seen. A KOH wet mount shows pseudohyphae and spores (see Figure 7-1).

Trichomoniasis

Trichomoniasis is asymptomatic in about half of the women affected and 90% of the men. It is usually transmitted by sexual contact but can also be spread by fomites. Women with chronic infections will have copious amounts of discharge and little or no inflammation of the vaginal tissues. When there is an acute infection, they will complain of vulvar itching, swelling, and redness. The pH is greater than 5; the discharge is white or grayish-green or yellow and sometimes frothy; infrequently there will be a "strawberry cervix" (cervical petechiae). If the woman has douched within the last 24 hours, the sensitivity of tests will be greatly decreased. Wet mount shows "gyrating" motile protozoa and often greater than 10 WBCs/HPF (see Figure 7-1).

Atrophic Vaginitis

In atrophic vaginitis, there is a dry (shiny), pale, thin vaginal wall caused by an insufficient amount of endogenous estrogen. During menopause, the vaginal mucosa and vulva, which lack glycogen, become fragile and are susceptible to injury and infection. Patients may experience burning, dryness, irritation, or dyspareunia. This also occurs in postpartum women, those who are breast-feeding, and in prepubertal girls. The pH is alkaline and ranges from 6.5 to 7.0. Wet mount reveals a few WBCs and is negative for pathogens.

Allergic Vaginitis

The causes for allergic vaginitis are different for the child and the adult. In the child, the most common offending agents are bubble baths and perfumed soaps. Adult vulvovaginitis involves any harsh or caustic substance that comes into direct contact with the area. Often a new brand of vaginal lubricant, douche, spermicide, or condom will cause the inflammation and edema. Vinegar douches stronger than 1 to 2 tablespoons per quart of water

may also irritate tissues. The wet mount is positive for WBCs and negative for pseudohyphae.

Foreign Body

The presenting symptom in foreign body retention is a very malodorous, whitish discharge. In children, the foreign body is as variable as those objects found in the ears and nose. However, children less than 12 months do not have the coordination to insert anything into their vagina, so suspect child abuse in such cases and inspect for bruising or excoriations. Wet mount reveals many WBCs.

Chlamydia

Chlamydia is the most prevalent STD in the United States. About 30% of infected women are asymptomatic. Gonorrhea and chlamydia coexist in up to 60% of patients. Women with chlamydia have an increasing amount of vaginal discharge and bleeding after intercourse. Those patients at greatest risk for infection are young (less than 25 years old), sexually active (3 or more partners), and not using barrier methods of contraception. Wet mount shows greater than 10 WBCs/HPF and few microscopic bacteria. Except for perinatal syndromes, nonsexual transmission has not been reported; therefore, suspect child abuse.

Gonorrhea

Gonorrhea is one of the most common reportable diseases. Women are asymptomatic 50% to 80% of the time. However, the patient may have a purulent discharge that originates from the endocervical columnar and transitional cells. Patients often experience inflammation of the Skene's glands, Bartholin's glands, or the urethra, which causes pain and dysuria. Culture or DNA probe confirms diagnosis. A finding of gonorrhea in children is considered specific evidence of sexual abuse.

ITCHING AND LESIONS

Syphilis

The chancre of primary syphilis is an ulcerative lesion that most often develops at the site of initial inoculation. The syphilitic chancre begins as a papule and progresses to a painless to tender, hard, indurated ulcer. The infection causes inguinal lymphadenopathy. Even without treatment, the lesion will heal in 3 to 6 weeks. Many chancres go unnoticed until the appearance of condylomata lata, the warty papule of secondary syphilis, or a maculopapular rash on the palms of the hands and soles of the feet. Diagnosis is confirmed by a serological test for syphilis.

Genital Warts

Genital warts (condylomata acuminata) are caused by the human papilloma virus and may be precursors to genital cancers. The warts may involve the vagina, cervix, perineum, or perianal areas. Condylomata can be flat or raised verrucous lesions. The patient usually notices a bump on the genital region, accompanied by itching and leukorrhea. A wet mount should be done to rule out any co-existing vaginal infections. An acetic acid test is helpful in identifying flat warts. Referral to a dermatologist or gynecologist is indicated for treatment of warts of the urethra or anus.

Herpes

Herpetic lesions can be difficult to distinguish from ulcerative lesions. The most typical presentation is that of grouped vesicles that rupture and leave an erosion. A prodrome of tingling or itching occurs before the outbreak of the vesicles. On the vulva, the erosions are covered with a whitish, exudative layer. Herpetic outbreaks can involve the cervix, vagina, vulva, anus, or extragenital organs, like the pharynx. Culture, DNA probe, or Tzanck smear confirm diagnosis.

If the mother has an active primary herpes simplex virus infection at the time of birth, the infant has a 50% risk of becoming infected. Recurrent maternal infections impart less than a 5% risk of transmission. Clinical signs of the infant's infection become apparent in the first week of life and pose the possibility of death.

Molluscum Contagiosum

Molluscum are small (2 to 5 mm in diameter), umbilicated, flesh-tone papules. These characteristic lesions are the hallmark of the diagnosis. Scratching can spread them. Molluscum is a sexually transmitted disease of adults and is a likely finding in HIV-infected patients. When children are found with genital molluscum, suspect child abuse.

Table 7-1

Differential Diagnosis of Common Causes of Vaginal Discharge and Itching

Condition	History	Physical Findings	Diagnostic Studies
Discharges			
Physiological discharge	Increase in discharge; no foul odor, itching, or edema	Clear or mucoid; pH <4.5	Up to 3-5 WBCs; epithelial cells, lactobacilli

Table 7-1

Differential Diagnosis of Common Causes of Vaginal Discharge and Itching—cont'd

Condition	History	Physical Findings	Diagnostic Studies
Discharges—cont'd			
Bacterial vaginosis	Foul-smelling discharge	Homogenous, thin, white or gray discharge; pH >4.5	Presence of KOH "whiff" test, presence of clue cells, <lactobacilli (see Figure 7-1)
Candida vulvovaginitis	Pruritic discharge	White, curdy, pH 4.0-5.0	KOH prep: mycelia, budding, branching yeast, pseudohyphae (see Figure 7-1)
Trichomoniasis	Watery discharge; foul odor	Profuse, frothy, greenish discharge; red friable cervix; pH 5.0-6.6	Round or pear-shaped protozoa; motile "gyrating" flagella (see Figure 7-1)
Atrophic vaginitis	Dyspareunia; vaginal dryness	Pale, thin vaginal mucosa; pH >4.5	Folded, clumped epithelial cells
Allergic vaginitis	New bubble bath, soap, douche, etc.	Foul smell, erythema, "lost tampon,"; pH <4.5	WBCs
Foreign body	Red and swollen vulva; vaginal discharge; past history of use of tampon, condom, or diaphragm	Bloody, foul-smelling discharge	WBCs
Chlamydia	Partner with non-gonococcal urethritis; asymptomatic	May or may not have purulent discharge	DNA probe; >10 WBCs/HPF
Gonorrhea	Partner with STD; often asymptomatic	Purulent discharge; Skene/Bartholin inflammation	Gram stain; culture; DNA probe
Itching and Lesions			
Syphilis	History of painless ulcerative lesion; rash on palms and soles of feet; warty growth on vagina or anus	Chancre: usually 1 but can be more, painless ulceration; condyloma lata: flat, whitish papule or plaque; maculopapular rash: palm, soles, body	VDRL, RPR, FTA-ABS

Continued

Table 7-1

Differential Diagnosis of Common Causes of Vaginal Discharge and Itching—cont'd

Condition	History	Physical Findings	Diagnostic Studies
Itching and Lesions—cont'd			
Genital warts	Mild-to-moderate itching, foul vaginal discharge; child: history of sexual abuse; adult: new or multiple partners; past history of warts	Moist, pale-pink, verrucous projections on base; located on vulva, vagina, cervix ,or perianal area	Acetic acid test: white
Herpes	History of prodromal syndrome, paresthesias, burning, itching, may have mucoid vaginal discharge	Grouped vesicles on a red base, erode to an ulcer; if on mucous membrane, exudate forms, if on skin, crusts form; redness, edema, tender inguinal lymph nodes	Viral culture; Tzanck smear
Molluscum contagiosum	History of contact with infected person; if inflamed: itching	Flesh-colored, dome-shaped papules, some with umbilication; usually 2-5 mm in diameter	None

Vaginal Bleeding

The average menstrual cycle is 28 days. It is considered abnormal if the cycle occurs less than every 21 days (polymenorrhea) or longer than every 35 days (oligomenorrhea). Bleeding at irregular intervals is known as metrorrhagia. Intermenstrual bleeding is bleeding between cycles. The average duration of menses is 4 days; if the duration is longer than 7 days or blood loss is heavier than 80 mL, it is considered excessive and is classified as menorrhagia. Hypomenorrhea occurs when the frequency of periods remains normal but the menstrual flow decreases in amount. Systemic disorders that cause an imbalance in the hypothalamic-pituitary-ovarian (HPO) axis may lead to menses that are too heavy (menorrhagia/hypermenorrhea), too often (polymenorrhea), or too heavy and irregular (menometrorrhagia).

Other systemic reasons for vaginal bleeding are blood dyscrasias, liver and kidney diseases, as well as medications (hormones, anticoagulants, and non-steroidal anti-inflammatory drugs [NSAIDs]). Organic causes for aberrant menstrual cycles are many and include problems like vaginitis, ectopic pregnancy, fibroids, and polyps. Vaginal bleeding in peri- and postmenopausal women may indicate gynecological cancer. When organic and systemic reasons for abnormal vaginal bleeding are not found, then the diagnosis of dysfunctional uterine bleeding (DUB) is warranted.

DIAGNOSTIC REASONING: FOCUSED HISTORY

Is this related to age? Where is the woman in her reproductive life cycle?

Key Question
- How old are you?

Age today. Knowing the woman's present age is the first step in determining the most common causes of vaginal bleeding. The majority of adolescents with abnormal bleeding are experiencing anovulatory cycles. This is caused by estrogen stimulating the uterine lining with no opposing progesterone. This condition leads to a thicker, more vascular, and less stable endometrium, predisposing the adolescent to dyssynchronous bleeding. A young woman's bleeding is most frequently caused by pregnancy, contraceptive methods, or infection. The woman over age 40 is more likely to have problems related to polyps, fibroids, or ovarian dysfunction. If the patient is over 50 years of age, the origin of bleeding irregularities is often hormone replacement therapy (HRT) or endometrial hyperplasia, which can potentially give rise to endometrial cancer.

Is this prepubertal bleeding?

Key Questions
- How old is the child?
- Is there a family history of early sexual development?
- Is there a family history of bleeding problems or blood dyscrasias?
- Did the child ingest any birth control pills or estrogens?

- Are there any accompanying symptoms?

Pediatric vaginal bleeding. In the United States, the average age of menarche is 12 years old. Vaginal bleeding before age 9 is abnormal and may indicate foreign body or injury. The presence of secondary sexual characteristics indicates sexual precocity. Newborn females may experience breast bud enlargement, galactorrhea, and a small amount of vaginal bleeding from maternal exogenous hormones. These symptoms resolve without intervention within a few weeks.

Although uncommon, malignant genital tract tumors in girls can cause vaginal bleeding. Vaginal adenosis and adenocarcinoma are the most common tumor types.

Bleeding problems. A family history of bleeding problems or a positive review of systems and physical examination indicating the presence of petechiae or bruises may suggest a bleeding tendency. Platelet counts or clotting studies are indicated.

Accompanying symptoms. Vulvovaginitis is the most common pediatric gynecological problem. A vaginal discharge, vaginal itching, vulvar erythema, and lesions often accompany vulvovaginal bleeding. A foul-smelling discharge is noted with bacterial vaginosis, trichomoniasis, and a foreign body. Wet mounts and cultures should be taken for all vaginal discharges of a child, including cultures for *gonorrhea* and *Chlamydia*. If a sexually transmitted disease and sexual abuse are suspected, syphilis and HIV testing should be done. Throat and rectal cultures for *gonorrhea* and *Chlamydia* should also be obtained.

Trauma to the perineum is more common in children because there is less subcutaneous fat of the vulva. Large lacerations and hematomas warrant referral for examination and repair under anesthesia.

Prolapse of the urethra may cause bleeding. It is accompanied by pain at the meatus and pain with urination.

What is the character of the bleeding?

Key Questions
- When did it begin?
- How long has it gone on?
- What is the flow like?
- How many pads do you use?
- Are there any accompanying problems?

Symptom analysis. Determine the amount of flow and its duration to establish if there is menorrhagia, metrorrhagia, or menometrorrhagia. Menorrhagia is considered to be 80 mL of menses, which is estimated as saturating a sanitary pad hourly, over several hours. Metrorrhagia is defined as bleeding at irregular intervals or intermenstrual bleeding. When the menstruation has an unpredictable schedule and lasts for a prolonged time, it is termed menometrorrhagia.

Associated complaints. Patients may experience postcoital bleeding with cervical infections, cervical polyps, or cervical cancer. Accompanying dyspareunia may indicate endometriosis. Dysmenorrhea can be caused by an intrauterine device (IUD) or adenomyosis. Pelvic pressure or pain is suspicious for persistent corpus luteum cyst. Uterine prolapse causes pelvic pressure, which is subjectively described as "something falling out of the vagina." Fever is associated with a pelvic infection. Menorrhagia, accompanied by fatigue, weight gain, hair loss, cold intolerance, decreased libido, and constipation, is a symptom of hypothyroidism. Bleeding disorders may become apparent for the first time in the teenager, with severe menorrhagia accompanied by bruising, petechiae, and gingival bleeding.

Is this an acute or chronic problem? How does it compare to usual menses?

Key Questions
- Has this kind of vaginal bleeding occurred before?

- Were your periods regular before this episode?
- How long did they last?
- What was the amount and pattern of bleeding?

Irregular menses. In anovulatory cycles, the endometrium proliferates under the influence of high estrogen levels until it can no longer be supported—then bleeding occurs. This results in a menstrual pattern that is longer than 28 days with a very heavy flow that lasts 7 to 14 days. If the patient's estrogen levels are fluctuating, she may have two periods a month. Both of these patterns are consistent with dysfunctional uterine bleeding (DUB). However, organic problems with any component of the reproductive tract must be ruled out.

Acute bleeding. One episode of acute bleeding in a woman with normally regular menstrual cycles suggests uterine fibroids or a complication of pregnancy such as threatened abortion.

Chronic bleeding. Chronic, irregular menstrual cycles coupled with obesity are likely to be caused by polycystic ovary syndrome (PCOS), also known as Stein-Leventhal syndrome. Chronic midcycle spotting can occur secondary to the normal midcycle drop in estrogen and usually is not bothersome to the patient because the amount of vaginal bleeding is very scant and the duration is short.

Could this be related to pregnancy?

Key Questions
- Could you be pregnant?
- When was your last normal menstrual period?
- What are you using for birth control?
- Do you have any symptoms of pregnancy? (e.g., missed period, breast tenderness, nausea/vomiting)
- Have you ever been pregnant? What

were the number of times and outcomes of your pregnancies?

Pregnancy complications. An estimated 10% to 15% of clinically recognized pregnancies result in first trimester loss. A patient with a history of three or more spontaneous abortions is considered to have habitual abortions, and referral to a fertility specialist is indicated. If the patient has recently delivered an infant, the abnormal vaginal bleeding could likely be from retained placenta, infection of the uterus (endometritis), or a laceration.

If she is pregnant, is it a spontaneous abortion, threatened abortion, or an ectopic pregnancy?

Key Questions
- Are you experiencing any pain or cramping?
- Have you ever had any sexually transmitted diseases?
- Have you ever had an infection of your tubes (PID)?
- Have you ever had an ectopic pregnancy?

Pain. If there is any pain associated with ectopic pregnancy. it will usually be described as "crampy," pelvic pressure, or "soreness" in the lower abdomen.

Sexually transmitted diseases (STDs). STDs may have gone unnoticed, untreated, or have been inadequately treated and caused scarring of the fallopian tubes, which would put the patient at greater risk for ectopic pregnancy.

Ectopic pregnancy. Ectopic pregnancy occurs in about 1 out of every 200 pregnancies. However, if the woman has had pelvic inflammatory disease (PID), it is as high as 1 out of every 40 pregnancies. Therefore, the provider should keep a high suspicion for this life-threatening diagnosis. Ectopic pregnancy is the second most common cause of maternal death in the United States.

Tubal pregnancy is the most common type of ectopic pregnancy. The menstrual pattern for these patients begins with a time of amenorrhea, followed by abnormal bleeding. They may have some symptoms of pregnancy (e.g., breast tenderness, nausea, and vomiting), have passed some tissue (decidual cast), or have experienced fainting or dizziness. Box 7-1 lists the risk factors associated with ectopic pregnancy.

Could this be caused by her birth control method?

Key Questions
- Do you use a birth control method?
- Which kind(s)?
- How do you use it?

Birth control. Menorrhagia from IUD contraception is accompanied by increased cramping and pain. If spotting or cramping is not of a usual pattern, ectopic pregnancy or infection must be considered. Displacement or perforation of the uterus by the IUD can be verified by pelvic ultrasound. Women who have recently discontinued use of oral contraceptive (OC) pills after several years of use may experience heavier menstrual bleeding than when they were on OCs. Breakthrough bleeding caused by OCs may occur in the first 2 weeks of the cycle because of low estrogen or in the last 2 weeks because of low progesterone. Long-acting progestin contraceptives (Norplant, medroxyprogesterone acetate) may cause irregular heavy menses

---

Box 7-1

Risk Factors for Ectopic Pregnancy

History of PID or ectopic pregnancy

History of tubal surgery or infertility

Intrauterine diethylstilbestrol exposure

Present use of IUD

because there is a lack of estrogen to stabilize the endometrium. Changes in bleeding patterns for progestin users necessitate ruling out pregnancy.

Is she experiencing anovulatory cycles?

Key Questions

- Have you experienced irregular menstrual cycles?
- Are you having symptoms of menopause—vaginal dryness, hot flashes, night sweats?
- At what age did your mother or grandmother go through menopause?

Irregular menstrual cycles. Anovulatory cycles are the most common cause of irregular bleeding patterns among females beginning (adolescent) or ending (perimenopausal) their menstrual cycles. It is estimated that 80% of young adolescents will be anovulatory during the first year of their menstruation. Regular ovulatory cycles are usually established by the second year of menses but may take up to 5 years.

Menopause symptoms. The hot flash is the most commonly experienced symptom of menopause. It is a sensation of increased upper body warmth that begins in the chest area and progresses upward to the neck and face. Sweating, which can be so profuse as to leave clothing wet, follows the hot flash. Hot flashes often lead to disturbed sleep patterns, insomnia, and fatigue. Vaginal atrophy is experienced by the patient as vaginal dryness, dyspareunia, and atrophic vaginitis (see Vaginal Discharge and Itching, p. 273). Atrophic changes can affect the urinary system, causing urinary frequency, urgency, and exacerbation of stress incontinence.

Menopausal syndrome. The frequency of monthly ovulation begins to become irregular at about 40 years of age, and this gives rise to intermittent symptoms of menopause. The time frame from onset of symptoms to complete cessation of menstruation is termed the perimenopause or climacteric phase. The perimenopause can last up to 10 years. If menopause is completed before age 40, it is considered premature ovarian failure. The age of menopause is genetically determined and will be similar to that of the woman's mother and grandmother. Menopause is unrelated to age of menarche, pregnancies, or contraceptive methods used.

Is she experiencing postmenopausal bleeding?

Key Questions

- How old were you at menopause?
- Did you have a hysterectomy? Why did you have surgery? Did they remove your ovaries?
- Have you been or are you currently taking hormone replacement therapy (HRT)?
- What is your regimen? Are you taking your medicine as prescribed?

Age at menopause. The average age for a woman in the United States to go through menopause is 51 years. Menopause is defined as 1 year without menstrual cycles. However, a diagnosis can be accurately made earlier by measuring the rising follicle-stimulating hormone (FSH) and the falling estradiol levels. Postmenopausal bleeding is any bleeding that occurs after the establishment of menopause. Vaginal bleeding after menopause warrants investigation to rule out endometrial cancer. Box 7-2 lists risk factors for endometrial cancer.

Hysterectomy. Any vaginal bleeding after hysterectomy justifies suspicion of endometrial cancer at the surgical site, but the bleeding will most likely be a symptom of atrophic vaginitis. If the ovaries were left in place at the time of the hysterectomy, the woman may not experience menopausal syndrome until about 8 to 10 years after the surgery. The ovaries become atrophic and nonfunctional over time, probably secondary to altered blood flow

Box 7-2

Risk Factors for Endometrial Cancer

Over age 40 with abnormal vaginal
  bleeding
Family history of endometrial
  cancer
Hypertension, diabetes mellitus,
  liver disease
Obesity
Chronic anovulatory cycles
Unopposed estrogen therapy
Tamoxifen therapy

---

resulting from the surgery. The bleeding of atrophic vaginitis occurs from the slightest trauma; even wiping the perineum with tissue after urination can cause spotting.

Hormone replacement therapy (HRT). There are multiple regimens for HRT that include the cycling of estrogen and progestin to continuous daily doses of both hormones. The cycled hormones produce a regular scheduled bleeding. However, the continuous daily combination therapy will often cause amenorrhea after 3 to 6 months of use. After a pattern of amenorrhea has been established, new bleeding should be investigated via endometrial biopsy and hysteroscopy. Discontinuation of HRT is common because of poor patient acceptance of the reinstatement or continuation of cyclic bleeding.

Unopposed estrogen therapy in a woman with an intact uterus predisposes her to endometrial cancer from a thick, built-up endometrium. Endometrial hyperplasia accounts for about 20% of postmenopausal women complaining of abnormal vaginal bleeding. Endometrial hyperplasia can be diagnosed by endometrial biopsy, ultrasonography, or dilatation and curettage (D & C).

Vaginal bleeding can also be caused by a cancerous cervical lesion (diagnosed by

colposcopy and biopsy), cervical polyps, or endometrial polyps. Ovarian tumors can excrete estrogens and progestins, causing vaginal bleeding. Fallopian tube cancer more commonly presents with scant vaginal bleeding or watery vaginal discharge with a pelvic mass.

Could this be from infection or inflammation?

Key Questions

- Have you noticed any sores, rashes, or lumps in the vaginal area?
- Do you have a vaginal discharge or vulvar itching or burning?
- What were the results of your last Pap test?

Lesions and lumps. Condylomata acuminata (genital warts) can cause bleeding secondary to trauma that has been induced. Typically, genital warts are located inferiorly from fossa navicularis to the fourchette and perineal area and internally on the walls of the vagina and cervix. A painless ulcer suggests syphilis and classically appears as a solitary lesion; however, there can be more than one chancre, especially if the patient is immunocompromised. Lesions secondarily infected by bacteria may bleed. Inguinal lymphadenopathy can signal a sexually transmitted infection of the genitourinary tract.

Vaginal discharge. Acute or chronic endometritis and pelvic inflammatory disease (PID) may cause heavy menstrual bleeding. An endometrial infection disturbs the clotting properties, resulting in painful, heavy bleeding. *Chlamydia* and *gonorrhea* are the most frequent causes of PID.

Last Pap test. The last Pap test result may give clues to a chronic vaginal infection revealing a predominance of coccobacilli or atrophy with inflammation; a progressive, low-grade, squamous, intraepithelial lesion; or a cancerous condition. However, the accuracy of a normal Pap test is unreliable if a cervical lesion or abnormal cervical vascular patterns are noted on physical examination.

What other causes of bleeding should I consider?

Key Questions
- Could this bleeding be from the urethra or rectum?
- What other medications are you taking?
- Do you have a history of anemia or do you bleed easily with dental work?
- Did your mother take any drugs when she was pregnant with you?

Urinary or rectal bleeding. Bleeding from the urethra or rectum can be misinterpreted as vaginal bleeding. A prolapsed cystocele or rectocele might be subject to drying, abrasion, and bleeding. These causes can be documented through physical examination, urinalysis, fecal occult blood testing (FOBT), and colonoscopy.

Medications. Antibiotics, phenobarbital, rifampin, phenytoin, carbamazepine, and other drugs that induce hepatic microsomal enzymes may produce lower estrogen levels and cause bleeding irregularities. Drugs containing aspirin can increase menstrual flow.

Blood dyscrasias. Some females with a coagulation defect have excessive menstrual bleeding as the first symptom of a blood disorder; also most platelet abnormalities will cause vaginal bleeding. If the patient has severe anemia (hemoglobin less than 10 g/dL) resulting from the vaginal bleeding, it is highly probable that a coagulopathy is present. If this occurs in the perimenarcheal or second or third decade of life, suspect von Willebrand's disease, a congenital bleeding disorder caused by deficiency in factor VIII.

Drug exposure in utero. In utero exposure to diethylstilbestrol (DES) has been associated with adenocarcinoma of the vagina in daughters.

DIAGNOSTIC REASONING: FOCUSED PHYSICAL EXAMINATION

Perform a General Assessment

Determine if the patient's general state of health includes problems of nutrition (e.g., obesity or muscle wasting), hirsutism, hypo- or hyperthyroidism, all of which may cause an endocrinopathy with consequential vaginal bleeding.

Determine Patient Weight and Calculate Body Mass Index (BMI)

A BMI of greater than 27% corresponds to being more than 20% overweight. See Amenorrhea, p. 303, for calculation of BMI. Obesity causes anovulatory cycles because the adipose cell stroma converts androstenedione to estrogen (estrone) as the body fat increases. Obesity also increases sex hormone binding globulin, thereby increasing free steroid levels. Both processes can cause an imbalance in the hypothalamic-pituitary-ovarian (HPO) axis and increase the probability of an anovulatory cycle and heavy vaginal bleeding. Amenorrhea in anorexia nervosa may precede weight loss by many months.

Perform a Lymph Node Examination

Lymph node examination should be performed to assess for leukemia or metastatic gynecological cancer. Inguinal lymph nodes can be enlarged from a sexually transmitted disease or vulvar infection (e.g., Bartholinitis).

Perform a Thyroid Examination

Observe and palpate the thyroid gland. Hypertrophy (enlargement) may be found in hypo-functioning glands. Hypothyroidism is known to be present in 22% of women with severe menorrhagia.

Perform a Breast Examination

The finding of clear or non-bloody nipple discharge on breast examination could be indicative of hyperprolactinemia, which may cause amenorrhea or irregular vaginal bleeding.

Perform a Pelvic Examination

If practitioners and patients believe bleeding to be uterine in origin, the external and internal pelvic examination can verify that etiology. Perform an examination of the external genitalia, noting whether the bleeding is coming from external hemorrhoids or a painless labial lesion like a squamous cell cancer or condyloma acuminata. Note bruising, lacerations on the vaginal walls, or other signs of sexual abuse. Observe the introitus for signs of a prolapsed uterus or cystocele or rectocele that might be subject to drying, abrasion, or bleeding. These signs are usually accompanied by pelvic pressure or urinary or bowel symptoms.

Observe the external genitalia for signs of estrogen deficiency: sparse hair distribution, graying or white hair color, clitoral atrophy, and thin, small labia minora. These signs strongly suggest atrophic vaginitis as the cause for bleeding.

Next perform a vaginal examination to determine if the bleeding may be caused by a vaginal infection. Note the color and condition of the vaginal walls. Pale non-rugated vaginal walls are a sign of an atrophic vagina, which is easily abraded to cause bleeding. Pale vaginal mucosa with splotchy red patches is also a sign of vaginal atrophy. Bleeding from atrophic vaginitis most commonly follows intercourse or douching. It often is a whitish-brown discharge with no particular foul odor. The patient may also have pruritus and a burning sensation of the vagina, labia, and urinary tract because of a lack of estrogen.

Note the amount, color, consistency and odor of the vaginal discharge. Take samples for wet mount examination from the pooled discharge in the lateral fornices. Note cervical friability and discharge from the cervical os. Take samples of the discharge and assess as noted in Vaginal Discharge and Itching, p. 270. Cervical polyps are red, glossy, nontender masses protruding from the cervical os. They are usually benign and can be removed by twisting them off with ring forceps. The specimen should be sent to pathology for evaluation.

If a threatened or spontaneous abortion is suspected, check the internal cervical os to determine if it is closed or open.

Ectopic pregnancy will cause adnexal or cervical motion tenderness. However, uterine enlargement is not often appreciated. Uterine size and contour can be grossly assessed via bimanual examination. Uterine leiomyomas (myomas, fibroids) typically feel firm and may make the uterus asymmetrical. These tumors can progress to a size that mimics an advanced pregnant uterus. The uterine size is measured in weeks like the pregnant uterus is measured. When the uterus reaches 12- to 14-week size, referral to a gynecologist for surgery (myomectomy or hysterectomy) is appropriate. The patient may experience urinary or bowel problems (e.g., urinary frequency and constipation) because the fibroid(s) is distorting or obstructing those systems. Carcinogenic tumors of the uterus are classically firm, hard, and rapidly growing, becoming fixed masses. Ultrasound is a valuable tool in documenting size and growth patterns of tumors.

The average-size adult uterus measures 8 cm long, 5 cm wide, and 2.5 cm deep for the nulliparous woman. Add 1 centimeter to each dimension for the average size of the multiparous uterus ($9 \times 6 \times 3.5$ cm). The uterus with adenomyosis is increased in size to 2 to 3 times that of normal, may be globular, and has a uniform consistency. Adenomyosis is accompanied by worsening menorrhagia and dysmenorrhea.

The rectovaginal examination can detect lesions or nodularity of the cul-de-sac, which is present with endometriosis or the presence of a primary rectal tumor.

Pediatric Examination: Perform a Breast and Genital Examination

Assess for signs of sexual precocity by determining the presence and stage of secondary sexual characteristics of the breasts and pubic hair. Assess development using Tanner staging (see pp. 298 and 299). Inspect the vulva, noting the hygiene status—presence of smegma in the labial folds, urine, fecal material, or erythema and lesions. Examine the urinary meatus. A prolapsed urinary meatus is noted by the presence of a dark red tissue surrounding the urinary opening. This tissue is usually tender. Use an appropriate pediatric size speculum, long otoscope, or nasal speculum. It may be necessary to refer the patient for a vaginoscopy or cystoscopy under anesthesia for a complete assessment of the vagina and uterus.

Consider the possibility of infection or sexual abuse. See Vaginal Discharge and Itching, p. 272, for assessment of vaginal discharges.

LABORATORY AND DIAGNOSTIC STUDIES

Serum Human Chorionic Gonadotropin (Beta hCG)

A beta hCG test is the first step in determining a complication of pregnancy. All women with a potential for childbearing should be tested. If the pregnancy test is positive, then ultrasound is the usual next step in determining abnormal implantation or threatened abortion.

The test is a fluorometric enzyme immunoassay that is highly specific for the beta receptors of hCG, with almost no cross-reactivity with other hormones. Results are provided as values. The reference ranges for determining an abnormal pregnancy are as follows:

Not significant	0-5.0 mU/mL
Borderline significance	5.0-25 mU/mL
Evaluate with serial determinations	>25 mU/mL

A rapid beta hCG test (with a sensitivity of at least 5 mU/mL) that measures less than 5 mU/mL is highly predictive in excluding ectopic pregnancy. The beta hCG levels have a doubling time of 58 hours with pregnancy. Ectopic pregnancy causes an increase in hCG levels at the same rate as a normal pregnancy but only up to a certain point. In ectopic pregnancy, that point is usually less than 4 to 6 weeks, at which time the hCG levels plateau or begin to fall. Therefore serial determinations are more useful than a single determination.

The beta hCG and ultrasound are used together to determine the possibility of ectopic pregnancy. If the discriminatory threshold of beta hCG is 1500 mU/mL and a vaginal ultrasound determines absence of a gestational sac (gestational age 35 days) or a value of 6500 mU/mL and negative transabdominal ultrasound (gestational age 42 days), the presumptive diagnosis of ectopic pregnancy can be made. A drop in serial hCG levels and an ultrasound that does not identify an intrauterine gestational sac supports the diagnosis of spontaneous abortion.

Hematocrit/Hemoglobin

Hematocrit and hemoglobin are used to determine anemia caused by blood loss from long-standing menorrhagia. Hematocrit and hemoglobin levels are not useful in evaluating acute blood loss from a single episode of heavy bleeding caused by a spontaneous abortion or ectopic pregnancy.

Complete Blood Count with Indices and Differential (CBC)

CBC with indices will give information about the degree and cause of anemia. Typically, the hematocrit and hemoglobin reflect the degree of anemia, with erythrocyte indices suggesting the cause. Microcytic hypochromic anemia is reflective of chronic blood loss, whereas normocytic normochromic anemia suggests acute hemorrhage. Microcytic hypochromic anemia is indicated by a mean corpuscular volume (MCV) less than 80 and a mean corpuscular hemoglobin (MCH) less than 27. The MCV and MCH values are within reference range in normocytic normochromic anemia.

An increased WBC count with a shift to the left (an increase in the number of bands that are immature neutrophils) points to infection as a cause of the vaginal bleeding. Additionally, the CBC can rule out leukemia and thrombocytopenia, both of which can produce abnormal vaginal bleeding.

Prothrombin Time/Partial Thromboplastin/Bleeding Time (PTT/PT/BT)

If the history and/or the physical examination are suggestive of a bleeding problem, these tests can differentiate between blood dyscrasias, hepatic or renal diseases, or iatrogenic causes (anticoagulants, nonsteroidal anti-inflammatory drugs).

Serum Progesterone

A serum progesterone level greater than 25 ng/mL is predictive of an intrauterine pregnancy; however, if the level is less than 15 ng/mL it suggests an ectopic pregnancy.

Serum Follicle-Stimulating Hormone (FSH) Levels

Ovarian failure, which causes a low estradiol secretion, will raise the FSH level above 40 mU/mL. If both the FSH and luteinizing hormone (LH) levels are greater than 50 mU/mL, primary ovarian failure is established. If the patient is older than 30 years, menopause is diagnosed; if she is younger than 30 years, a chromosomal karyotype should be done. A FSH measurement of less than 40 mU/mL denotes a hypothalamic-pituitary dysfunction and secondary ovarian failure.

Serum Luteinizing Hormone (LH) Levels

A serum LH level greater than 35 mU/mL is frequently seen in patients with polycystic ovarian syndrome (PCOS). An LH/FSH ratio higher than 2:1 is suggestive of PCOS, while a ratio greater than 3 is considered diagnostic of PCOS.

Serum Estradiol Levels

Serum estradiol levels less than 15 pg/mL are found with menopause.

Fecal Occult Blood Test (FOBT)

A negative FOBT rules out the cause of bleeding being located in the colon or rectum (see Chapter 5, Rectal Pain and Bleeding, p. 208).

Vaginal/Lower Abdominal Ultrasound

Ultrasonography is helpful in identifying cystic enlargement of the uterus and the presence or absence of the products of conception. When the intrauterine sac is identified within the uterus by ultrasound, an ectopic pregnancy is rarely the diagnosis, even though it is possible to have simultaneous intrauterine and ectopic pregnancies. Ultrasonography can determine endometrium thickness. A thickness greater than 3 mm indicates hyperplasia. In postmenopausal women, 5 mm is the cutoff for a normal unilateral stripe.

Endometrial Biopsy (EMB)

EMB is used to exclude cancer in any woman over 40 years of age who is experiencing abnormal vaginal bleeding. EMB should also be performed on women who are in their 30s if they are at increased risk for endometrial cancer (see Box 7-2). The sensitivity of this biopsy for endometrial carcinoma is from 95% to 97%. If the test results are abnormal or inadequate in terms of amount of tissue, the next diagnostic test would be dilation and curettage. If the test is normal and abnormal bleeding continues, further work-up is indicated to exclude neoplasia.

Dilation and Curettage (D & C)

D & C is useful in determining the cause of abnormal uterine bleeding and for the removal of retained products of conception. The curetting of the entire uterus provides specimens to send to pathology to rule out carcinogenic causes for the uterine bleeding.

Hysteroscopy

Hysteroscopy allows for visualization of the uterine cavity. Endometrial biopsies, endometrial polyps, and submucosal leiomyomas can be obtained and/or removed by hysteroscopy.

DIFFERENTIAL DIAGNOSIS

ORGANIC CAUSES OF VAGINAL BLEEDING

Pregnancy

A small amount of bleeding can occur at the time of implantation. The blastocyst burrows into the endometrium and invades the maternal blood supply; the formation and implantation of the placenta follow this. If bleeding occurs from implantation, it happens about 1 week before the expected menstrual cycle.

Spontaneous Abortion

A spontaneous abortion (or miscarriage) is the natural termination of a pregnancy before fetal viability (before 20 weeks). Approximately 15% of diagnosed pregnancies abort spontaneously. It is a complete spontaneous abortion if the fetus and the placenta are completely expelled and incomplete if partial tissue remains within the uterus. Most often the woman will present with persistent uterine cramping and bleeding that is increasing in severity and amount. She may have experienced passage of tissue. The typical patient experiencing a spontaneous abortion presents to the clinic at about 10 to 12 weeks of gestation. The pregnancy test may remain positive for weeks after fetal demise. Serial serum hCG and ultrasound are useful in establishing the diagnosis.

Threatened Abortion

Threatened abortion produces menstrual-like cramping and bleeding but the cervical os remains closed. The pain is often midline or suprapubic. Perform a sterile speculum examination to inspect the external cervical os. Only if the facility is prepared to deal with the possibility of surgical intervention, should a cotton-tipped applicator or ring forceps be passed through the os to verify its closed status. In addition to the bleeding and cramping, if the cervical os is open or if tissue is in the cervical canal, the woman is diagnosed with an inevitable abortion.

Placenta Previa

Placenta previa occurs in the third trimester of pregnancy and presents with bright red painless bleeding. The placenta is implanted in the lower segment of the uterus. When the cervix begins to dilate, the placenta is pulled away from the endometrial wall, and bleeding can occur. Any significant bleeding that leads to hemorrhage can endanger the mother and may interfere with uteroplacental sufficiency. Fetal activity is present. The uterus is nontender with a normal resting tone. Diagnosis is made by sonogram. Pelvic examination should not be performed in order to avoid dislodging any clot that may have formed at the cervix.

Placenta Abruptio

Placenta abruptio can occur any time after 20 weeks of gestation. As the placenta detaches from the uterine wall, the patient experiences dark-red, painful bleeding. The amount of bleeding varies from scant to profuse. On physical examination, vaginal bleeding is apparent, and the uterus may be tender and demonstrate increased tone. Signs of fetal distress may be apparent. Vaginal examination is not done until placenta previa is ruled out as a diagnosis through the use of ultrasound.

Ectopic Pregnancy

Ectopic pregnancy occurs in about 1 out of 200 pregnancies. Ninety percent of ectopic pregnancies are implanted in the fallopian tube. About half of these women will have an adnexal mass. Ectopic pregnancy symptoms can be the same as normal pregnancy symptoms. Therefore, any pregnancy accompanied by bleeding or pain must be considered high risk for ectopic pregnancy and must be worked up to rule out this life-threatening diagnosis. Persistent one-sided pain or pain that radiates toward the midline of the abdomen is indicative of ectopic pregnancy. The patient experiencing an ectopic pregnancy typically presents at about 6 to 8 weeks of gestation.

Leiomyomas (Myomas or Fibroids)

Fibroids are found in about 1 out of 4 women over age 35. They are more frequently found in black women than in white women, and they usually decrease in size after menopause. Depending on location, they are associated with infertility in 2% to 10% of patients. These benign tumors are estrogen dependent and may grow during hormone replacement therapy (HRT). The most frequent symptom of leiomyomas is bleeding, which ranges from slightly heavier menstrual flow to continuous bleeding. Fibroids may occur as single or multiple tumors within the uterine layers, or they can be pedunculated. Pain is not a common complaint of women with fibroids unless there has been strangulation of a pedunculated fibroid, degeneration of a large fibroid, or compression of other organ systems.

Adenomyosis

Adenomyosis is a condition in which there are endometrial glands and stroma within the myometrium of the uterus. It is a condition, more common in multiparous women, that occurs in the later reproductive years. The uterus is 2 to 3 times its normal size, and there is often dysmenorrhea and infertility. Adenomyosis often coexists with uterine fibroids. Ultrasound may not identify this diffuse intramural lesion. Adenomyosis is found in 20% of hysterectomy specimens.

Uterine/Endometrial Cancer

Endometrial cancer is presently the most common female genital cancer in the United States. The average age at diagnosis is 61 years, but it occurs throughout the reproductive and postmenopausal years. Uterine cancer risk factors are anovulatory states (e.g., obesity), endometrial hyperplasia (e.g., unopposed estrogen), and family history (see Box 7-2). Classic symptoms include painless vaginal bleeding and a rapidly enlarging uterus. Late symptoms are those of systemic disease, like weight loss and weakness.

SYSTEMIC CAUSES OF VAGINAL BLEEDING

Anovulatory Cycles

Perimenopause

The perimenopausal years occur from ages 40 to 50 and last about 7 to 10 years. The perimenopausal woman experiences irregularities in her menstrual flow. Often she has spotting, followed by a day or two of heavy bleeding, or has her regular menstrual flow and a few days of spotting at the end of the cycle. These types of irregular patterns are characteristic of a degenerating corpus luteum function. A woman who has had a year of irregular periods and who has missed the past 3 cycles can be clinically diagnosed as being in perimenopause (another synonymous term is climacteric). The perimenopause progresses to menopause when the FSH is elevated above 40 mU/mL, or there has been an absence of periods for 1 full year. An FSH level of 30 mU/mL is typical of perimenopause.

Perimenarche

With perimenarche, the patient has a history of beginning her menstrual cycles and then experiencing months of amenorrhea, followed by resumption of regular cycles. The menstrual flow may be heavier, more frequent, or longer in duration. The young adolescent has appropriate secondary sexual characteristics and sexual maturity ratings. These symptoms are characteristic of anovulatory cycles.

Newborn

A bloody vaginal discharge may occur normally in the female newborn because of maternal estrogen hormone withdrawal during the first few weeks of life.

Endocrinopathies

Polycystic Ovary Syndrome (PCOS)

In PCOS, the patient typically is obese, hirsute, has oligomenorrhea, and large cystic ovaries. However, women with chronic anovulatory cycles and hyperandrogenemia meet the criteria for PCOS even if they are slim and without hirsutism. The LH:FSH ratio is greater than 3:1.

Thyroid Dysfunction

Both hypothyroidism and hyperthyroidism are associated with abnormal menstrual bleeding. Menorrhagia can occur with hypothyroidism, whereas oligomenorrhea or scant menses may occur with hyperthyroidism.

With hypothyroidism, the patient may also experience delayed growth, weight gain, fatigue, constipation, and cold intolerance. On physical examination, you may note dry skin, coarse hair, and galactorrhea. The TSH level will be high.

With hyperthyroidism, the patient may experience weight loss, nervousness, heat intolerance, and palpitations. On physical examination, the skin may be moist and sweaty, the hair thin, and the pulse rapid. The thyroid gland may be enlarged or nodular. The TSH level will be low, with high T3 and T4 levels.

Hyperprolactinemia

Prolactin inhibits gonadotrophin release and causes anovulatory cycles that may be associated with irregular and sometimes heavy bleeding or with amenorrhea (see Amenorrhea, p. 293). Galactorrhea often accompanies hyperprolactinemia. Nipple discharge will be negative for RBCs. Prolactin levels will be elevated. Thyroid function tests can rule out hypothyroidism. MRI or CT scan along with a cone view of the sella turcica assists in diagnosis of pituitary tumor.

Vaginal Infection

Atrophic Vaginitis

In atrophic vaginitis, there is a dry (shiny), pale, thin vaginal wall caused by an insufficient amount of endogenous estrogen. During menopause, the vaginal mucosa and vulva, which lack glycogen, become fragile and are susceptible to injury and infection. The patient may experience burning, dryness, irritation, dyspareunia, or atrophic vaginitis. This also occurs in the postpartum woman, the woman who is breast feeding, or the prepubertal girl. The pH is alkaline and ranges from 6.5 to 7.0. Wet mount reveals a few WBCs and is negative for pathogens.

Endometritis

Endometritis is an infection of the endometrium, in which *Chlamydia* is the cause about 25% of the time. Group A or B *Streptococcus* produces puerperal sepsis and may lead to peritonitis, abscess, thrombophlebitis, disseminated intravascular coagulation, septic shock, and infertility. The woman has a slight vaginal discharge (lochia) that is bloody or purulent. The bleeding is accompanied by fever (39° C to 39.8° C; 102° to 103° F) and uterine tenderness often within the first 24 hours after delivery. Endometritis should be suspected in a woman with these symptoms, especially if she has undergone an emergency cesarean section or an intrauterine manipulative procedure. Other contributing factors for endometritis are premature rupture of membranes and prolonged labor.

Pelvic Inflammatory Disease (PID)

PID is most commonly caused by *Chlamydia* and *N. gonorrhea* (see Chapter 5, Abdominal Pain) and can produce bleeding, abdominal pain, fever, and vaginal discharge. Women with PID have an increasing amount of vaginal discharge and bleeding after intercourse. Infection begins intravaginally in most cases and then spreads upward, causing salpingitis. In the early stages, women may be asymptomatic. Patients may have a purulent discharge that originates from the endocervical columnar and transitional cells. With *gonorrhea,* patients often experience inflammation of Skene's glands, Bartholin's glands, or the urethra, which causes pain and dysuria. On examination, abdominal tenderness, CMT, and adnexal tenderness is present. As with peritonitis, patients may also have guarding and rebound tenderness. WBC and ESR are usually elevated. Cultures and Gram staining can assist with diagnosis (see Vaginal Discharge and Itching, p. 270).

Genital Warts

Genital warts (condylomata acuminata) are caused by the human papilloma virus and may be precursors to genital cancer. The warts may involve the vagina, cervix, perineum, or perianal areas. Condylomata can be flat or raised verrucous lesions. The patient usually notices a bump on the genital region accompanied by itching and leukorrhea. A wet mount should be performed to rule out any coexisting vaginal infections. An acetic acid test is helpful in identifying flat warts. Refer to a dermatologist or gynecologist for treatment of warts of the urethra or anus.

Foreign Body

In foreign body retention, the presenting symptom is a very malodorous, whitish discharge. In children, the foreign body is as variable as those objects found in the ears and nose. Children less than 12 months do not have the coordination to insert anything into their vagina. So suspect child abuse in those cases and inspect for bruising or excoriations. Wet mount reveals many WBCs.

Blood Dyscrasias

von Willebrand's Disease

von Willebrand's disease is a congenital autosomal dominant bleeding disorder. Altered factor VIII activity and deficient platelet function characterize it. The patient has a prolonged bleeding time. Hypermenorrhea may occur at menarche or may begin in women 20 to 30 years of age.

Leukemia

Hypermenorrhea may be one of the chief complaints of the woman presenting with leukemia. Other symptoms may include fatigue, bruising, and lymph node enlargement. The CBC and bleeding times will direct the work-up for this diagnosis.

Other

Medications

Drugs such as rifampin, phenytoin, carbamazepine, and phenobarbital reduce the efficacy of oral contraceptives. If the woman is on a low estrogen oral control pill, these medications are likely to be the cause of irregular vaginal bleeding. Changing the oral contraceptive to one of higher estrogenic potency will alleviate the bleeding.

Table 7-2			

Differential Diagnosis of Common Causes of Vaginal Bleeding

Condition	History	Physical Findings	Diagnostic Studies
Organic Causes of Vaginal Bleeding			
Pregnancy	Implantation bleeding; breast tenderness, nausea and vomiting	Internal cervical os closed; minimal spotting; globular, enlarged uterus; soft, bluish color cervix	Pregnancy test; beta hCG positive
Spontaneous abortion	Vaginal bleeding following a time of amenorrhea; cramping, passage of tissue; history of miscarriages	Internal cervical os open; blood from cervical os	Serial beta hCG declining levels; ultrasound negative
Threatened abortion	Vaginal bleeding, following a time of amenorrhea; mild cramping	Fetal activity present; internal cervical os may be open	Beta hCG positive; ultrasound positive
Placenta previa	Late pregnancy: bright red, painless bleeding	Fetal activity present; uterus is nontender, normal resting tone	Ultrasound
Placenta abruptio	Dark-red, painful bleeding; any time after 20 weeks of gestation	Vaginal bleeding; uterus tender with tone; signs of fetal distress	Rule out placenta previa with ultrasound
Ectopic pregnancy	Painless vaginal bleeding; multiparity, older gravida, multiple gestation; history of PID, infertility, STDs	Internal cervical os closed; bloody discharge present	Beta hCG positive; ultrasound negative; laparoscopy
Leiomyomas	Heavier menstrual bleeding; menorrhagia	Enlarged uterine size; firm, spherical masses; nontender	Pelvic examination; ultrasound
Adenomyosis	Worsening menorrhagia; dysmenorrhea	Pelvic enlargement (2-3 times normal size)	Pelvic examination; ultrasound not always helpful
Uterine/ endometrial cancer	Rapidly enlarging uterus; painless menorrhagia; pelvic pressure; weight loss, weakness	Enlargement of uterus, often symmetrical; fixed with advanced disease	Endometrial biopsy; D & C; ultrasound; CT or MRI

Table 7-2

Differential Diagnosis of Common Causes of Vaginal Bleeding—cont'd

Condition	History	Physical Findings	Diagnostic Studies
Systemic Causes of Vaginal Bleeding			
Anovulatory Cycles			
Perimenopause	Irregular menses, amenorrhea coupled with heavier and longer menstrual cycles; hot flashes, night sweats, insomnia, mood changes	Pale, dry vaginal mucosa, few rugae	FSH and LH high; estradiol low
Perimenarche	History of beginning menses within last 1-2 years; has period of amenorrhea followed by irregular menstrual cycles that are of heavy, frequent, or long duration	Physical exam normal; secondary sexual characteristic present	History and examination
Newborn	Less than 2 months old	Small amount of vaginal spotting	History and examination
Endocrinopathies			
Polycystic ovary syndrome	Infertility; irregular menstrual cycles	Hirsute; obese; enlarged ovaries	Pelvic exam; ultrasound: enlarged ovaries with multiple fluid-filled cysts
Thyroid dysfunction	Hypothyroid: menorrhagia, delayed growth, weight gain, fatigue, constipation, cold intolerance	Hypothyroid: dry skin, fine hair, galactorrhea	TSH high
	Hyperthyroid: oligomenorrhea, weight loss, nervousness, heat intolerance, palpitation	Hyperthyroid: moist skin, hyperpigmentation over bones, thin hair, goiter	TSH low; T_3 high; T_4 high

Continued

Table 7-2

Differential Diagnosis of Common Causes of Vaginal Bleeding—cont'd

Condition	History	Physical Findings	Diagnostic Studies
Endocrinopathies—cont'd			
Hyperprolac- tinemia	Menometrorrhagia, oligomenorrhea	Bilateral, multi-duct, clear-to-white nipple discharge	Wet mount or hemoccult of nipple discharge: negative for RBCs; prolactin high; cone-down view of sella turcica; MRI or CT with contrast
Vaginal Infection			
Atrophic vaginitis	Dyspareunia; vaginal dryness	Pale thin vaginal mucosa; brown or bloody discharge; pH > 4.5	Folded, clumped epithelial cells
Endometritis	History of emer- gency cesarean section, PROM, prolonged labor, intrauterine ma- nipulative proce- dures	Tenderness of the uterus on bi- manual examina- tion; fever 102- 103° F; discharge or lochia may be purulent	WBC >10,000/mm^3
Pelvic inflam- matory disease (PID)	History of past PID; chronic vaginitis; STDs	Bilateral abdominal pain following menses; pelvic mass; cervical motion tender- ness; vaginal discharge temperature >100.4° F	WBC, ESR; Gram staining, cultures
Genital warts	Mild-to-moderate itching; foul vaginal discharge; child: history of sexual abuse; adult: new or multiple partners; past history of warts	Moist, pale pink, verrucous projec- tions on base; located on vulva, vagina, cervix or perianal area; bleeding with trauma	Acetic acid test— white
Foreign body	Red and swollen vulva; vaginal discharge; past history of use of tampon, condom, or diaphragm	Foreign body present (tampon, condom); bloody, foul-smelling dis- charge	Wet mount: many WBCs, no patho- gens; history and examination

	Table 7-2		
Differential Diagnosis of Common Causes of Vaginal Bleeding—cont'd			
Condition	**History**	**Physical Findings**	**Diagnostic Studies**
Blood Dyscrasias			
von Willebrand's disease	Menorrhagia, adolescent	Bruising; petechiae; gingival bleeding	Bleeding time, factor VIII deficiency, decreased platelets
Leukemia	Menorrhagia; fatigue usually less than 3 months duration	Fever, bruising, pallor; lymph node enlargement; hepatic or splenic enlargement	WBCs: 1000-400,000/mm³ leukocytosis with immature blasts or cells; anemia, thrombocytopenia, decreased factors V or VIII
Other			
Medications	Taking rifampin, phenytoin, carbamazepine, or phenobarbital while on low-estrogen dose oral contraceptives	Normal GYN exam	Bleeding stops with higher estrogen dose oral contraceptive

Amenorrhea

Amenorrhea is a lack of menstruation that may be the result of primary or secondary causes. Primary amenorrhea can be defined as absence of menarche by 16 years of age with normal pubertal growth and development, absence of menarche by 14 years of age with lack of normal pubertal growth and development, or absence of menarche 2 years after sexual maturation is complete. Primary amenorrhea is a rare condition with constitutional puberty delay the most common cause. The etiology of one third of primary amenorrhea is genetic, such as Turner's syndrome or abnormality of the X chromosome.

Secondary amenorrhea is defined as the absence of menstruation for at least 3 cycles or 6 months in females who have already established menstruation. The most common causes of secondary amenorrhea are the physiological events of pregnancy, lactation, and menopause. Traditionally the primary care provider would begin investigation of etiological reasons for amenorrhea and use that knowledge to determine the type of amenorrhea. In turn, the suspected cause would guide diagnostic tests, treatment, and referrals. This method of classification looks first at the lower genital tract and then for a dysfunction of any component of the hypothalamic-pituitary-ovarian (HPO) axis.

The normal menstrual cycle begins with the pulsatile delivery of gonadotropin-releasing hormone (GnRH) by the medial-basal hypothalamus. In response, the pos-

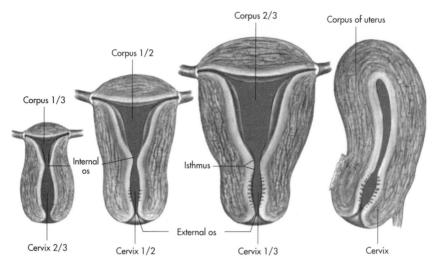

Figure 7-3 Comparative sizes of prepubertal, adult nonparous, and multiparous uteruses. (From Thompson JM et al: *Mosby's clinical nursing*, ed 4, St. Louis, 1997, Mosby.)

terior pituitary releases luteinizing hormone (LH) and follicle-stimulating hormone (FSH). These influence the growth and development of a follicle and its release of estradiol, which causes the uterine endometrium to proliferate, and initiates the LH surge, which is followed by ovulation and menstruation (Figures 7-3, 7-4, and Table 7-3).

The hypothalamus is also affected by the central nervous system and the thyroid gland, which can determine the amount of GnRH received by the pituitary. Alterations in the pattern of GnRH pulsatile release will decrease circulating LH and FSH; the consequence will be an anovulatory menstrual cycle and amenorrhea.

About 66% of all amenorrheic women are hypoestrogenic because of either hypothalamic-pituitary hypofunction or end-organ failure. Determining whether the patient is hypoestrogenic can expedite finding the reason for her amenorrhea and determining the sequencing of laboratory tests. The progesterone challenge test will cause withdrawal bleeding if there is estrogen production and an adequate outflow tract. The functional status of the pituitary-ovarian unit is assessed by measuring the gonadotropins.

DIAGNOSTIC REASONING: FOCUSED HISTORY

Is there a pregnancy?

Key Questions
- Are you sexually active?
- Are you using any birth control methods?
- Are you trying to become pregnant?

Pregnancy. For any female with a uterus, it is important to rule out pregnancy as the first step in determining the etiology of amenorrhea. It is rare, but a young girl can become pregnant before the onset of menses. Pregnancy should be ruled out before the administration of androgenic challenge tests. If the woman is pregnant and there is accompanying bleeding, determination of whether the pregnancy is uterine or ectopic is the next priority (see Vaginal Bleeding, p. 287). Be cognizant of domestic violence and sexual abuse, with consequent unintended

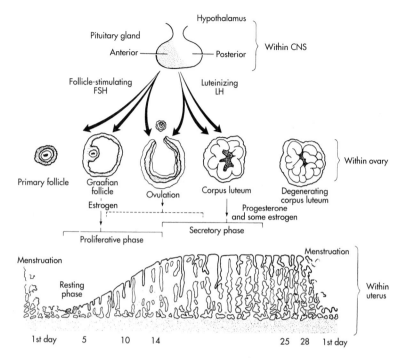

Figure 7-4   Interrelationships among cerebral hypothalamic, pituitary, ovarian, and uterine functions throughout the menstrual cycle. (Modified from Lowdermilk DL, Perry SE, Bobak IM: *Maternity and women's health care,* ed 6, St. Louis, 1997, Mosby.)

pregnancy. Ask direct questions in private about being hit, pushed, slapped, or nonconsensual sex.

Contraceptive use. The type and use patterns of contraceptives is important in the search for the cause of amenorrhea. Contraceptive failures may account for an unintended pregnancy. Amenorrhea can occur after discontinuing oral contraceptives. Measurement of serum gonadotropins is affected by long-acting contraceptives like depo-medroxyprogesterone acetate (DMPA), implants, or intrauterine devices (IUD) containing progestogens; these must be discontinued before testing.

Seeking pregnancy. Knowing that the patient is seeking pregnancy or, if the patient is pregnant, whether it is intended or unintended, will allow the interview to be structured appropriately. It will also aid in proper counseling and referral. Amenorrheic patients seeking pregnancy who do not bleed following androgen challenge tests are most successfully treated by an infertility specialist. Young maternal age and early referral to a specialist increases a woman's conception rate.

Is this primary or secondary amenorrhea?

Key Questions

- Have you ever had a menstrual cycle?
- Have you started your pubertal development? Can you show me how your breast and pubic hair look compared to these pictures? (use Tanner Sexual Maturity Rating Scales, pp. 298 and 299)
- At what age did you start your periods?

Table 7-3

Correlation of Ovarian and Endometrial Cycles (Ideal 28-Day Cycle)

	MENSTRUAL (1-3 TO 5 DAYS)	EARLY FOLLICULAR (4 TO 6-8 DAYS)	ADVANCED FOLLICULAR (9 TO 12-16 DAYS)	OVULATION (12-16 DAYS)	EARLY LUTEAL (15-19 DAYS)	ADVANCED LUTEAL (20-25 DAYS)	PREMENSTRUAL (26-32 DAYS)
Ovary	Involution of corpus luteum	Growth and maturation of graafian follicle		Ovulation	Active corpus luteum		Involution of corpus luteum
Estrogen	Diminution	Progressive increase		High concentration	Secondary rise		Decreasing
Progesterone	Absent	Absent	Absent	Appearing	Rising	Rising	Decreasing
Endometrium	Menstrual desquamation and involution	Reorganization and proliferation	Further growth and watery secretion		Active secretion and glandular dilation	Accumulation of secretion and edema	Regressive
Pituitary secretion							
Follicle-stimulating hormone (FSH)	Fairly constant until just before ovulation			Moderate increase just before	Rapid decrease in previous levels		
Luteinizing hormone (LH)	Fairly constant until just before ovulation			Marked increase just before	Rapid decrease in previous levels		

From Thompson JM et al: *Mosby's clinical nursing*, ed 4, St. Louis, 1997, Mosby.

- When was your last normal menstrual period?
- What is the nature of your periods? (frequency, duration, amount of flow)

Onset of menstruation. The age range for menarche in the United States is 11 to 15 years. If the woman has had established menses at intervals of every 21-38 days, then the classification of secondary amenorrhea would apply. Established menses indicate that there is not an outlet flow problem and that the hypothalamic-pituitary-ovarian (HPO) axis and endometrium are functioning.

Pubertal development. Female pubertal development begins with a growth spurt 1 year before the development of breast buds (thelarche) at the age of 11. Then there is continued growth for 1.1 years until the peak height velocity is achieved. Pubic hair appears (pubarche), followed by axillary hair and the beginning of menarche. The average age of menarche for American girls is 12 years and 4 months (age range is 9 to 17). The length of time from thelarche to menarche is 2 to 3 years.

A thorough review of pediatric growth charts is helpful in determining the young girl's norm of growth and development and the centimeters attained by her latest growth spurt. Most adolescent girls have a mean height gain of 29 cm (64.8 inches) and the growth spurt lasts approximately 4 years. Asking adolescents to self-identify their Tanner Sexual Maturity Ratings (SMR) scales for breast and pubic maturity provides very accurate staging (Figures 7-5 and 7-6). Additionally, it gives the opportunity for insight into their feelings about their body and self-esteem.

Age of menarche. The lack of menstrual periods and secondary sex characteristics by age 14 or the lack of menses by age 16 in the presence of secondary sex characteristics is considered primary amenorrhea. Fifty-six percent of all adolescents start menses when pubic hair (PH) devel-

opment is at PH stage 4 and 19% at PH stage 3 (see Figures 7-5 and 7-6). If the adolescent is PH stage 4 but has not had a menses, then primary amenorrhea should be diagnosed. However, if the adolescent does not meet the age and maturation criteria, then suspect she is experiencing delayed puberty or is a so-called "late bloomer." She is likely to have a family history in her mother and sisters of delayed menarche. Almost 80% of amenorrheic adolescents with intact female genitalia and developed breasts have an inappropriate LH feedback, anovulatory cycles, or high levels of androgenic hormones. They will bleed after a progesterone challenge test and should be monitored for continued menses to avoid endometrial hyperplasia.

Menstrual history. Absence of a menstrual period for the past 6 months or a cycle interval exceeding 35 days (a time frame that is equal to 3 missed cycles) is considered secondary amenorrhea. Sudden cessation of menstruation is more likely to indicate pregnancy or stress as a cause, whereas a gradual cessation suggests PCOS or premature ovarian failure.

Are there any constitutional delays causing the amenorrhea?

Key Questions
- Has there been a change in weight, percentage of body fat, or athletic training intensity?
- Are you under unusual stress at school, home, or work?
- Do you or your family have any congenital disorders or chronic diseases?

Change in weight, percentage body fat, athletic training intensity. Underweight persons typically have a low body fat to lean muscle ratio. Body fat can be assessed by measuring the body mass index (BMI). The severe stress of anorexia nervosa can produce prolonged amenorrhea. Exercise from various sports—jogging,

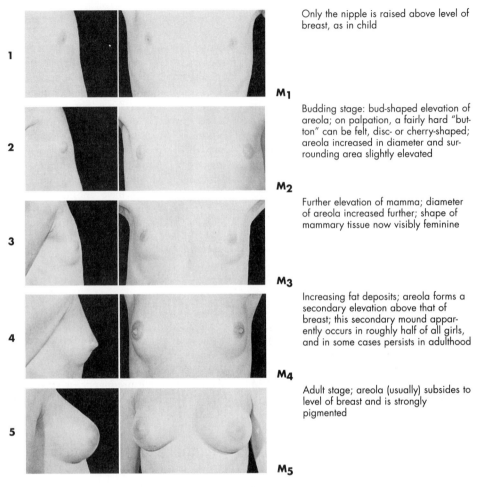

1

M₁

Only the nipple is raised above level of breast, as in child

2

M₂

Budding stage: bud-shaped elevation of areola; on palpation, a fairly hard "button" can be felt, disc- or cherry-shaped; areola increased in diameter and surrounding area slightly elevated

3

M₃

Further elevation of mamma; diameter of areola increased further; shape of mammary tissue now visibly feminine

4

M₄

Increasing fat deposits; areola forms a secondary elevation above that of breast; this secondary mound apparently occurs in roughly half of all girls, and in some cases persists in adulthood

5

M₅

Adult stage; areola (usually) subsides to level of breast and is strongly pigmented

Figure 7-5 Five stages of breast development in females. (Photographs from Van Wieringen JC: *Growth diagrams 1965 Netherlands Second National Survey on 0 to 24-year-olds,* Groningen, Netherlands, 1971, Wolters-Noordhoff; reprinted by permission of Kluwer Academic Publishers.)

middle and long distance running, ballet dancing, gymnastics, and track and field events—can lower body fat sufficiently to cause menstrual aberrations. Long distance runners and ballerinas are more apt to be amenorrheic than are swimmers; however, even moderate exercise can cause one or two missed periods a year. The mechanism of action on the HPO axis is unknown but is expressed by delayed puberty, shortened luteal phase, anovulation, and amenorrhea. Obesity may be the cause of amenorrhea or be a sign of PCOS.

PCOS will cause ovarian dysfunction—elevated androgens, hirsutism, low sex steroid-binding globulin (SSBG), and an elevated LH:FSH ratio.

Emotional state. The stress of athletic competition, family situations, school performance, peer relations, and work can disrupt normal cyclic menses. The HPO axis of a teenager is more sensitive to physical and psychological stress than that of an adult female.

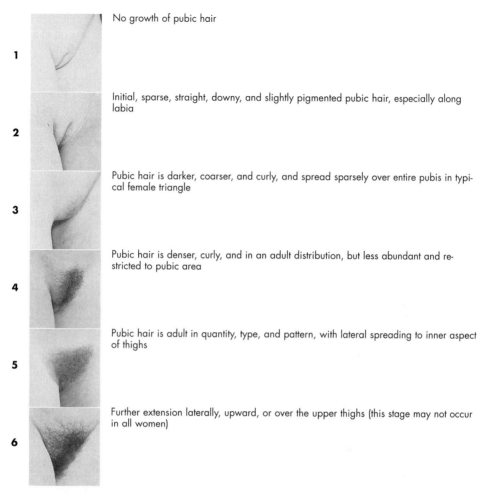

1   No growth of pubic hair

2   Initial, sparse, straight, downy, and slightly pigmented pubic hair, especially along labia

3   Pubic hair is darker, coarser, and curly, and spread sparsely over entire pubis in typical female triangle

4   Pubic hair is denser, curly, and in an adult distribution, but less abundant and restricted to pubic area

5   Pubic hair is adult in quantity, type, and pattern, with lateral spreading to inner aspect of thighs

6   Further extension laterally, upward, or over the upper thighs (this stage may not occur in all women)

Figure 7-6   Tanner sexual maturity development in females. (Photographs from Van Wieringen JC: *Growth diagrams 1965 Netherlands Second National Survey on 0 to 24-year-olds,* Groningen, Netherlands, 1971, Wolters-Noordhoff; reprinted by permission of Kluwer Academic Publishers.)

Congenital or chronic diseases. Turner's syndrome stigmata (see physical examination) or similar physical findings suggest the probability of an abnormality of one or all components (CNS, structural, or HPO axis) necessary for menstruation. Most structural anomalies that would prevent outflow of the menstrual blood are detectable on physical examination. Chronic diseases like anorexia nervosa, diabetes mellitus, Crohn's disease, systemic lupus erythematosus, glomerulonephritis, cystic fibrosis, pituitary adenoma, adrenal diseases, or thyroid dysfunction can cause amenorrhea.

Could this be thyroid dysfunction?

Key Questions
- Have you noticed changes in the texture of your hair or skin?
- Are you bothered by hot or cold temperatures?

- Have you had any changes in your energy level?
- Have you had any changes in your bowel function?

Hair and skin changes and temperature intolerance. Hypothyroidism and hyperthyroidism is expressed by changes in hair and skin texture. Hyperthyroidism often makes women intolerant of the heat, and this is sometimes confused with menopausal syndrome symptoms. Cold intolerance is frequently exhibited by persons with low-functioning thyroids.

Energy and bowel changes. Increased functioning of the thyroid causes restlessness and diarrhea, while decreased functioning results in constipation and fatigue. Even mild thyroid dysfunction can cause menstrual irregularities; therefore, a thyroid function test (i.e., TSH) is needed to assess the thyroid status.

Could this be caused by hyperprolactinemia?

Key Questions
- Are you able to express a discharge or liquid from your nipples?
- Is there increased stimulation to your nipples?
- Has there been any surgery or disease of the breasts or chest wall?

Galactorrhea. Women may notice breast nipple discharge that is not associated with breast feeding or medications. Offensive medications are listed in Box 7-3 and include primarily the dopamine antagonist agents and estrogens.

Nipple stimulation and chest wall stimulation. Nipple stimulation from clothing irritation during jogging or nipple manipulation during sexual activity may cause galactorrhea. Surgical interventions like lymph node dissection or disease processes like herpes zoster may also lead to galactorrhea, triggered by peripheral neural stimulation.

> **Box 7-3**
>
> # Drugs That May Cause Amenorrhea
>
> **Prolactin Increase**
> Antipsychotics: Phenothiazines, haloperidol, pimozide, clozapine
> Antidepressants: Tricyclic antidepressants, monoamine oxidase inhibitors
> Antihypertensives: Calcium channel blockers, methyldopa, reserpine
>
> **Estrogenic Effect**
> Digitalis, marijuana, flavonoids, oral contraceptives
>
> **Ovarian Toxicity**
> Busulfan, chlorambucil, cisplatin, cyclophosphamide, fluorouracil

Modified from Kiningham RB et al: Evaluation of amenorrhea, *Am Fam Phys* 53(4):1186, 1996.

Could the hyperprolactinemia be caused by medications?

Key Questions
- What prescription medicines are you taking?
- Have you used any street drugs? What kind?

Medication history. Medications such as phenothiazines or contraceptives may cause amenorrhea. These drugs either increase prolactin levels, estrogenic effect, or are toxic to the ovaries (see Box 7-3). Illicit drugs such as heroin and methadone also lead to menstrual abnormalities.

Is a pituitary tumor causing the amenorrhea?

Key Questions
- Have you experienced any visual changes?
- Are you having an increased number of headaches?

Visual changes and headaches. A pituitary tumor may be responsible for the hyperprolactin state. Enlarging pituitary tumors cause headache. As the tumor grows out of the sella, it compresses the optic chiasm and nerves. The common visual defect is bitemporal hemianopia, although other defects may occur. Changes in visual fields are often self-diagnosed when the patient recognizes vision problems while reading or driving a car. Clinical changes in vision warrant a referral to an ophthalmologist and work-up for a tumor of the sella turcica by CT or MRI. A high prolactin level will indicate a pituitary adenoma that presents with or without galactorrhea.

Is this a problem of the HPO axis?

Key Questions

- Have you experienced any problems with infertility?
- Do you have excess hair on your face or chest?
- Are you having any menopausal symptoms (e.g., hot flashes, vaginal dryness)?

Infertility. Many cases of infertility are caused by failure of ovulation. PCOS affects women between the ages of 15 to 30 years. Basal body temperature charts and endometrial biopsies can reveal anovulatory cycles. Vaginal ultrasound will show enlarged ovaries with multiple small, fluid-filled cysts. Infertility can be caused by low or high estrogen levels. Measurement of gonadotropins, vaginal maturation index, and progesterone levels will all give insight into the functioning of the HPO axis.

Androgen excess. About 50% of women diagnosed with PCOS are hirsute, obese, and have difficulty conceiving. Seldom are other signs of masculinization noted. LH is elevated with PCOS. Truncal obesity, acne, and male pattern baldness can signify androgen excess.

Estrogen deficiency. Hot flashes or flushes, changes in mood, and difficulty sleeping are common menopausal symptoms that women with low estradiol may experience. A dry vagina is often accompanied by dyspareunia and sometimes dysuria. The dysuria may be secondary to the hypoestrogenic state of the urethra and not be the result of a urinary tract infection. Prolonged hypoestrogenic status leads to osteopenia, regardless of age.

Is this a problem of the uterus or reproduction?

Key Questions

- When was your last pregnancy?
- Have you had a miscarriage, dilation and curettage, or uterine infection?

Recent pregnancy. Amenorrhea can occur subsequent to a pregnancy if, at the time of delivery, there had been severe hemorrhage. Obstetric hemorrhage causes pituitary ischemia and infarction and results in pituitary insufficiency. This pathological process is known as Sheehan's syndrome. In this instance, refer the patient to an endocrinologist.

Gynecological problem. Endometritis, incomplete abortion, or aggressive curettage of the uterus can lead to denuding of the endometrial layer, scarring, and Asherman's syndrome. The patient with Asherman's syndrome will not bleed after the progesterone challenge test, nor will she bleed after priming the uterus with estrogen and challenging with medroxyprogesterone acetate. The diagnosis can be made by performing weekly serum progesterone tests to determine if any value is within the ovulatory range (greater than 3 ng/mL) yet there are no periods. The diagnosis can also be made by the gynecologist via hysteroscopy, hysterosalpingography, or measuring endometrial thickness by ultrasonography.

What symptoms support a structural outflow problem?

Key Questions
- Do you have cyclic abdominal bloating or cramping?
- Have you been amenorrheic since you had a cervical procedure?

Presence of premenstrual symptoms or dysmenorrhea. Cyclic symptomatology of dysmenorrhea in the absence of menses may be caused by an incomplete outflow tract. Physical examination will validate a vaginal opening, imperforate hymen, intact uterus, or congenital imperforate cervical os. If there is no indication of a uterus by examination or lower abdominal ultrasound, a karyotype is needed to determine the congenital disorder. A referral to an endocrinologist or gynecological surgeon may be indicated for removal of any abdominal male gonads, which would be a risk for cancerous degeneration.

Cervical os stenosis. Stenosis of the cervical os can occur after gynecological office surgeries like cervical biopsies and cryotherapy. However, it is more common after cone biopsies of the cervix— such as the loop electrosurgical excision procedure (LEEP) or carbon dioxide laser treatment.

DIAGNOSTIC REASONING: FOCUSED PHYSICAL EXAMINATION

Note General Appearance

The body morphology of the patient can provide clues to the etiology of amenorrhea; often diseases can be diagnosed secondary to short stature, underweight, or overweight. A height less than 5 foot (short stature) in a girl who is 14 plus years may indicate a congenital chromosomal problem. Assess the woman's general state of health to determine if there are signs of systemic, chronic, or congenital disease.

Assess Nutritional Status and Plot Measurements on Growth Chart in Adolescents

Assess nutritional status, looking for signs of under-nutrition or over-nutrition. Measure the height, weight, and arm span of the adolescent. Plot on a growth chart if delayed puberty is a consideration. Anorexia nervosa is often found while evaluating an adolescent who has both short stature and underweight.

Assess Sexual Maturity

Use the Tanner Sexual Maturity Rating (SMR) Scales to assess and rate the stage of breast and pubic hair development. An SMR may be calculated by averaging the girl's stage of public hair and breast development. The stage of breast and public hair development in the adolescent girl is related to her chronological age, age at menarche, and evidence of height spurt. The breasts often develop at different rates, so some asymmetry is common. Menarche generally occurs at SMR 4 or breast stage 3 to 4. Plot there physiological events on the growth curve.

Screen for Eating Disorders

If you suspect anorexia nervosa or bulimia, administer a screening instrument to help determine the diagnosis. Refer to the DSM-IV for diagnostic criteria. About half of the females with eating disorders will have short stature.

Calculate the Body Mass Index (BMI)

Seventeen percent body fat is needed for most females to be menarchal and about 22% body fat is necessary for ovulation. Calculate the Body Mass Index (BMI) (Box 7-4). A BMI of 19 kg/M^2 compares to a 17% body fat, which may cause amenorrhea. A weight loss of 10% to 15% of the woman's body weight corresponds to a loss of approximately a third of her body

---

Box 7-4

Body Mass Index (BMI)

BMI is helpful in assessing the nutritional status and total body fat of the patient.
You can calculate the BMI by using the following formula:
Multiply the patient's weight in pounds by 704. Take that number (product) and
divide by the height in inches. Once again, divide by the height in inches.

_____ pounds × 704 = _____

Divide by the height in inches _____

Again, divide by the height in inches _____ = patient's BMI

Example: WT: 75 pounds; HT: 4 foot 2 inches or 50 inches

75 × 704 = 52800; divided by 50 = 1056; divided by 50 = 21.12 or 21 BMI

---

fat and consequently a BMI of less than 22% and anovulatory cycles.

Obesity causes amenorrhea secondary to ovarian dysfunction. A BMI of greater than 27% corresponds to being more than 20% overweight. Adipose cell stroma convert androstenedione to estrogen (estrone) as the body fat increases. Obesity also increases sex hormone binding globulin, thereby increasing free steroid levels. Both processes may cause an imbalance in the HPO axis and lead to amenorrhea.

Examine the Skin and Hair

Observe for signs of thyroid dysfunction or adrenal excess. Features of hypothyroidism include dry, coarse, flaky skin; coarse hair that tends to break; and thick, brittle nails. Hyperthyroidism is characterized by fine, warm skin that is hyperpigmented at pressure points. The nails of these women will often separate from the nail plate (onycholysis), and their hair will be fine, thin, and limp. Cushingoid features include truncal obesity, striae, and moon face. Observe for other signs of androgen excess, which include hirsutism, acne, and male pattern baldness.

Perform a Head and Neck Examination

During the head and neck examination, note any visual changes, including visual field defects that might indicate a pituitary tumor. Anosmia might denote a congenital absence of LHRH, producing no secretion of LH or FSH from the pituitary. **Without LH or FSH production, there is no ovulation; anovulatory cycles are amenorrheic.** Also look for Turner's syndrome stigmata—webbed neck and low-set ears (other signs are shield-like chest and short fourth metacarpal).

Palpate the Thyroid Gland and Lymph Nodes

Palpate the thyroid gland for diffuse enlargement, asymmetry, and nodules. Auscultate for thyroid bruits and count the pulse rate. Assess for supra- and infra-clavicular lymphadenopathy or carcinogenic masses of the sternal notch and abdomen, which might arise from a tumor of germ cell, adrenal, or pituitary origin.

Perform Clinical Breast Examination

Physical examination verifies sexual maturation level. The growth spurt occurs before breast development (thelarche), which is followed by the appearance of axillary hair. Perform a breast examination and assess breast maturity level using Tanner staging. More than 95% of adolescents are menarchal 1 year after they reach a breast maturity rating of 4. Check for galactorrhea (see Chapter

8, Breast Lumps and Nipple Discharge, p. 311).

Perform a Pelvic Examination

Observe for maturation of the female genitalia and secondary sex characteristics. Assign a Tanner stage for pubic hair development (sexual maturity P1-P6). A congenital problem might manifest as vaginal or uterine agenesis and is identified by the absence of a vagina, cervix, or uterus. There may be a small invagination of the perineum below the urinary meatus. It can be explored using a cotton-tipped applicator and otoscope with a large ear speculum or nasal speculum to determine the dimensions of the vault and presence of a cervix. A clitoris larger than 1 cm is suggestive of androgen excess.

Assess for other outlet problems, including an imperforate hymen (painful, bluish bulging of the perineum), stenotic cervix (bulging os or inability to pass a cotton-tipped applicator through the os), or a transverse vaginal septum. The development of hematocolpos or hematometra or hematoperitoneum from menses behind an obstructed outflow tract needs immediate intervention to prevent inflammatory changes and endometriosis. Needle aspiration is NOT recommended because it might potentiate infection. Refer to a reconstructive gynecological surgeon for MRI and often extensive surgery.

If the introitus is small, use a pediatric Pedersen, Huffman-Graves, or Graves speculum (which measures approximately ½ inch wide and 3¾ inches long) or a Huffman vaginoscope. Vaginal walls that are pale, dry, have few rugations, and may be friable are estrogen deficient. Low estrogen will cause scant cervical mucus. Vaginal cytology for women exhibiting such symptoms will report a maturation index (MI) lacking or low in estrogen.

The bimanual examination can be performed with only an index finger in the vagina if the vaginal vestibule is small. Or if the hymen is rigid, a rectal bimanual examination may be completed instead of the usual vaginal bimanual examination. On pelvic bimanual examination, enlarged ovaries will be palpated about half the time in patients with PCOS. Assess for position, size, shape, and consistency of the cervix, uterus, and ovaries.

DIAGNOSTIC STUDIES

Pregnancy Test: Radioimmunoassay for Beta Subunit of hCG

The pregnancy test is used to identify or rule out pregnancy and is an essential test on all females presenting with amenorrhea.

Thyroid-Stimulating Hormone (TSH)

A serum TSH identifies hypothyroidism. When hormonal supplementation is provided, menses usually will resume for these patients. If the amenorrhea is associated with galactorrhea and hyperprolactinemia, the prolactin level will need to be measured again after the thyroid function levels have become normal.

Prolactin Levels

The prolactin level is most reliable when it is a fasting measurement. When the patient's fasting prolactin level is normal (less than 50 ng/mL), a progesterone challenge test is indicated. If the patient's level is high (greater than 50 ng/mL) or if she has galactorrhea, a cone-down view of the sella turcica is taken to rule out a pituitary adenoma. An adenoma greater than 10 mm is unlikely if the cone view is normal and the prolactin is less than 100 ng/mL. A prolactin elevation less than 100 ng/mL but higher than normal is most frequently caused by prescribed or illicit drugs. The hyperprolactinemia usually subsides a few weeks after stopping the offending drug.

Microscopic examination of breast discharge will reveal fat globules and no red blood cells (see Chapter 8, Breast Lumps and Nipple Discharge, p. 321).

Serum Follicle-Stimulating Hormone (FSH) Levels

Ovarian failure, which causes a low estradiol secretion, will raise the FSH level higher than 40 mU/mL. If both the FSH and LH levels are greater than 50 mU/mL, then primary ovarian failure is established. If the patient is older than 30 years, menopause is diagnosed; if she is younger than 30 years, a karyotype should be done. A FSH measurement of less than 40 mU/mL denotes a hypothalamic-pituitary dysfunction and secondary ovarian failure.

Serum Luteinizing Hormone (LH) Levels

A serum LH level greater than 35 mU/mL is frequently seen in patients with PCOS. The LH/FSH ratio higher than 2:1 is suggestive of PCOS, while a ratio greater than 3:1 is considered diagnostic of PCOS.

CNS Imaging

If both FSH and LH levels are low, indicating a problem of the pituitary, imaging of the central nervous system is warranted. Either contrast computed tomography (CT) or magnetic resonance imaging (MRI) of the sella turcica will determine an abnormality. If the prolactin level is greater than 100 ng/mL or the cone-down view of the sella turcica is abnormal, a CT or MRI with contrast enhancement should be obtained.

Pelvic Ultrasound and Vaginal Ultrasound

Pelvic and vaginal ultrasound are used to determine the presence of a uterus, its anatomical size, endometrial thickness, and whether there are fibroids or other tumors. Ultrasound measures ovarian size, identifies cysts, and evaluates follicular development. In primary amenorrhea, ultrasound is helpful in assessing mullerian agenesis and gonadal dysgenesis because there may be internal organs and no conduit to the perineum. A third of these patients also have urinary tract abnormalities. So, an abdominal ultrasound can be obtained at the same time to evaluate that system.

Progesterone Challenge test (PCT) (Progesterone Withdrawal Test)

PCT consists of administration of oral medroxyprogesterone acetate 10 mg daily for 5 days or parental progesterone in oil 200 mg intramuscularly. The patient will respond to the medication within 2 to 7 days. If there is a positive PCT, the patient will bleed. This demonstrates that there is sufficient endogenous estrogens to prepare the endometrium and confirms that there is a functioning outflow tract. It substantiates an intact HPO axis.

Estrogen and Progesterone Challenge Test (E and PCT)

E and PCT consists of administration of conjugated estrogens 1.25 mg daily for 21 days and medroxyprogesterone acetate 10 mg for the last 5 days of the regimen (days 17 through 21). If there is no menstrual flow, administer the regimen a second time. If there is no flow after both courses of therapy, the cause is either the outflow tract or the uterine endometrium. The E and PCT is positive if there is menstrual flow within 2 to 7 days. A positive test denotes that there is inadequate estrogen production either from inadequate functional ovarian follicles or there is inadequate pituitary gonadotropic stimulation.

Chromosome Analysis (Karyotyping)

A buccal smear or vaginal smear of epithelial cells is stained with cresyl violet and examined microscopically. Karyotyping is done to delineate probable chromosomal abnormalities. It is used in the work-up for ambiguous genitalia, primary amenorrhea, oligomenorrhea, delayed puberty, or abnormal development at puberty.

Endometrial Biopsy

Endometrial biopsy may be used to reveal the hormonal response of the uterine endometrium.

Basal Body Temperature Charting (BBT)

A woman can take her awakening body temperature each day and chart it to determine if ovulation is occurring. This test is based on progesterone's effect on raising body temperature by 0.5° to 0.8° for 11 days during the luteal phase. If this rise occurs, ovulation has occurred, and a positive estrogen component is inferred. Digital read-out thermometers are quick and easy to use.

Maturation Index (MI)

A vaginal cytological smear (Papanicolaou smear) for evaluation of ovarian function can determine the hormonal status of the vagina:

- Lack of estrogen effect is demonstrated by *predominance of parabasal cells*
- Low estrogen effect is demonstrated by *predominance of intermediate cells*
- Increased estrogen effect is demonstrated by *predominance of intermediate cells*

Both increased and decreased estrogen effect can be reflective of a hormonal imbalance of the HPO axis.

Progesterone Levels

Serum progesterone levels collected at weekly intervals can establish whether ovulation has occurred. A value greater than 3 ng/mL is found with ovulation.

DIFFERENTIAL DIAGNOSIS

Pregnancy

Pregnancy is the most common reason for amenorrhea of the childbearing woman. Determining the pregnancy status of the patient is the first step in the amenorrhea work-up.

CONSTITUTIONAL

Delayed Puberty

A pituitary adenoma must be ruled out for all patients with delayed puberty. Yearly prolactin levels should be performed for those with delayed puberty because of the possibility of occult pituitary adenomas.

Anorexia Nervosa and Bulimia

Anorexia nervosa and bulimia are disorders that are psychiatric in origin. Affected women have such a fear of being fat that they do not eat or they purge after eating. Often these women are over-achievers and have low self-esteem. The majority are adolescents with a mean age of 13 to 14. Amenorrhea is caused by extreme weight loss and/or cachectic state.

Exercise-Induced Amenorrhea

This amenorrhea is common in competitive athletes, but exercise can also cause skipped menses in the casual trainer. Gymnasts, ballerinas, and long distance runners are at high risk, especially if they started their training at a very early age. Body fat of 17% is needed for menarche, whereas 22% body fat is necessary for ovulation. BMI estimates the woman's body fat level.

CONGENITAL OR CHRONIC DISORDERS

Turner's Syndrome

Turner's syndrome causes primary amenorrhea because of ovarian agenesis. The stigmata is short stature, webbed neck, shield-like chest, and delayed secondary sex characteristics.

Cushing's Syndrome

Cushing's syndrome is caused by an excess secretion of ACTH from a pituitary or adrenal adenoma. Classically patients present with a moon face, acne, hirsutism, kyphosis, purplish striae of the abdomen, and hypertension. CT may reveal pituitary or adrenal adenoma.

Thyroid Dysfunction

Amenorrhea from thyroid dysfunction will subside as soon as serum thyroid levels return to normal. Hypothyroidism frequently causes amenorrhea and is characterized by fatigue, constipation, cold intolerance, and dry skin.

Polycystic Ovary Syndrome (PCOS)

PCOS typically causes infertility in women ages 15 to 30 years. Half of these women will exhibit hirsutism and obesity. The ovaries are often large and contain multiple fluid-filled cysts. The diagnosis is established by ultrasonography.

UTERINE AND OUTFLOW TRACT PROBLEMS

Imperforate Hymen

The woman with an imperforate hymen may present with a painful, bulging perineum. There is lack of an intact outflow tract, which causes the primary amenorrhea.

Stenotic Cervical Os

Stenotic cervical os can be either the cause for either primary or secondary amenorrhea. It is often caused by therapeutic procedures of the cervix such as cryotherapy or cone biopsies. These procedures cause scarring and stenosis of the os, obstructing the outflow tract.

Asherman's Syndrome

Asherman's syndrome occurs when the uterine endometrial lining is denuded or scarred, usually by infection or curettage. The patient will not respond to either a progesterone challenge or an estrogen and progesterone challenge test.

HYPOTHALAMIC-PITUITARY-OVARIAN AXIS PROBLEM

Menopause

The average age of menopause in the United States is 51 years. The cause is primary ovarian failure. It is a state of hypoestrogenemia. The gonadotropins rise (FSH—above 40 mU/mL), and the estradiol levels fall (less than 15 pg/mL). Clinical symptoms are hot flashes, night sweats, insomnia, mood changes, and amenorrhea for 12 months.

Sheehan's Syndrome

Sheehan's syndrome is brought on by severe obstetrical hemorrhage, which causes pituitary ischemia and infarction. The pituitary gland becomes dysfunctional.

Medications

Prescription and illicit drugs may increase prolactin levels, which in turn promote galactorrhea. Offending drugs are primarily the dopamine antagonist agents and estrogens as well as marijuana.

Chest Wall or Nipple Stimulation

Prolactin inhibits the pulsatile secretion of GnRH, unbalancing the HPO axis and possibly causing amenorrhea. The higher the prolactin level, the greater the chance that the patient will be amenorrheic.

Pituitary Adenoma

Pituitary macro- and microadenomas should be suspected if the prolactin level is greater than 100 ng/mL or if there are any abnormalities of the cone-down view of the sella turcica. Patients with pituitary adenomas should be referred to an endocrinologist. Those patients with prolactin levels exceeding 1000 ng/mL probably have an invasive tumor.

Table 7-4

Differential Diagnosis of Common Causes of Amenorrhea

Condition	History	Physical Findings	Diagnostic Studies
Pregnancy			
Pregnancy	Breast tenderness, morning sickness, urinary frequency	Globular, enlarged uterus; soft, bluish color cervix	Beta HCG pregnancy test positive; ultrasonography positive
Constitutional			
Delayed puberty	No menstruation at age beyond 16 years; more than 5 years between initiation of breast growth and menarche	Breast stage 1 persists beyond age 13.4; pubic hair stage 1 persists beyond age 14.1	Prolactin normal; TSH, T_4 normal; CBC, UA normal; chemistry profile normal; bone age normal; skull x-ray normal
Anorexia nervosa/ bulimia	Mean age 13-14; fear of being fat; low self-esteem; depression; isolation; over-achiever; food is a parental battleground; preoccupation; hair loss; abdominal bloating, pain, constipation	Amenorrhea before or after weight loss; cachexia; low body fat; short stature; yellow, dry, cold skin; acrocyanosis—increased lanugo hair; hypotension, systolic murmurs often with mitral valve prolapse	TSH normal; prolactin normal; FSH and LH usually low; glucose normal; ECG bradycardia, low-voltage changes, T-wave inversions, and occasional ST segment depression
Exercise-induced amenorrhea	Began athletic training at young age; more common with long-distance runners, ballerinas, gymnasts	BMI <17% body fat	TSH normal; prolactin normal

Table 7-4

Differential Diagnosis of Common Causes of Amenorrhea—cont'd

Condition	History	Physical Findings	Diagnostic Studies
Congenital or Chronic Disorders			
Turner's syndrome	Congenital; short stature; infantile sexual develop-ment	Characteristics: webbed neck, low-set ears, shield-like chest, short fourth metacarpal	Karyotype (45,X)
Cushing's syndrome	Weight gain; weak-ness; back pain	Moon face, acne, hirsutism, purple striae of abdomen	Cortisol increased; 17-ketosteroids increased; CT adenoma
Thyroid dysfunction	Hypothyroid: delayed growth, weight gain, fatigue, con-stipation, cold intolerance; hyper-thyroid : weight loss, nervousness, heat intolerance	Hypothyroid: dry skin, fine hair, galactorrhea; hy-perthyroid: moist skin, hyper-pigmentation over bones, thin hair, goiter	Hypothyroid: TSH high; hyperthyroid: TSH low; T_3 high; T_4 high
Polycystic ovary syndrome	Infertility	Hirsutism; obese; enlarged ovaries	Ultrasonography: enlarged ovaries with multiple fluid-filled cysts; testos-terone high
Uterine and Outflow Tract Problems			
Imperforate hymen/ stenotic cervical os	Monthly bloating, cramping and pelvic pressure; no menses; cryo-therapy or other procedure to cervix	Fibrotic hymen without patent opening; stenotic cervical os	Clinical diagnosis by history and findings
Asherman's syndrome	History of uterine infection; tubercu-losis, schistosomia-sis; uterine iatrogenic scarring: curettage, irradiation	Pelvic exam normal	PCT negative; E and PCT negative; hysteroscopy adhesions
Hypothalamic-Pituitary-Ovarian Axis Problem			
Menopause	Hot flashes, night sweats, insomnia, mood changes	Pale, dry vaginal mucosa, few rugae	FSH and LH high; estradiol low

Continued

Table 7-4

Differential Diagnosis of Common Causes of Amenorrhea—cont'd

Condition	History	Physical Findings	Diagnostic Studies
Hypothalamic-Pituitary-Ovarian Axis Problem—cont'd			
Sheehan's syndrome	Recent history of postpartum hemorrhage and shock during delivery	Hair loss, depigmentation of skin, mammary and genital atrophy	Pituitary and end-organ hormones low; hemoglobin low
Medications/ chest wall or nipple stimulation	Breast nipple discharge; history of dopamine antagonists, estrogens, or illicit drugs; stimulation to nipples: exercise or sexual; history of chest wall surgery or herpes zoster	Nipple discharge: bilateral; multi-duct; milky, clear, or yellowish discharge	Wet mount or hemoccult of nipple discharge: negative for RBCs; prolactin high; cone-down view of sella turcica; MRI or CT with contrast
Pituitary adenoma	Delayed puberty; history of visual changes, increasing headaches	Visual field defects; galactorrhea	Prolactin high; cone-down view of sella turcica positive; MRI or CT with contrast positive

Chapter 8

Common Problems of the Breasts

Breast Lumps and Nipple Discharge, 311

Breast Lumps and Nipple Discharge

Eighty to 90% of all breast lumps are found by the woman or her partner before diagnosis by clinical breast examination or mammography. The three most common breast lumps are fibroadenomas, fibrocystic breast change, and breast cancer. Fibroadenomas are benign solid tumors most frequently seen in young women less than 30 years old. Fibrocystic breast changes can include cysts, fibrosis, adenosis, duct ectasia, hyperplasia, and papilloma. Fibrocystic symptoms are seen with great frequency in women ages 30 to 50 years but less often in those who are menopausal.

Breast cancer is the most common cancer in women and the second leading cause of death. The risk of breast cancer in women rises steadily with age and accelerates rapidly after the age of 50. While benign conditions that affect the breast are more common, the presence of a lump raises legitimate fears. The goal of the assessment process is to reach a diagnosis that addresses the possibility of breast cancer because it is presently the leading cause of death in women 40 to 50 years old.

Another condition of the breast that may be of concern to women across the age range is nipple discharge. Nipple discharge is a complaint commonly elicited from post-menarchal female clients. It is often related to pregnancy, recent breast feeding, or the taking of estrogenic medications. In women who are not lactating, nipple discharge is most frequently caused by intraductal papilloma, fibrocystic changes with duct ectasia, or cancer. Fortunately, nipple discharge is more commonly caused by benign lesions than cancerous ones.

Lactation depends on the anterior pituitary hormone lactogen and the ovarian and placental hormones estrogen and progesterone. Physiological stimulation (sucking, pregnancy, mechanical stimulation) of the breasts may produce lactation as can breast trauma and inflammation (e.g., herpes zoster, mammoplasty), pituitary disorders (e.g., irradiation of pituitary), or tranquilizing drugs (e.g., phenothiazines, methyldopa).

DIAGNOSTIC REASONING: FOCUSED HISTORY FOR BREAST LUMPS

Is this lump likely to be malignant?

Key Questions

- How long has the lump been present?
- Is the lump changing (getting bigger, worse, or more painful)?
- Is the lump in one breast only or are there lumps in both breasts?
- When was your last menstrual period? Are you going through menopause or are you past menopause?
- Is there any discharge from the nipple?
- Have you recently been treated for a breast infection?

Duration and growth. The primary presenting complaint of a malignant lesion is that of a single, hard, painless lump in the breast that is unchanged by the cyclic hormonal milieu. A change from the patient's normal physical findings is the most persuasive criteria for considering a diagnosis of breast cancer.

Malignant lumps are more likely to be new lumps that show progressive increase in size. The lump grows until there is an alteration in the contour of the breast tissue. An unchanged lump of long duration (years) is almost always benign. Half of all newly appearing benign cysts resolve within 2 to 3 menstrual cycles.

Unilateral versus bilateral. Breast lumps found bilaterally in identical quadrants of the breast are more likely to be benign. A solitary unilateral lump, while usually a cyst, fibroadenoma, or lipoma (rare), raises more suspicion for malignancy.

Postmenopausal. Cyclic cysts of the breast are more rare after menopause and necessitate diagnostic investigation. A postmenopausal woman with unilateral mastodynia (breast pain) has a greater risk for a diagnosis of breast cancer. Perimeno-

pausal and postmenopausal women are also at greater statistical risk for breast cancer because of the higher incidence of breast cancer as they grow older. A breast lump in a postmenopausal woman warrants a high degree of suspicion for cancer.

Nipple discharge with a lump. The occurrence of nipple discharge with the presence of a lump is worrisome because it may represent a ductal cancer. One example is Paget's disease, which may present as a breast mass with a bloody nipple discharge. This condition demands further investigation, such as an occult blood test, Papanicolaou test, mammogram, ductogram, or biopsy.

Infection. Any residual masses in the breast following antibiotic therapy are suspicious for malignancy and must be biopsied.

Does the person have additional risk factors for breast cancer?

Key Questions

- Have you ever had breast cancer?
- Do you have a family history of breast cancer? (first-degree relative)
- Have you ever had ovarian, endometrial, colon, or thyroid cancer?
- Do you have a family history of ovarian, endometrial, colon, or prostate cancer?

Risk factors. The presence of risk factors in a woman who has a lump raises the index of suspicion for malignancy. It is important to remember that the absence of such risk factors is not cancer protective. About 70% to 80% of all breast cancer patients have no risk factors for malignancy prior to their diagnosis. Patients with a personal history of epithelial hyperplasia, ductal carcinoma in situ (DCIS), or lobular carcinoma in situ (LCIS) are usually evaluated every 6 months by a breast spe-

Box 8-1

Primary Risk Factors for Breast Cancer

Female Gender

Age
80% of all cases occur after age 50; no plateau effect with age

Personal History of Breast Cancer or Cancer in Situ
DCIS increases the risk for cancer by 11 times; LCIS increases the risk by 10 to 11 times

Previous History of Breast Biopsies for Benign Breast Disease
Biopsy-proven proliferative changes or atypical epithelial hyperplasia; fibrocystic histological findings that increase the risk of breast cancer are moderate or severe hyperplasia (1.5 to 2 times the risk), atypical hyperplasia (5 times the risk), and carcinoma in situ (8 to 10 times the risk)

Laboratory Evidence of Specific Genetic Mutation
Increases susceptibility to breast cancer; i.e., mutation in BRCA1 or BRCA2 gene

Personal History of Cancer
Ovarian, endometrial, colon, or thyroid cancers

Family History of Breast Cancer
In first-degree relatives (mother, sister, or daughter) or in two or more close relatives

---

cialist because of their increased risk for malignancy. See Box 8-1 for a summary of characteristics that might increase a woman's risk for breast cancer.

Is this condition more likely benign?

Key Questions
- How old are you today?
- Have you had any lumps before? Do you have a history of cystic breast changes or lumpy breasts?
- Does this lump feel like other lumps you've had?
- Do the lumps come and go or change with your periods?
- Have you ever had a mammogram or ultrasound? Why was it done? What were the results?
- Have you ever had a lump drained or biopsied? What was the diagnosis?

Age. Any woman older than 25 years who has a breast lump should be evaluated by clinical breast examination (CBE), mammography, and fine needle aspiration (FNA). Fibrocystic breast changes occur predominantly between the ages of 20 and 30. Fibroadenomas are more frequent in women aged 15 to 39. Intraductal papilloma and ductal ectasia occur in the age range of 35 to 55 years, while breast cancer is most prevalent in women from 40 to 71 years of age.

Timing, consistency, and duration. The most frequent breast complaint is that of a painful, mobile lump that increases in size and tenderness as the menstrual cycle approaches. The lump commonly has discrete borders that allow for measurement of the length, width, and depth of the lesion by the patient (e.g., size of a pea). The lump remains prominent on breast self-examination, is almost always painful to palpate, and frequently causes pain with changes in position of the arm on the affected side. Fibrocystic breast changes exist on a continuum that correspond with the menstrual cycle. There is tenderness and size variations throughout the month.

Previous mammograms or biopsies. History or documentation of cyclic changes in lumps or the presence of glandular breast tissue on a mammogram or ultrasound supports a clinical diagnosis of benign disease. More convincing evidence of benign disease occurs when there is a clear fluid aspirate from the cyst with no residual or recurring breast lump, with the caveat that both benign and malignant disease can occur simultaneously.

Could this lump be mastitis related to lactation?

Key Questions
- Have you recently had a baby?
- Are you currently breast feeding or breast suckling?
- Are your nipples sore and cracked?
- Is your breast painful or hot? Are there any areas of redness?
- Have you had a fever?

Recently had a baby or breast feeding. A breast mass in a lactating woman is usually associated with mastitis, an inflammation of breast tissue, and a blocked duct. It occurs most often in primiparous nursing mothers and is usually caused by coagulase-positive *Staphylococcus aureus*. It can also occur during periods of weaning when the flow of milk is disrupted. Engorgement or congestive mastitis begins on day 2 or 3 after delivery and affects both breasts. Inflammatory breast cancer in lactating women is rare but must be considered.

Sore or cracked nipples. Cracked nipples may be a site for introduction of infection.

Painful or hot breast. Mastitis is characterized by a breast that is painful, hot, and red. In lactating women, the most frequent symptom is a painful erythematous lobule in an outer quadrant of the breast. Although mastitis is most common in lactating women, it can also occur in non-lactating women, usually as the result of a generalized dermatitis occurring from insect bites, sunburn, or allergic reactions. However, the most common cause of an inflamed breast in non-lactating women is inflammatory breast cancer. In inflammatory breast cancer, the entire breast is swollen, heavy, and edematous.

Fever. Fever is a sign of infectious mastitis and occurs most often associated with lactation and breast feeding. High fever does not occur because of simple breast engorgement in the postpartum period. Also fever does not usually occur in inflammatory breast cancer and is rare in dermatitis reactions.

DIAGNOSTIC REASONING: FOCUSED HISTORY FOR NIPPLE DISCHARGE

A focused history can help sort out the causes of the most frequently presenting cases of nipple discharge. Questioning should address normal lactation, high circulating levels of prolactin, and malignancy.

Is this normal lactation?

Key Questions
- When was your last normal menstrual period? How frequent are your cycles?
- Is it possible that you are pregnant? What are you using for birth control?
- When was your last delivery or miscarriage? How long were you pregnant?
- Did you breast feed? How long? When did you stop?
- Is the nipple discharge clear or milky in color?
- How long have you had the nipple discharge?

Menstrual cycle. Frequently, fibrocystic breast changes are most marked just before menses and manifest as a spontaneous multiple duct discharge that can be either unilateral or bilateral.

Pregnancy and lactation. Pregnancy is the number one cause of breast tenderness (mastodynia) and clear or milky nipple discharge (galactorrhea). A bloody nipple discharge during pregnancy is usually the result of vascular engorgement and clears within weeks. Recent pregnancy and/or breast feeding (within 8 weeks) may account for a prolonged clear or milky discharge that is successfully suppressed by decreased breast stimulation or by administration of dopamine agonist therapy (bromocriptine or pergolide). If the patient has had prolonged lactation, there may be milk formation even though prolactin levels are normal.

Color of discharge. Normal lactation produces a discharge that is milky and nonpurulent. Mastitis associated with breast feeding may produce purulent discharge. A subareolar abscess may also produce a purulent discharge. Mastitis and abscesses that produce purulent nipple discharge MUST be distinguished from inflammatory breast cancer by evoking remission with antibiotic therapy or biopsy. Oral contraceptives may cause a clear, serous, or milky discharge from single or multiple ducts. Ductal ectasia and papillomatosis produce a greenish or brownish nipple discharge. A serous or serosanguineous discharge from a single duct is usually indicative of an intraductal papilloma, but on rare occasion it may be found to be an intraductal cancer. A bloody nipple discharge is suggestive of cancer.

Duration of discharge. Women who breast feed sometimes experience a milky discharge long after the termination of nursing. New-onset discharge in a woman who is not pregnant or lactating requires further investigation (see the following discussion).

Is the discharge related to high prolactin levels?

Key Questions
- What medications are you taking?
- Do you jog or run? If yes: Do you wear a sports bra? Do your nipples rub on your clothing?
- Are your breasts fondled, squeezed, or suckled during sexual activity?
- Do you have a thyroid condition?
- What medical conditions or health problems do you have?
- If newborn: has the discharge been present since birth?

Medicines. Patients taking multiple tranquilizing medications are often found to have nipple discharge. Discontinuation of the medication(s) will eliminate most clear or milky bilateral nipple discharge. However, the condition may not warrant a drug cessation trial. See Box 8-2 for medications that can produce nipple discharge.

Box 8-2

Drugs That May Produce Nipple Discharge

Estrogens or Drugs That Increase Estrogen
Digitalis
Marijuana
Heroin

Dopamine Receptor Blockers
Phenothiazines
Haloperidol
Metoclopramide
Isoniazid

Central Nervous System (CNS) Dopamine Depleters
Tricyclic antidepressants
Reserpine
Methyldopa
Cimetidine
Benzodiazepines

Behavioral activities. Nipple stimulation (sexual or during jogging) increases prolactin levels, as does the use of marijuana. Only about 13% of men with hyperprolactinemia will develop gynecomastia and galactorrhea. Women commonly experience both galactorrhea and amenorrhea.

Other causes of galactorrhea. Certain genetic disorders, medical conditions, and central nervous system lesions can be responsible for the production of galactorrhea:

- *Genetic disorders:* Chiari-Frommel syndrome, Argonz-Del Castillo (Forbes-Albright) syndrome
- *Medical conditions:* Chronic renal failure, sarcoidosis, Schuller-Christian's disease, Cushing's disease, hepatic cirrhosis, hypothyroidism
- *Central nervous system lesions:* pituitary adenoma, empty sella, hypothalamic tumor, head trauma

Newborn. The breasts of a newborn may be abnormally enlarged secondary to the effects of maternal estrogens. A discharge that is usually white may be present that is commonly referred to as "witch's milk."

Can the nipple discharge be a sign of malignancy?

Key Questions

- Is the nipple discharge colored or bloody?
- Must it be expressed from the nipple or is the discharge spontaneous?
- Does it come from one or both nipples?
- Does it come from one or multiple nipple ducts?
- Do you also have a breast lump?
- Are you postmenopausal?

Discharge characteristics. Ductal ectasia and papillomatosis produce a greenish or brownish nipple discharge. A serous or serosanguineous discharge from a single duct is usually indicative of an intraductal papilloma, but on rare occasions it may indicate an intraductal cancer. A bloody nipple discharge is suggestive of cancer.

Spontaneous versus expressed discharge. Spontaneous discharge is likely related to fibrocystic breast changes, lactation, or systemic causes (e.g., hyperprolactinemia).

Unilateral versus bilateral discharge. Unilateral discharge is usually associated with an intraductal papilloma or cancer. Bilateral breast findings are seldom cancerous.

Single duct versus multiple duct discharge. Single duct involvement is more suspicious for intraductal papilloma or cancer. Multiple duct discharges usually are caused by hyperprolactinemia or duct ectasia.

Associated mass. An associated mass may be benign or malignant. Further evaluation is mandatory. Ultrasonography is helpful in differentiating solid from cystic lesions and is often the first step in the evaluation of a cyst or a mass in the woman with firm, dense breast tissue.

Postmenopausal women. Postmenopausal women have a higher incidence of breast cancer. Other risky signs for a cancerous cause of nipple discharge are presence of a mass or lump, unilateral nipple discharge, abnormal cytology, and an abnormal mammogram.

Nipple discharge that is unilateral, single duct, bloody, and not associated with pregnancy or a medication use is highly suspicious for a cancerous etiology. Because of the malignant potential of bloody or purulent discharge, these two findings demand further investigation via biopsy.

DIAGNOSTIC REASONING: FOCUSED PHYSICAL EXAMINATION

Perform a multi-position physical examination of the breasts and nipples.

Inspect Breasts and Nipples

Inspect the breasts while the patient is sitting with arms at sides, arms pushing down on hips (to contract the pectoralis muscles), arms elevated above head, and while the patient is bending forward from the waist (gravity pulling on breast tissue). Look for changes in breast shape or contour, a lump, or dimpling. Contraction of underlying muscles in the different arm positions will accentuate skin findings caused by a fixed adherent lesion, characteristic of cancer. The skin over the lesion may then flatten, dimple inward, or the nipple might be directed differently than the nipple of the opposite breast. Normal nipples are everted and point in like directions. A nipple lump may be revealed by nipple retraction. Engorgement (congestive mastitis) involves both breasts, which are enlarged and tense. Infectious mastitis usually involves one lobe or a quadrant of one breast.

Look for breasts that are notably asymmetrical—if no lump is found during the clinical breast examination (versus the patient finding a lump on self-examination), the patient should be followed more carefully. Re-examination is warranted every week for a month, and, if no mass is found on clinical breast examination (CBE), then reevaluate every 3 months for a year.

Observe Skin of Breasts and Nipples

Observe skin color for erythema and unilateral prominent blood vessels, which may be a presentation of breast cancer. Prominent vessels plus a tender cord-like vein suggests thrombophlebitis of the superficial veins of the breast. Both conditions demand a CBE and a mammogram to look for a mass. Paget's disease begins as a scaling eczematoid area on the nipple and progresses to a deep lump behind the nipple well. Paget's disease can produce darkly pigmented lesions that are suspicious for malignant melanoma. An excisional or punch biopsy is recommended to distinguish Paget's disease from malignant melanoma or other ulcerative lesions like Bowen's disease, eczema, or papillomatosis. Observe condition of the skin of the nipples for cracks or dried exudate or the presence of nipple flattening or retraction.

Palpate Breasts and Nipples With Patient Sitting

Perform a complete and systematic examination of the breasts, using a grid or concentric circle pattern of palpation. For large pendulous breasts, sandwich the breast between the hands, sweeping the breast tissue, and use circular, gliding motions of the superior finger pads to capture a lump, nodule, or thickening. If the woman has augmentation of breast tissue, small masses, including those from ruptured implants, may best be felt with the patient in the sitting position. Gently compress each nipple to observe for discharge. Mastitis causes the breast tissue to become swollen, tense, and warm.

Look for "Dimpling Sign"

Compression of the breast will accentuate dimpling of the skin if there is a malignancy or inflammation. Compress the breast by pushing inferiorly with one hand toward the suspected area of the lump and pushing superiorly with the other hand. The area will better reveal dimpling of the skin if the tissue is pushed inward from either side.

Transilluminate Breast Masses

Transillumination of a breast mass (best performed in a darkened room) may sometimes provide diagnostic clues. A fluid-

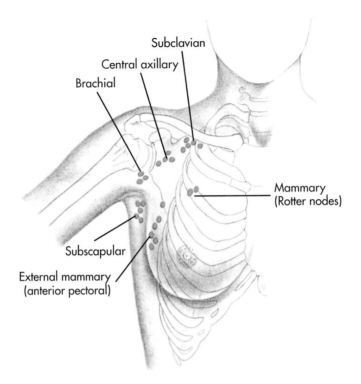

Figure 8-1   Six groups of lymph nodes may be distinguished in the axillary fossa. (From Seidel HM et al: *Mosby's guide to physical examination,* ed 3, St. Louis, 1995, Mosby.)

filled cyst will transilluminate whereas a solid mass will not. A solid lump is more frequently a malignant mass, whereas a cystic, fluid-filled lump is more commonly benign.

Examine Nipple Well

Place 1 or 2 finger pads over the nipple and apply pressure to invaginate the nipple and palpate for lumps in the cup-like nipple well. A normal nipple well is a smooth concave structure. Most lumps in this area will be found at the areola border.

Examine Nipple for Discharge

Place the thumb and first finger 1 to 2 cm outside the border of the areolar complex and gently compress, sliding the fingers toward the nipple in a milking fashion. Repeat this maneuver twice, cephalocaudally and laterally. Palpation of a single site on the areola border may reproduce the discharge and reveal the responsible duct. Specimen collection is often easier and of a larger quantity when the patient is sitting.

Look for blood in the nipple discharge; a positive finding has a high correlation with malignancy. Inflammatory symptoms and a purulent nipple discharge are suggestive of a breast abscess.

Palpate Lymph Nodes

Palpate the supraclavicular, infraclavicular, and axillary lymph nodes (Figures 8-1 and 8-2). The supraclavicular lymph nodes can be palpated easily by having the patient shrug her shoulders; then feel deep in the supraclavicular hollow. Feel for lymph nodes, noting their size, shape, consistency, and mobility. The presence of a small (less than 1 cm), single, rubbery, and

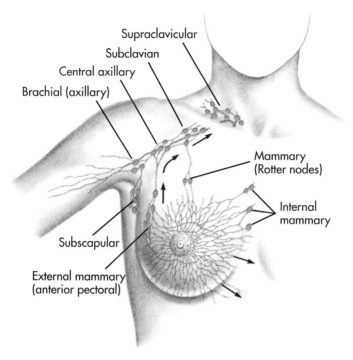

Figure 8-2   Lymphatic drainage of the breast. (From Seidel HM et al: *Mosby's guide to physical examination,* ed 4, St. Louis, 1998, Mosby.)

mobile lymph node can be a sign of in-flammation: rarely is it a sign of early malignancy. On the other hand, finding one or more lymph nodes in the same region that are greater than 1 cm, firm, fixed to the chest wall, or that have a matted consistency is highly suggestive of metastatic disease.

Palpate Breasts and Nipples With Patient Supine

With the patient supine, ask her to position one arm above her head. Place a small towel behind the scapula to aid in flattening the breast tissue. With your finger pads, palpate the breast tissue. Compress the breast against the chest wall. Examine the axillary tail (tail of Spence) of the breast, as well as accessory breast tissue (supernumerary nipples or breast tissue). Repeat with the other breast.

Characterize Lumps

Accurately measure any lumps by marking the edges with a pen and measuring the width and length with a centimeter ruler. Estimate the depth of the lesion, contour, shape, fluctuation, firmness, and mobility.

Fluctuation can be determined by holding the edges of the mass against the chest wall and pressing the center with finger pads. Fluctuation ("bouncy" consistency) occurs with cysts, lipomas, and abscesses. Cysts are frequently tender, especially premenstrually. Re-examination in a week or two will usually demonstrate cyclic hormonal changes of the tissue, and lump size and tenderness will have changed. In the postmenopausal woman, hormone replacement therapy may stimulate similar symptoms of breast lumps and pain (mastodynia). A single, firm, asymmetrical, immobile mass in a postmenopausal woman will, when biopsied, prove to be cancerous 75% of the time.

LABORATORY AND DIAGNOSTIC STUDIES

The diagnostic accuracy of ultrasound, mammography, and aspiration biopsy ranges from about 70% to 80% and varies with the training and skills of the clinician or technician. Therefore a high degree of suspicion for cancer and excellent patient follow-up should be sustained for a breast lump or nipple discharge.

Ultrasound

Ultrasound is helpful in differentiating solid from cystic lesions. Ultrasound is often the first step in the evaluation of a cyst or a mass in the adolescent or young woman with firm, dense breast tissue. It can also confirm that densities found on a mammogram are indeed cystic. The ultrasound finding of a cystic lesion should then be followed by aspiration of the cyst, eliminating it to make sure it is not concealing another abnormal breast finding. The ultrasound identification of a solid mass should be followed by needle localization, open biopsy, or stereotactic biopsy.

Mammography

Mammography is the radiographic examination of breast tissue for identification of nonpalpable breast lesions. Serial mammography is helpful in identifying breast architectural changes that may suggest malignancy. Mammography should never be used as the "gold standard" tool in the evaluation of a mass; there are too many false-negative studies. All clinically identifiable discrete masses should be diagnosed by cytological evidence. A mammogram is necessary for the woman who will have an open biopsy. It will define the size and location of the lump and note if there is bilateral involvement. However, if a woman is less than 35 years old and does not re-

quire a biopsy, a mammogram is of little diagnostic value because of the density of the breast tissue.

Fine Needle Aspiration (FNA)

FNA is a safe, routinely performed office procedure used to evaluate a breast lump. It is a procedure that is both diagnostic and therapeutic. It immediately determines if the lump is a cyst or a solid tumor. FNA facilitates breast examination by removing cysts that may be hiding a cancerous tumor. If the FNA aspirate is nonbloody, and the mass completely goes away and is not present on follow-up examinations, no further treatment is necessary. Bloody FNA aspirate should be cytologically evaluated, and the mass removed by excisional biopsy.

Fine Needle Aspiration (FNA) Cytological Examination

FNA cytological examination, when positive for malignancy, can eliminate excisional biopsy before the therapeutic regimen (e.g., lumpectomy and radiation). However, if the cytology is negative, continued investigation by open biopsy is mandated as the sensitivity of the test is not absolute.

Excisional Biopsy or Open Biopsy

Excisional biopsy is indicated if there is a breast mass whose FNA is bloody or is unproductive. The surgical specimen is evaluated histologically.

Stereotactic or Needle Localization Biopsy

Stereotactic biopsy is performed to assist in the complete excision of the tumor. A wire is placed at the site of the lesion, it is verified by mammography, and the surgeon uses this three-dimensional mammographic placement to identify the surgical tissue to be removed.

Ultrasonography

Ultrasound is useful in determining if mammogram-identified lesions are cystic or solid. It is not helpful in determining the cause of a palpable mass; FNA is the diagnostic study of choice.

Microscopy

Microscopy of nipple discharge can reveal "fat cells" of galactorrhea, leukocytes of infection, or red blood cells. The presence of red blood cells is a "red flag" to rule out malignancy. Care must be taken to prevent the slide from drying out. Place a cover slip on the slide immediately after obtaining the specimen and review the slide shortly after it is prepared.

Occult Blood Testing

Occult blood testing by either a fecal occult blood test (e.g., Hemoccult) or a urine hemoglobin test (e.g., Hemastix) is a quick, inexpensive, and readily available indicator for the presence of red blood cells in nipple discharge.

Cytological Smear

A cytological specimen of discharge is placed directly from the nipple onto the slide, or, if there is only a small amount of discharge, it can easily be collected with a saline-saturated cotton-tipped applicator and spread onto the slide. The slide is then fixed in the same manner as a cervical specimen (Papanicolaou smear). This technique may reveal cancerous cells. However, a negative smear is not conclusive, and additional work-up is mandated.

Ductography (Ductogram)

A ductogram is useful in evaluating the cause of nipple discharge. Contrast medium is injected by the radiologist into the discharging duct, and a mammogram is taken, which can reveal a filling defect (commonly an intraductal papilloma), a dilated or cystic appearance (duct ectasia or fibrocystic disease), or an abrupt obstruction (malignancy).

Serum Prolactin Level

Hyperprolactinemia should be suspected when the prolactin level exceeds 20 to 25 ng/mL. Prolactin elevation secondary to medications is generally less than 100 ng/mL. Prolactinomas are found when the prolactin level exceeds 150 ng/mL. Elevated serum prolactin levels can produce nipple discharge.

Thyroid Function Testing (TSH)

TSH is high in hypothyroidism. About 20% of patients with hyperprolactinemia are hypothyroid. TSH testing is done to rule out primary hypothyroidism as a cause of the hyperprolactinemia and associated nipple discharge.

DIFFERENTIAL DIAGNOSIS

SINGLE BREAST MASS

Cancer

Breast cancer can occur anytime after puberty but occurs more frequently with increasing age. Classically, breast cancer is a single lump that is hard, nontender, and immobile with borders that are not clearly delineated from the rest of the breast tissue. It most commonly occurs in the upper outer quadrant of the breast. Malignant tumors will eventually affix to the skin, ligaments, or chest wall and cause retractions. Cancers hardly ever cause pain or tenderness on palpation, but some do. They continually increase in size (although at varying rates) and do not come and go. Other suspicious signs of cancer include nipple inversion, dimpling of the breast, bloody nipple discharge, and axillary lymphadenopathy. Occasionally, breast cancer presents as diffuse swelling, pain, or breast erythema. Unilateral breast pain in a postmenopausal woman is suggestive of cancer. A mammographic finding of a nonpalpable mass or preinvasive lesion associated with macrocalcifications may be the only evidence of a malignant breast mass. Benign lumps are usually smooth, round, and freely movable. However, colloid, medullary, and expansive intraductal cancers can feel like benign tumors.

Fifteen percent of women under age 40 with breast cancer are diagnosed during pregnancy or the postpartum period. Pregnant and postpartum breast cancer patients make up about 2% of total breast cancer patients. The normal physiological changes of the breast tissue during these times necessitates a thorough history and physical examination. A breast lump during pregnancy or lactation is more difficult to biopsy because of the increased vascularity of the breasts. Additionally, the lactating breast can act as a ideal medium for bacterial infection and is slower to heal.

Cysts

Benign cysts occur with higher frequency than any other type of breast lump. They are typically round or elliptical, soft or fluctuant, and mobile. Cysts are not attached to the surrounding breast, nipple, or chest wall, so there is no dimpling of breast tissue or nipple retraction. There are often multiple cysts, frequently in the upper outer quadrants of each breast. Cysts vary in size throughout the menstrual cycle and are usually at their smallest and least tender stage at the end of menses (end of the secretory phase). Transillumination of a cyst allows light to pass through the lump and supports the clinical diagnosis.

Fibroadenoma

Fibroadenoma usually occurs as a single, nontender, rubbery, firm, ovoid or lobulated mass that measures 1 to 5 cm in diameter. This lump is freely mobile; thus there is no dimpling or retractions. It also does not vary in size with the menstrual cycle. Fibroadenomas can be multiple or

bilateral about 25% of the time. They are the most commonly occurring breast mass in adolescence. Only biopsy can distinguish them from dysplasia, cancer, or cystosarcoma phylloides.

Cystosarcoma phylloides is a type of fibroadenoma in which the tumor grows rapidly and reaches a large size. Surgical removal of the tumor with a margin of normal breast tissue or simple mastectomy is sometimes necessary to prevent recurrence. The tumor is rarely malignant.

Abscess

Abscesses often follow systemic signs of mastitis. If mastitis is not treated early with antibiotics, it can progress to an abscess. A peripheral abscess is found more than 1 cm away from the areola and is usually caused by *Staphylococcus aureus* or streptococcal organisms. A subareolar abscess is located in the nipple complex and may be associated with duct ectasia. Anaerobic organisms are the likely cause for subareolar abscesses. A chronic abscess can be encapsulated by fibrous tissue, causing the mass to be an irregularly shaped, firm mass that is nontender. An abscess should be incised and drained, and breast feeding stopped.

Fat Necrosis

Fat necrosis occurs as the result of thickened and retracted scar tissue from an injury and subsequent hematoma. A biopsy alone can differentiate this single, fixed, often irregular tumor from cancer.

Lipoma

A lipoma is a rare finding, a fatty tumor of the breast, whose borders are smooth and well defined. The mass has a fluctuant consistency and is usually nontender and mobile.

Tuberculosis

Tuberculosis is an uncommon breast finding but should be considered, especially in immunocompromised patients. In early stages, tuberculosis may appear as a solitary, firm, irregular, nontender mass.

Ruptured Implant

With a ruptured implant, augmented breast tissue is pushed away from the chest wall by the implant. Masses found in these patients often are best palpated with the patient in the sitting position. The definitive diagnosis is made by mammogram, ultrasound, or magnetic resonance imaging.

INFLAMMATORY BREAST MASS

Mastitis and Acute Abscess

An acute abscess typically follows lactational mastitis. It is exquisitely tender on palpation and is very warm to the touch. The breast is erythematous and swollen, and the abscess usually involves only one fourth of the breast. The mass has a fluctuant consistency. Chills and fever may be present. Axillary lymphadenopathy suggests an abscess, but inflammatory breast cancer must be considered.

Inflammatory Breast Cancer

Inflammatory breast cancer presents similarly to acute mastitis but differs from mastitis in that the entire breast is swollen and fever is rarely present. Axillary lymphadenopathy is present. Inflammatory breast cancer is a rapidly progressing disease; therefore, close follow-up and prompt referral is necessary.

MULTIPLE OR BILATERAL BREAST LUMPS

Fibrocystic Breast Changes

Fibrocystic breast changes usually present as multiple bilateral painful masses, which frequently intensify premenstrually during the luteal phase of the menstrual cycle. The masses often rapidly fluctuate in size, are transient in appearance, and cause cyclic mastodynia. They occur most often in young women aged 30 to 50 and are rare in postmenopausal women. Fibrocystic histological findings that increase the risk of breast cancer are moderate or severe hyperplasia (1.5 to 2 times the risk), atypical hyperplasia (5 times the risk), and carcinoma in situ (8 to 10 times the risk).

NIPPLE DISCHARGE

Intraductal Papilloma

Intraductal papillomas are the most common benign lesions to cause a bloody nipple discharge. They usually are unilateral, subareolar lesions occurring in perimenopausal women. Solitary papillomas do not increase breast cancer risk.

Fibrocystic Breast Changes

Fibrocystic breast change symptoms can include nipple discharge. See earlier section on fibrocystic breast changes for a more detailed discussion (p. 322).

Duct Ectasia

Duct ectasia is an inflammatory response to ductal dilatation and stasis of ductal contents. The discharge may be greenish in color.

Neonatal Discharge ("Witch's Milk")

Newborns may have breast enlargement and a white nipple discharge secondary to maternal estrogens. This condition will disappear within 1 to 2 weeks after birth.

Hyperprolactinemia

A frequent cause of pituitary hyperfunction is hyperprolactinemia. It is present in up to 25% of infertile women. It should be suspected when prolactin levels exceed 20 to 30 ng/mL. It often causes amenorrhea in women. It can also cause headaches, decreased libido, gynecomastia, and galactorrhea in men and women. The nipple discharge is usually bilateral, milky, and from multiple ducts.

MALE BREAST DISEASE

Acute Mastitis

Acute mastitis in males occurs from trauma (e.g., nipple chafing from jogging) and presents as previously discussed in the preceding section on mastitis.

Cancer

Male breast cancer is extremely rare and represents about 1% of all breast cancers. It begins as a painless induration, retraction of the nipple, and an attached mass. It progresses to include lymphadenopathy and skin and chest wall lesions.

Table 8-1

Differential Diagnosis of Common Causes of Breast Lumps and Nipple Discharge

Condition	History	Physical Findings	Diagnostic Studies
Single Breast Mass			
Cancer	Usually over age 35; unilateral new lump	Single, hard, non-tender, fixed lump; borders are irregular or not discrete; there may be erythema, dimpling, increased vessel patterns; may have bloody nipple discharge	Clinical exam; FNA: bloody or noncystic; Hemoccult positive; microscopy: positive RBCs
Cysts	Younger age, often younger than age 35; often multiple	Round or elliptical; soft or fluctuant; mobile	Clinical exam; FNA: clear aspirate; mammogram; ultrasound: cyst(s)
Fibroadenoma	Common in adolescence	Single, sharply circumscribed, mobile lump	Ultrasound; biopsy
Abscess	History of mastitis	Single mass; irregular shape; chronic abscess may be nontender	Biopsy
Fat necrosis	May have a history of injury at the site	Single fixed and often irregular tumor	Biopsy

Table 8-1

Differential Diagnosis of Common Causes of Breast Lumps and Nipple Discharge—cont'd

Condition	History	Physical Findings	Diagnostic Studies
Lipoma	May have others on arms, trunk, buttocks, or back; usually nontender	Singular tumors; smooth, well defined; fluctuant consistency	Biopsy
Tuberculosis	History of tuberculosis, positive PPD or chest x-ray; immunocompromised patient status	Single; irregular shaped; nontender	Biopsy
Ruptured implant	History of augmentation; change in size or shape of breast	Nodule palpated best when patient is sitting	Mammogram; ultrasound; MRI
Inflammatory Breast Mass			
Mastitis and acute abscess	Primigravidas more often than gravidas; >1 week after delivery; breast feeding; tender nipples	Red, warm, tender; usually unilateral, one fourth of the breast or 1 lobule; breast engorgement; fever; nipple discharge: pus	Culture: positive for *S. aureus, E. coli,* streptococcus; elevated WBCs
Inflammatory breast cancer	History of mastitis or inflammatory process of breast	Entire breast swollen, fever rarely present; axillary lymphadenopathy	Biopsy
Multiple or Bilateral Breast Lumps			
Fibrocystic breast changes	Multiple breast lumps of both breasts; cyclic changes that worsen at time of menses	Bilateral nodularity, dominant lumps; tender, mobile	FNA: clear fluid; biopsy: hyperplasia, atypical hyperplasia, or CIS increases risk for cancer; ultrasound; mammogram
Nipple Discharge			
Intraductal papilloma	Bloody nipple discharge; usual age is 40-50 years	Unilateral, subareolar	Occult blood test: positive

Continued

Table 8-1

Differential Diagnosis of Common Causes of Breast Lumps and Nipple Discharge—cont'd

Condition	History	Physical Findings	Diagnostic Studies
Nipple Discharge—cont'd			
Fibrocystic breast changes	Milky nipple discharge; cyclic changes that worsen at time of menses	Spontaneous, clear or milky, bilateral, multiduct nipple discharge; multiple breast lumps of both breasts	Occult blood test: negative; microscopy: no RBCs
Duct ectasia	Green nipple discharge	Greenish or brownish nipple discharge	Occult blood test: negative
Neonatal discharge (witch's milk)	Milky discharge 1-2 weeks after birth	Enlarged breast tissue, milky discharge lasting 1-2 weeks after birth	None
Hyperprolactinemia	Milky or clear nipple discharge; history of medications: estrogenic, dopamine blockers, or depleters; hypothyroidism; pregnancy; postabortion; nipple stimulation; visual changes	Spontaneous, unilateral or bilateral, multiduct clear or milky nipple discharge	Prolactin levels: >20-30 ng/ml
Male Breast Disease			
Acute mastitis	History of clothing rubbing nipple (jogging); swelling or lump of chest wall; tenderness of site	Red, warm, tender; usually unilateral, one fourth of the breast or 1 lobule; breast engorgement; fever; nipple discharge: pus	Culture: positive for *S. aureus, E. coli,* streptococcus; elevated WBCs
Cancer	Family history of male breast cancer; painless lump of chest wall	Induration, retraction of nipple or a mass in the nipple well, fixed, nontender; lymphadenopathy	Mammogram; FNA: positive; open biopsy

Chapter 9

Common Problems of the Musculoskeletal System

≣ Limb Pain

Complaints of pain in a limb present a diagnostic challenge because of the many possible pathophysiological causes. Because of the broad range of differential diagnoses, it is best to use a framework of differentiating the pain as a symptom of musculoskeletal injury, musculoskeletal or joint disease, systemic disease, or a mixture of factors. Pain can be the result of a direct reaction in tissues, secondary reaction in adjacent tissues, or referral from a proximal or distal lesion or from organs such as the heart or kidney. In children, aches and pains in limbs are common; however, presence, location, and intensity of the pain are often difficult to assess. Interpretation of the symptom is often made by the parents.

It is helpful to distinguish between limb pain that affects the bones, muscles, and tendons and injury/inflammation of a joint that can affect surrounding musculature, nerves, and blood vessels. For example, lower extremity pain is often referred from the low back and emanates from irritated nerve roots or is secondary to myofascial syndromes of the low back, pelvic, and hip musculature.

DIAGNOSTIC REASONING: FOCUSED HISTORY

Is the pain caused by an acute musculoskeletal injury? What is the precipitating event?

Key Questions
- Have you had a recent injury?
- Describe exactly how the injury occurred.

Injury. Injuries to the musculoskeletal system can range from simple muscular strain to a significant fracture associated with nerve or vascular injury. Therefore, when a patient presents with a history of trauma, the priority is to assess the vascular integrity of the limb. Neurological integrity is next. Symptoms of coldness, severe pain, or paresthesia are signals that physical examination should begin immediately to assess the extent of injury and the need for emergency treatment. Acute pain and swelling that follows trauma usually indicates injury to a previously normal structure.

If the injury does not warrant urgent attention, obtain further history. Ask questions that specify the mechanism of injury, such as a direct blow or impact, landing position after a fall, twisting, jumping, running, overstretching, or overuse. When discussing the precipitating event, ask the patient to describe any noise such as snapping, popping, or breaking that may have occurred with the injury.

Could this be caused by a sprain or strain?

Key Questions
- Describe how the injury occurred.
- Did you hear a noise with the injury, such as a ripping or cracking sound?

Strain. A strain involves injury to muscles and tendons, whereas sprains involve injury to ligamentous structures. Both types of injuries can produce a ripping or tearing sound and range in severity from minor damage to a complete tear. Injuries are generally classified as mild, moderate, or severe. A moderate to severe strain/sprain may involve some loss of joint or ligament stability. Strains may be acute or chronic. Injury commonly occurs when lateral stress is applied while the joint is plantar flexed. This position is the least stable position of the ankle, and the overstretched ligaments are more susceptible to eversion or inversion forces.

Sprain. Sprains cause minimal to moderate pain increasing 1 to 2 days after the trauma when the inflammatory process begins. A complete disruption that severs the sensory nerve fibers within the structure will cause little pain, while a partial injury

irritates sensory fibers and may produce intense pain.

In children, ligaments and joint capsules are 2 to 5 times stronger than the epiphysis; therefore, growth plate injuries are more common than sprains.

Fracture. A fracture produces diffuse swelling around the injured bone soon after injury. A patient may report hearing a crack and being disabled by the increased severity of pain with weight-bearing or movement of the limb.

If there is no history of trauma or a precipitating event, is the pain caused by overuse?

Key Question
- Describe your usual daily activities at home, work, and with hobbies.

Overuse. Repetitive microtrauma results from cumulative injury or overuse. This type of trauma most often affects the fingers, wrists, and upper extremities. Persons who work on keyboards for long periods may complain of paresthesia of the fingers and pain and soreness of the wrists and fingers. Weekend hobbies or participation in sports may result in overuse of certain muscle groups associated with those activities.

What does the location of pain tell me?

Key Questions
- Where does it hurt?
- Is the pain localized to one area or does it radiate?

Location. Location of pain provides a clue for identifying the site where the pain originates. There are general characteristics to keep in mind when seeking the location of pain. Local pain receptors signal the site of irritation, and an increase in sensitivity (hyperesthesia) results. Referred pain generally involves the muscle chains, nerve pathways, and vessels. Unilateral, circumscribed limb or quadrant pain involves autonomic nerve fibers. Bilateral pain is more likely to originate from systemic involvement. Diffuse pain with inconsistent distribution may be the result of psychosomatic conditions such as depression and anxiety. Collagen diseases and connective tissue diseases can affect one or more joints.

The more vaguely defined the boundaries of the pain, the deeper or more central the location of the somatic irritation.

In joint pain with injury, what do I need to know about the specific joints involved?

UPPER EXTREMITIES: SHOULDER, WRIST, ELBOW

Key Questions

- Is the pain in your dominant limb?
- Did you fall on an outstretched hand or arm?
- Did you overuse a joint?

Pain in the dominant had may indicate repetitive microtrauma or overuse. Breaking a fall with an outstretched arm is a common mechanism of injury for a fracture or dislocation of the hand or wrist.

LOWER EXTREMITIES: KNEE, ANKLE

Key Questions

- How is the pain affected by weight bearing or activity?
- Did you feel a sense of "giving way?"
- Did you hear a pop, tear, or other sound?
- What position was your leg in when you hurt your knee?

Continuing with an activity means the injury did not totally disrupt any ligamentous structures. An inability to straighten or bend the knee suggests a mechanical blockage, such as a patellar dislocation or meniscus tear. In chondromalacia, the pa-

tient can bend the knee, but the movement is usually painful.

A loud pop is virtually diagnostic of an anterior cruciate ligament tear. A ripping sound suggests a meniscus injury. A cracking sound may signify a bony injury or dislocation of the patella.

A sudden change in direction or sudden stop may put more force on the ligaments than they can dissipate, resulting in acute rupture. A sudden twisting injury is likely to represent a meniscus tear and a serious ligament disruption. Running or jumping activities are commonly associated with knee and ankle injuries.

Ten percent to 20% of knee symptoms in children are the result of a problem in the hip joint.

Could this be musculoskeletal joint disease?

Key Question

- What does the pain feel like?

Musculoskeletal joint disease. Generally, sharp, piercing, stabbing, cutting, pinching, gnawing pain is most common with lesions of the nerves and skin. Dull, tearing, boring, burning, and cramping are common terms used to describe pain arising from deeper structures such as muscles, joints, and internal organs. Pulsating, pounding, throbbing, or hammering are common descriptions of vascular pain. Gradually increasing sensations of pressure, tension, heaviness, and calf pain indicate venous obstruction. Severe pain that develops over 1 to 4 days is typical of osteomyelitis or septic arthritis in children.

Muscle pain is caused by receptors located in bursa, muscle fibers, ligaments, and tendon attachments. It is a diffuse, dull, gnawing, boring, or tearing pain that increases with use and decreases with rest.

Intra-articular pain arises from receptors of the synovial membrane, joint capsule, or the fibrochondreal layers of the articular surfaces. Joint pain is either inflammatory or degenerative. Inflammatory joint pain radiates diffusely to surrounding tissues. It is intense, sharp, burning, boring, or pulsating (effusion) pain. It persists during rest and is evident especially at night, worsening in the morning with morning stiffness that lasts more than 45 minutes, and then improves throughout the day.

Degenerative joint pain radiates to the soft tissue structures around the joint (muscles, ligaments, tendons). It is dull, boring, and gnawing when associated with muscle pain, or it can be a sharp acute pain that increases with overuse.

Bone lesions cause a dull ache; periosteal pain is sharp, not well localized and increases in intensity with dependency of the extremity.

Neuralgic pain occurs in the distribution of a peripheral nerve or nerve root. The pain is stabbing or cutting and can also present as pricking or lacerating.

What does the history of swelling tell me?

Key Questions
- Is there any swelling?
- When did the swelling begin?

Swelling. Swelling around a joint is always abnormal. Children do not always recognize swelling; they often report that they can't squat down or flex their knee fully because it feels "full or tight."

Generally, swelling that develops immediately or within 2 hours after an injury is the result of a fracture or hemarthrosis and indicates a severe injury. Swelling 6 to 24 hours after an injury is usually of synovial origin, such as a meniscal tear, subluxation, dislocation, or ligamentous damage. Swelling after 24 hours implies an inflammatory reaction.

Is this an acute or chronic problem?

Key Questions
- When did the pain first occur?
- When did you first notice a problem?

Pain experienced hours after an injury or physical activity is usually caused by acute extensor injury or overuse. Severe ligament sprain is manifested as an immediately disabling pain at the moment of the injury.

Determining if the complaint is acute or chronic helps to differentiate the cause. Chronic joint problems compound each other, whereas intermittent or episodic pain is characteristic of diseases of the musculoskeletal system. In children, limping or not using the extremity may be a signal that the child is experiencing pain. Parents will often note the loss of motion in an extremity or note an awkward gait or report that the child is not able to do activities he or she could previously do.

Patients may report noticing pain, weakness, or difficulty in activities of daily living, such as using a hair dryer, opening jars, holding a pen, or handling eating utensils.

How is activity affected?

Key Questions
- What are your usual activities?
- What activity makes the pain worse?
- What movements make the pain worse?

A large percentage of musculoskeletal injuries are caused by repetitive motion that leads to microtrauma and eventually cumulative damage. Repetitive microtrauma in the lower extremities from inappropriate rate and intensity of training, shoe wear, or playing surfaces can cause stress fractures of the weight-bearing bones of the lower limbs. Pain is worse over the site of the fracture.

In children, pain in the groin or referred to the knee and anterior thigh, occurring intermittently after activity and gradually becoming constant, may indicate Legg-Calve-Perthes disease (LCPD).

Intra-articular lesions usually worsen with joint motion and sports activities. Intraosseous tumors are less sensitive to joint motion.

In children with a septic hip, pain increases with movement.

What does joint stiffness or locking tell me?

Key Questions
- Have you had any joint stiffness?
- Does activity make the stiffness worse or better?
- Do you have locking of the knee?

Joint stiffness or locking. Stiffness is felt after being in one position for a long time. This complaint gets confused with locking of the knee, which is an abrupt occurrence where the patient complains that something "gets in the way" and is unable to fully extend the knee. Manipulation of the leg often results in an equally abrupt unlocking. This is usually a sign of a chronic unstable meniscus tear.

Stiffness is a common feature of any inflammatory arthropathy. It is important to know if it is localized or generalized. The length of time the stiffness lasts in the morning is a useful index of active synovitis in disease states such as rheumatoid arthritis or systemic lupus erythematosus. With most inflammatory arthropathies, stiffness and pain are alleviated by activity, whereas mechanical problems are aggravated by activity. Musculoskeletal tumors commonly present with mild joint stiffness because of muscle involvement but rarely demonstrate instability.

What does the history of a limp tell me?

Key Questions
- Is there pain with the limp?
- Did the limp come on suddenly?
- Is the limp constant or intermittent?
- What is the effect of running or climbing stairs?

Limp. Limping is a pathological alteration of a smooth, regular gait pattern and is never normal. Gait can be divided into two phases: stance and swing. The stance phase starts with the foot in contact with the floor and ends with the toe being brought off the floor; the limb supports all the body weight. The swing phase begins with the toe off the floor and ends with the heel strike. During the swing phase, the foot is not touching the floor; the pelvis rotates forward and tilts slightly while the trunk maintains a neutral position. Limp after strenuous running may indicate a stress fracture.

Quadriceps weakness causes difficulty in climbing stairs. During ambulation, this weakness causes the knee to be unstable on heel strike, and assistance is needed to push the knee manually into an extended position.

Neuromuscular diseases can result in progressive and painless muscle weakness or spasticity that affect ambulation in a variety of ways.

Symptoms of pain and limping in children may often be incorrectly attributed to trauma instead of indicating a more serious problem such as neoplastic tumors or bone infections.

Could this be caused by systemic disease?

Key Questions
- Have you been treated with any antibiotics lately?
- Have you had any recent immunizations?
- Have you had a fever? Have you taken your temperature?
- Has the fever been constant or intermittent?
- Does the pain awaken you at night?
- Is the pain worse at night?
- Do you have a skin rash?

Medications. Certain antibiotics can cause serum sickness in children, producing joint pain and fever.

Transient arthralgia may occur 6 to 8 weeks after receiving MMR immunization. Recurrent or permanent arthritis may follow rubella vaccination, especially in adult females.

In adults, quinolone antibiotics can produce tendinitis or tendon rupture.

Fever. Fever related to joint problems can be the result of hematogenous seeding by an organism, direct invasion as a result of trauma or puncture, or spread from an adjacent area of infection. In rheumatic fever, a beta-hemolytic streptococcal infection precedes the initial joint pain by 1 to 3 weeks. Often the hip joint may be the first of many joints affected before polyarticular migratory involvement occurs. The fever is sustained, not intermittent. Fever spikes are seen with chronic forms of arthritis in children.

Other systemic infections associated with polyarthritis include bacterial endocarditis, Lyme disease, syphilis, and viruses such as hepatitis B, rubella, cytomegalovirus, human immunodeficiency virus (HIV), Epstein-Barr virus, and varicella zoster.

Night pain. Intense pain may occur at rest and during the night. At first the pain may occur only when the patient changes position while sleeping; however, as the pain increases, it will disrupt sleep. Report by an adolescent of night pain is a red flag for the intraosseous pain of a bone tumor. Pain in the lower limbs in children 6 to 12 who are in a rapid linear growth period may awaken a child at night. The cause of these "growing pains" is unknown, but they are thought to result from muscle structures that have to catch up with bone growth. They are usually bilateral, and no objective findings are found.

Could the pain be caused by Lyme disease?

Key Questions
- Have you been camping or out in the woods?
- Have you noticed any skin rash?

Lyme disease. Lyme disease is an infection caused by the tick-borne spirochete *Borrelia burgdorferi*. Early symptoms include diffuse arthralgias, myalgias, fever, chills, and a characteristic target-like rash. Although the arthralgia may involve multiple joints, usually the knee

is the affected joint. Joint manifestations occur 1 week to 2 years following the initial illness. Patients may or may not recall the antecedent tick bite or exposure.

What does past medical history tell me?

Key Questions
- Have you had anything like this before?
- Do you have a history of any chronic disease?
- Could you have been exposed to any sexually transmitted disease?
- Have you been treated with cortisone for longer than a few weeks?
- Have you had a recent cold or upper respiratory infection?

Chronic diseases, such as sickle cell anemia, inflammatory bowel disease, Crohn's disease, hypo- and hyperthyroidism, or collagen vascular diseases, are frequently associated with skin rashes, psoriasis, and limb and joint pain.

Gonorrhea may disseminate to the musculoskeletal system in 1% to 3% of individuals with the disease. Of these, over 80% develop arthritis.

Patients with chronic illness that requires long-term administration of corticosteroids are at risk for cortisone-induced necrosis of the hip. Sickle cell anemia can cause hip pain during a sickle cell crisis. Viral infections may cause diffuse myalgia.

Is this likely a mixed condition?

Consider the possibility that a patient may have a condition that is a mix of factors, for example, a systemic disorder that has resulted in an acute injury. Clues to mixed etiology might include an injury that seems out of proportion to the extent of the precipitating activity or the presence of a chronic condition or other symptoms that might point to an undetected chronic condition. It is important to evaluate the limb pain in the context of the whole person.

DIAGNOSTIC REASONING: FOCUSED PHYSICAL EXAMINATION

Evaluation of musculoskeletal injuries should include examination of joint stability, deformity, and function. Examination should be done as soon after an injury as possible for an accurate diagnosis. Always observe for symmetry, and then functionally assess limbs and joints bilaterally, beginning with the unaffected side. Order the examination so that the most painful tests will be done last.

Observe Patient Walking, Removing Coat/Jacket, Getting into a Sitting Position

Subtle clues of child abuse must be considered when the patient history is not consistent with the type or extent of injury. Abuse should always be considered in an infant within the first year when symptoms and history suggest a fracture, multiple injuries, rotational injuries, or multiple bruises in different states of healing. X-rays may show previous fractures.

Persons who have septic joints appear ill, and movement of the joint will increase the pain. Inspect the patient with minimal clothing obstructing your view of movements. A child with a septic hip lays with the thigh in a position of flexion, abduction, and external rotation and cries when lower limb is moved.

In adults, an internally rotated abducted leg is the posture assumed with a posterior hip dislocation. An externally rotated hip and shortened lower extremity are signs of hip fracture.

General stiffness or limitation of motion of a single joint forces the surrounding joints to accommodate by moving with greater excursion or range of usual movement. This makes the gait appear irregular or jerky.

Look for Limp

Pain, weakness, and deformity cause limping. Limping will be accentuated if the patient is asked to walk on the heels or tiptoes.

Common abnormal gaits related to limping are Trendelenburg gait, antalgic gait, and circumduction gait. Trendelenburg gait is a duck-like gait that reflects unilateral weakness of the gluteus medius muscle. The pelvis drops on the unaffected side during weight bearing on the affected side. In antalgic gait, there is an acute one-sided limp because the patient takes quick soft steps to shorten the period of weight bearing on the involved extremity. Stance time on the affected limb is decreased while stride length of the opposite side is shortened, allowing a quicker return of weight bearing to the normal limb. This is a reflex response to weight bearing on a painful limb.

Circumduction gait is seen with pathology of the foot or ankle and reduces discomfort by limiting movement of the ankle. The gait is characterized by a circular outward swing of the leg and external rotation of the foot that requires less ankle movement. External rotation of the entire extremity is seen with slipped capital femoral epiphysis.

Have the patient stand on one foot, then the other. When standing on one leg, the gluteus medius on that side maintains the opposite side of pelvis level, balancing the trunk over the weight-bearing hip. If the hip abductors are weak or painful, the opposite side of the pelvis dips down during the stance phase. With each step, the trunk shifts toward the side of a painful or weak extremity to decrease the force transmitted through the extremity to the hip.

Assessment of gait is best done either before or after examination when patients are less aware that they are being observed.

Ankle plantar flexion and dorsiflexion are necessary for normal gait. If plantar flexion is restricted, there is no push off and the forefoot and heel come off the floor at the same time. The result is a higher knee lift and the forefoot may slap against the floor. This condition is seen with weakness from peroneal nerve injury or with painful dorsiflexors associated with shin splints.

Observe the patient walking with and without shoes. If a child walks without difficulty with shoes off, the shoes are probably the problem. Inadequate shoe width is a common source of foot pain in children.

Have Patient Locate the Pain

Have the patient point to the area of pain. Location of pain and actual area of pathology may not be consistent. Hip pain often is referred to the knee area because the anterior branch of the obturator nerve passes close to the hip joint and, if irritated, provides a painful sensation to the medial side of the knee. True hip joint pain arises in the trochanteric bursa and is perceived in the groin area.

Shoulder pain from rotator cuff tendinitis is felt over the lateral aspect of the deltoid.

Swelling of the elbow may compress the ulnar nerve, producing a tingling sensation in the fourth and fifth fingers.

Pain in the groin, lateral hip, or knee in a child may indicate Legg-Calve-Perthes disease.

Pain in the groin, buttocks, or lateral hip in a child may indicate slipped femoral capital epiphysis.

Vague, nebulous discomfort in the front of the thighs, in the calves, and behind the knees located outside of the joints in a child may indicate growing pains.

Note Any Deformities

Fractures generally produce unilateral deformities or swelling in the extremities. Inflammatory and degenerative joint disease produce observable joint swelling and deformity that usually occurs bilaterally.

Osteoarthritis typically involves the distal interphalangeal (DIP) and proximal interphalangeal (PIP) joints, spine, hips, knees, and first metatarsophalangeal (MTP) joints. Joints are enlarged with He-berden's (DIP joints) and Bouchard's (PIP joints) nodes.

Joints affected by rheumatoid arthritis include PIPs, metacarpophalangeal (MCP), wrists, knees, elbows, cervical spine, and MTPs. Joints are swollen with a fusiform-shaped swelling of the PIP joints. Subluxation, ankylosis, and ulnar deviation may be observed as a result of joint destruction from chronic inflammation.

Assess Vital Signs

Elevated temperatures are seen with neoplastic, systemic, and infectious processes such as osteomyelitis and septic hip in children. Neonates may not exhibit a fever with a septic hip but may refuse to feed and will exhibit other symptoms of septicemia, such as lethargy and subnormal temperature. Palpate for quality and presence of pulses in any injured limb and compare to the opposite side.

Inspect the Skin and Nails

Inspect the skin for redness and inflammation.

Lyme disease usually presents with a rash before joint involvement; however, rash may occur concurrently. The rash, often characteristically found on the trunk, is an erythematous papule that develops into an annular lesion with a clear center. Concentric rings may develop, giving it a bull's eye appearance (erythema migrans).

Look for a puncture or abscess that could be the source of infection and seeding if a septic joint or osteomyelitis is suspected. Swelling and redness in a joint or in the midshaft of the tibia may be caused by osteomyelitis.

Look for an ingrown toenail that may alter gait. When the nails are trimmed by rounding off the edges, the hypertrophied and inflamed soft tissue-fold can overlap the nail, and ingrowth at the distal margin will occur. Ingrown toenail is enhanced when tight-fitting shoes compress the soft tissues around the nail.

Look for ecchymosis and bruising.

These indicate trauma as a source for pain as well as raise a suspicion of abuse. Ecchymosis indicates underlying bleeding and disruption of soft tissue or bone. Ecchymosis changes color over a period of days. Initially the color is dark red or violet, in 1 to 3 days the bruise is blue-brown, in 1 week it is yellow-green, and after a week it is light brown. Ecchymosis resolves within 2 to 4 weeks.

Ecchymosis in the popliteal fossa after dislocation of the knee may be a sign of arterial disruption. Hemarthrosis, or bleeding into a joint, usually occurs within 1 to 2 hours of an injury and can occur secondary to hemophilia or other bleeding disorders, or it can be associated with visible ecchymoses caused by blood leaking into soft tissues.

Swelling and redness of a joint means underlying infection or inflammation. Edema will present as an asymmetrical area of swelling. Effusion, or fluid in the joint capsule, always distends the joint in a smooth symmetrical manner.

Observe the muscles around the painful limb area. Decreased muscle tone or atrophy from disuse begins immediately after injury; however, it will not be clinically apparent for approximately 1 week.

Inspect for symmetrical gluteal folds. A congenital dislocated hip produces asymmetrical gluteal folds.

Measure Limb Circumference and Length

Use a tape measure to locate points at which to measure and compare limb circumference. Differences may be the result of muscle atrophy or edema. To measure leg length, have the patient lie supine with legs in comparable positions and measure the distance from the anterior iliac spines to the medial malleoli of the ankles. If a discrepancy is found, ask the patient to lie supine with knees flexed 90 degrees and feet flat on the table. If one knee is higher, the tibia of that extremity is longer. If one knee projects further anteriorly, the femur of that extremity is longer.

Palpate Extremities and Joints

Always palpate those areas that are suspected to be painless first and then compare to the affected limb.

Determine if there is edema (e.g., presence of interstitial fluid). Induration is interstitial swelling that has progressed and is now firm. An effusion is a collection of fluid in the joint capsule, which can be the result of rupture of a vascular structure or a synovial secretory response to an inflammatory process. The consistency of the fluid is noteworthy. Pus has a thick consistency and is less fluctuant than synovial fluid. Hematoma has a more gel-like consistency. Swelling in an ankle sprain is diffuse and nonfluctuant. Knee ligament sprain is much more fluctuant. Fluid in the knee is detected by pressing above the knee and watching the concave or shallow areas of the joint become distended with fluid and bulge on either side of the knee cap. Note that swelling can extend above and below the point of pathology.

In severe knee trauma, rupture of the capsule allows fluid to escape into surrounding tissues, and less distention may be apparent than with lesser injuries.

Palpate for fluid bulge if the knee is painful. Milk the fluid up into the suprapatellar pouch and then bring the hand down the lateral aspect of the knee looking for a medial fluid bulge. Palpate deeply to detect muscle fibrillation, fasciculation, or tumors.

Feel for heat in the affected joint, which can indicate an inflammatory or infectious process. Evaluate the joint for crepitus, both palpable and auditory. Tendinitis can produce a grating sensation on palpation of the ligament or a grating sound with movement.

Perform Passive/Active Range of Motion of All Limbs

Range of motion may be limited because of pain, weakness, or deformity.

If pathology is in the joint, pain will be the same with active and passive motion. If

---

Table 9-1

Muscle Strength Test

GRADE	MUSCLE STRENGTH	TERM
0	No palpable contraction	Zero
1	Muscle contracts but part does not move	Trace
2	Muscle moves the part but not against gravity	Poor
3	Muscle moves part through range against gravity	Fair
4	Muscle moves part even with resistance	Good
5	Normal strength against resistance present	Excellent

---

the disease is outside the joint, or extra-articular, passive motion may be painless while active motion produces pain. During passive tests, move the joint until an end point or end range is felt to help determine the affected structure and the severity of the injury.

There are six end points to note when assessing joint movement: (1) bone to bone sensation, felt with an osteophyte or abnormal bone development; (2) spasm, which can indicate severe ligamentous injury; (3) capsular feel or a firm arrested movement, with some give to it, which can indicate chronic joint effusion, arthritis, or capsular scarring; (4) spring block, or joint rebound at the end of range of movement, caused by an articular derangement or an intraarticular body; (5) tissue approximation, a normal end feel caused by tissue limiting further movement, such as the biceps muscle limiting elbow flexion; and (6) empty end feel, present when there is no tissue resistance, but the patient stops the movement because of pain. This last condition indicates bursitis, extra-articular abscess, or tumor.

Test for Muscle Strength

Test for flexor and extensor strength against resistance of both the proximal and distal muscle groups. Proximal muscle weakness is seen in myopathic disorders. Distal muscle weakness is seen secondary to a neuropathic process. Generally, if the opposite side is normal, strength should be compared to it. A scale of 0 to 5 is used to rate muscle strength (Table 9-1).

In the presence of significant pain, muscle strength may be unreliable. If the contraction is strong and painful, the pathology is caused by mild musculotendinous damage. If the contraction is weak and painful, the pathology is the result of severe musculotendinous damage. If the contraction is weak and painless, the pathology results from a neurological lesion (paresis).

Perform a Neurological Examination

A complete assessment of sensory and motor function and deep tendon reflexes should be done on the affected and contralateral limbs. If systemic illness is suspected, perform a complete neurological examination.

LABORATORY AND DIAGNOSTIC STUDIES

Complete Blood Count (CBC)

A CBC is done to evaluate for anemia associated with chronic disease, infection, or neoplasm. An altered white cell count may indicate infection or leukemia.

Erythrocyte Sedimentation Rate (ESR)

An ESR is elevated when inflammation is present. It is a non-specific test.

Joint Aspiration

Joint aspiration is done to assess synovial fluid for elevated white blood cell count, Gram stain, culture and sensitivity, crystal analysis, presence of glucose, and consistency or "string test." This procedure is performed using local anesthesia under sterile technique. Synovial fluid will flow easily when the joint capsule is penetrated.

X-Ray

Obtain at least two x-ray views, anteroposterior and lateral, because injuries are not always apparent on a single view. Any evidence of fracture or dislocation will require orthopedic attention, which is beyond the scope of this chapter. Sometimes radiographic comparisons with the opposite limb may be useful. Traumatic knee injuries should include four x-ray views: anteroposterior, lateral, tunnel (intracondylar notch) view, and a 30-degree sunrise (patella) view. Other diagnostic imaging techniques such as MRI, CT, or bone scan are usually ordered by specialists. MRI is usually used in spine, joint, and soft tissue imaging. CT scans are usually used for bone visualization.

Antinuclear Antibody (ANA)

ANA tests are positive with high titers in rheumatoid arthritis and systemic lupus erythematosus; however, other conditions such as aging, medications, and other connective tissue disease can produce positive antibody titers.

Rheumatoid Factor (RA)

RA is the single most useful test to confirm a diagnosis of rheumatoid arthritis. The RA is positive in 80% of patients with this disease.

C4 Complement

C4 complement determines serum hemolytic complement activity, a protein that binds antigen-antibody complexes for purposes of lysis. Complement is increased in active inflammatory disease and in autoimmune disorders such as juvenile rheumatoid arthritis.

C-Reactive Protein (CRP)

CRP indicates the presence of abnormal plasma protein or a nonspecific response to inflammation caused by both infectious and non-infectious processes. CRP is elevated in rheumatoid arthritis and infection.

Lyme Titer Enzyme-Linked Immunosorbent Assay (ELISA) Serology

ELISA detects antibodies against *Borrelia burgdorferi*, which causes Lyme disease. However, the ELISA may not detect antibodies for several weeks following onset of infection.

DIFFERENTIAL DIAGNOSIS

MUSCULOSKELETAL INFLAMMATION

Tenosynovitis (Tendinitis)

Soft tissue disorders of tendinitis, bursitis, and fibrositis tend to co-occur. Tenosynovitis is a term that refers to inflammation of the tendon and tendon sheath. In an acute inflammation, usually caused by trauma related to recreational or occupational activities, effusion may accumulate and result in swelling; with chronic inflammation, range of motion will be limited by fibrosis of the tendon sheath.

The patient's chief complaint will be pain that is worse with movement, and swelling around the affected area. Occupational and recreational history will provide vital clues to a traumatic or overuse cause of pain. Persons with arthritis may have tendinitis secondary to joint disease. Crepitus may be felt on palpation of the tendon.

Bursitis

Bursitis is inflammation of a sac lined with synovial fluid, most often secondary to traumatic tenosynovitis of the shoulder, hip, knee, and elbow. Numerous bursae lie over bony prominences and reduce friction from motion of fascial planes. Bursitis is caused by overuse and trauma and may be associated with rheumatoid arthritis. If isometric contraction of a group of muscles causes pain, the muscles or tendons or both may be involved. Bursitis causes an aching pain that radiates to points of tendon insertion or further along the limb. Muscle weakness may also be present. Palpation reveals local tenderness and swelling without full range of joint motion.

Fibrositis (Myofasciitis, Fibromyositis)

Fibromyositis is a response to underlying conditions, such as polymyalgia rheumatica, rheumatoid arthritis, ankylosing spondylitis, hypothyroidism, neuritis, and viral infection, that generate major muscle tension around a large, weight-bearing proximal joint. Fatty and fibrous nodules may be palpable, and painful trigger sites can be located throughout the shoulder and pelvic girdles or lower extremities. Patients complain of stress and anxiety, sleep disturbance, painful trigger points, and joint stiffness.

Osteomyelitis

The presentation of osteomyelitis, a pyogenic infection of bone, depends on the age of the patient as well as the bone involved. This condition should be suspected in any patient who complains of pain in long or flat bones and walks with an antalgic limp. Fever, chills, and vomiting are usually present in acute osteomyelitis but may not occur in the neonate or young infant. Chronic osteomyelitis is characterized by relapse of pain, erythema, swelling, or evidence of purulent discharge. The hallmark is a constant local pain that progressively worsens. The slightest motion of the limb aggravates the pain. The child keeps the limb motionless. Laboratory findings show increased WBCs, ESR, and C-reactive protein. X-rays may show bone destruction or deep soft tissue swelling at the site of infection.

JOINT INFLAMMATION

Osteoarthritis (OA)

Osteoarthritis is a degenerative disease of joint cartilage that results in osteophyte (spur) development and synovial inflammation. It is the most common form of arthritis and is present to some extent in all elderly persons. Patients will complain of joint stiffness, pain, and limited movement, most often of the spine (cervical and lumbar), large proximal joints (e.g., knee, hip), and proximal interphalangeal (PIP) joints. Symptoms may be asymmetrical. Heberden's nodes develop on the distal interphalangeal (DIP) joints. Patients at increased risk have a history of performing repetitive weight-lifting tasks, joint trauma, obesity, and diabetes mellitus. Acute arthritis is associated with an increased ESR, and x-rays will reveal spurs, joint deformity, and erosive changes.

Rheumatoid Arthritis (RA)

Rheumatoid arthritis is a systemic polyarthritis with a wide spectrum of clinical presentation. Symptoms of RA include morning stiffness of symmetrical small joints in the hands and feet, swelling, and progressive fatigue. Other symptoms may include fever, weight loss, anorexia, and diaphoresis. Rheumatoid nodules are soft and spongy and appear on the elbows, forearms, and hands. Pericarditis, pleuritis, and vasculitis are associated conditions. Laboratory data may reveal a normochromic, normocytic anemia, elevated ESR, and a positive rheumatoid factor in 75% to 90% of patients. X-rays may show bony erosion at the joint margins and joint deformities. Box 9-1 lists criteria for the diagnosis of RA.

Box 9-1

Criteria for Diagnosis of Rheumatoid Arthritis (Four Criteria Must Be Present)

At Least 6 Months' Duration
Morning stiffness at least 1 hour before improvement
Arthritis of three or more joints
Arthritis of hand joints
Symmetrical arthritis of same joint
Rheumatoid nodules
Positive serum rheumatoid factor
X-ray changes showing erosions or bony decalcification

Modified from Uphold CR, Graham MV: *Clinical guidelines in adult health,* 1994, Gainesville, FL, Barmarrae Books, p 547.

Juvenile Rheumatoid Arthritis (JRA)

JRA, the most common connective tissue disease in children, presents with fatigue, low-grade fever, weight loss, and failure to grow. Night pain and morning stiffness that improves with activity are common symptoms. Younger children may present with irritability, refusal to walk, or guarding of a joint. The disease may be systemic, affect fewer than four joints (pauciarticular), or affect more than four joints (polyarticular). Laboratory findings show anemia, leukocytosis, and thrombocytosis. Rheumatoid factor and antinuclear antibodies may be negative. ESR is elevated.

Septic Arthritis

Septic arthritis is a sudden pain and inflammation of a single joint, sometimes associated with systemic signs such as fever, malaise, and diaphoresis. The hip is a common site of blood-borne joint infection in neonates, infants, and young children. The presentation depends on the age of the child. A neonate may be afebrile but irritable, refusing to feed and failing to gain weight. In the older child, the onset of pain and fever is acute, and the child refuses to bear weight. Range of motion of the hip is markedly restricted and very painful.

In adults, migratory joint pain and tenosynovitis may follow 2 to 4 weeks after a mucosal site infection with *Neisseria gonorrhea*. Knee, wrist, ankle, and hand joints are most commonly affected. Joint aspiration shows increased WBCs, and culture of fluid or pus may reveal bacterial, tubercular, fungal, syphilitic, and viral organisms. The ESR and C-reactive protein are also elevated. With hip involvement, ultrasound shows marked distention of the hip joint, with varying degrees of femoral hip displacement. Septic arthritis is an emergency situation, and treatment must be initiated immediately.

Gout

Gout is a joint inflammation caused by deposits of urate crystals and is associated with an inborn error of uric acid secretion or with metabolic disorders (e.g., hemolytic anemia, renal insufficiency, sarcoidosis). Males over 30 years and persons with a family history of gout are most often affected. The patient reports a recurrent, sudden onset of pain early in the morning that subsides over several days, especially of the first metatarsophalangeal (MTP) joint. The joint is warm, tender, and red; tophi, chalky subcutaneous deposits of sodium urate, may be present on extensor surfaces. Gout can be differentiated from pseudogout by the presence of calcium pyrophosphate crystals, involvement of large joints, and secondary osteoarthritis. Laboratory findings during an acute attack show elevated serum uric acid levels, ESR, and WBC levels. The joint may be aspirated for fluid to observe uric acid crystals and cultured to exclude septic arthritis.

MUSCULOSKELETAL PAIN RELATED TO TRAUMA OR OVERUSE

Shoulder

Dislocation (glenohumeral joint instability)

A patient with shoulder dislocation presents with anterior and/or posterior joint pain, periarticular muscle spasm, anxiety, and limited movement. An anterior dislocation causes inability to internally rotate and abduct the humerus. Posterior dislocation causes limitation of external rotation, arm abduction, and hand supination with the shoulder flexed forward. X-rays of the shoulder (anteroposterior, lateral, and axillary views) will exclude fracture of surrounding bones.

Acromioclavicular (AC) joint injury

AC joint injuries usually result from sports injuries or motor vehicle accidents. Injury occurs when the acromion, scapula, and upper extremity are driven inferiorly, and the supporting ligamentous structures are sprained or torn. The severity of injury is classified into three grades: partial tear (dislocation) of the AC ligament (I), partial tear of the AC and coracoclavicular (CC) ligament (II), and complete rupture of the AC and CC ligaments and joint separation (III). History will reveal the nature of the injury. The patient will have pain and limited shoulder movement and may present with obvious deformity if there is a severe injury.

Bicipital tendinitis

Bicipital tendinitis is an overuse syndrome of the biceps brachii muscle, which ends in two tendons, one attached to the radial tuberosity (arm adduction) and one to the forearm fascia (arm abduction and internal rotation). The syndrome may be associated with other shoulder disorders, such as impingement syndrome. Children may have anomalies of the intertubercular groove, and younger individuals report repeated trauma from swimming, volleyball, baseball, or golf. Pain is localized to the intertubercular groove, is aggravated by the offending movement, and subsides with rest. Yergason's test can indicate bicipital tendinitis. A positive test is characterized by pain in the intertubercular groove with resistance to supination of the forearm while the elbow is flexed 90 degrees. A Fisk x-ray view enables the examiner to determine the size of the intertubercular groove.

Rotator cuff tear

Rotator cuff tears are acute injuries in children and young adults but occur as chronic injuries in older adults. In acute tears, the shoulder pain is severe, and the patient is unable to raise the arm sideways because of pain. In a complete tear, attempts to raise the arm laterally will produce a shoulder shrug. In a partial tear, the patient can raise the arm but cannot maintain the position with any resistance. Inflammation secondary to injury can cause rotator cuff tendinitis that produces shoulder pain, weakness, and a grating sound with movement.

Chronic rotator cuff tears are most common in persons over 50 years of age, the result of cumulative and repeated impingement processes. The onset of pain is insidious and is made worse with the arm in an overhead position. Patients experience shoulder pain with sleep and tenderness over the AC joint. Examination may reveal minimal restriction in movement, crepitus, and weakness in external rotation of the shoulder. X-rays will reveal any bony abnormality such as an acromial spur.

Elbow

Olecranon bursitis

Olecranon bursitis is commonly seen in patients who engage in contact sports, repetitive motion, rubbing or pressure to the elbow, or overuse. Pain is localized over the bursae, and swelling may be the result of hemorrhage in a traumatic injury. Range of joint motion is usually normal. The joint may be warm and red. When these signs are present, carefully examine the skin over the elbow to ensure intactness, because a penetrating injury may cause a septic bursitis. Radiography will exclude underlying bone infection and show the plane of soft tissue swelling.

Lateral humeral epicondylitis (tennis elbow)

Epicondylitis is an aseptic inflammation of the bone-tendon junction, resulting from repetitive concentric contractions that transmit force via the muscles to the origin on the lateral epicondyle. Persons most at risk for tennis elbow are the nonathletes who have occupations that require repeated contractions of extensor and supinator muscles. Athletes at risk are tennis players, bowlers, and hockey players. Patients present with gradual onset of pain and tenderness over the lateral epicondyle, that progresses in intensity. Palpation over the lateral epicondyle produces point tenderness although elbow movement is not limited. Resisted forearm supination with the elbow flexed at 90 degrees will intensify symptoms.

Wrist and Hand

Wrist fracture

Wrist fractures usually are the result of falling on an outstretched hand and may involve a number of types of fracture. Patients present with a painful, swollen distal forearm and wrist and may complain of numbness if the median nerve is involved. Gently palpate to locate the site of maximal pain, particularly the navicular ("snuffbox") area located between the extensor pollicis longus and the extensor pollicis brevis tendons when the mechanism of injury is hyperextension of the wrist. Pain localized here indicates a scaphoid (navicular) fracture. Assess pulses, pain sensation, and motor function (range and strength). X-ray views (PA, lateral, and oblique) will reveal the bone involved. In a Colles' fracture, the distal radius is displaced dorsally and shows up as a "silver fork" deformity on lateral view x-ray.

Finger fracture

The most common fractures of the fingers are those of the metacarpals and phalanges, commonly seen in sports injuries. Older persons usually sustain fractures as a result of falls. Correct diagnosis of a fractured finger is important in preventing long-term disability of use. Patients will present with a history of trauma or injury. Physical examination includes assessment of vascular and neurological function, tenderness and swelling, range of motion of each joint, and signs of joint instability or deformity. Three x-ray views (PA, lateral, and oblique) are needed for a complete evaluation.

Ganglion

Ganglions are cysts that contain a gelatinous fluid formed by outpouching of a joint capsule or tendon sheath. They most often occur on the dorsum of the wrist. A ganglion can be distinguished from a tumor by its soft consistency and transillumination.

Hip

Slipped capital femoral epiphysis

In children undergoing a rapid growth spurt, the onset of knee pain, an antalgic limp, and leg weakness may indicate slipped capital femoral epihysis (SCFE). Pain may be of several weeks' or months' duration and is exaggerated by strenuous physical activity. Examine the child in a prone position and assess the symmetry of medial rotation of the hip. A reduction of medial rotation may indicate SCFE. A widening of the epiphyseal plate can be visualized in a lateral view x-ray.

Transient synovitis of the hip

A nonspecific inflammatory condition of the hip, transient synovitis is the most common cause of a painful hip in children less than 10 years of age. History may reveal a recent upper respiratory infection or minor injury. The child complains of pain in the anteromedial aspect of the thigh and knee and walks with an antalgic limp; there is tenderness on palpation over the anterior aspect of the hip joint. Movement of the hip causes pain and is limited. There may be a low-grade fever. Ultrasound should be used for diagnosis, comparing it to the good hip. WBC is usually normal although the ESR may be elevated.

Legg-Calve-Perthes disease

This disease occurs as osteochondritis of the femoral head epiphysis and is characterized by a period of avascular necrosis of the femoral head, followed by revascularization and bone healing. It occurs most commonly in boys between the ages of 3 and 11 years. The child has groin or medial thigh pain and a limp. The pain may be recurring, and the child may have been limping for several months. The loss of medial hip motion is an early sign. There is a high incidence of hernia, undescended testicles, and kidney abnormalities in children with this condition. X-rays show the ossific nucleus of the femoral head combined with the widened articular cartilage space compared with the opposite hip.

Iliopsoas tendinitis

This tendinitis is caused by frequent repetitive flexions of the hip joint and is common in weight lifters, oarsmen, and football players. The patient complains of mildly intense groin pain on the anterior hip, which worsens with movement. An acute injury involves forced extension of a flexed leg, and, in younger age groups, x-ray evaluation is done if evulsion of the epiphysis is suspected. Test for iliopsoas tendinitis by having the seated patient place the heel of the affected leg on the knee of the other leg. This movement will create pain and a tense iliopsoas muscle.

Knee

Chondromalacia patellae

Chondromalacia of the patella is a change in the patellofemoral joint cartilage, which most often occurs in adolescent females. The condition can be caused by trauma, anatomical anomalies, and mis-alignment of the patella. Softening of joint cartilage, tufts of patellar cartilage, fissures, or ulcers occur. Patients present with anterior knee pain that is worse while climbing stairs or biking. X-ray studies of the knee, including tangential and sunrise views, show irregularities of the patellofemoral joint.

Patellar tendinitis (jumper's knee)

This overuse syndrome is characterized by inflammation in the distal extensors of the knee joint. Patellar tendinitis is more common in athletes who habitually place excessive strain on their knees from jumping or running. Determine the quadriceps (Q) angle by measuring the angle between the center of the patella to the anterior superior iliac spine and from the center patella to the tibial tubercle. An angle greater than 10 degrees in males and 15 degrees in females suggests patellar tendinitis. Persons affected complain of dull, achy knee pain that may have associated clicking or popping. Associated malalignment from femoral anteversion or ankle varus may be present.

Medial collateral ligament sprain

Medial collateral ligament injuries are common and are the result of valgus stress to the knee. The patient limps soon after the injury and may or may not have pain. On physical examination, there is mild effusion and point tenderness over the medial collateral ligament. To test for stability of the medial collateral ligaments, the knee is flexed about 30 degrees with the patient supine, and one hand is placed over the lateral knee with the other around the ankle. Apply medial pressure to the knee while pulling the ankle outward. An instability of the medial collateral ligament produces a sensation of opening the medial aspect of the joint. Apply lateral pressure in the same knee position tests for lateral ligament sprain. An x-ray is done to rule out fracture.

Medial meniscus tear

Medial meniscus injuries, more common than lateral meniscus injuries, occur after a twisting injury to the knee. The patient has pain, difficulty flexing the knee, and difficulty bearing weight. There is often a clicking or catching in the knee joint, and the joint may be swollen and tender. To examine for medial meniscus injury, perform the McMurray test to assess for clicking, locking, or a springy end point of motion. With the patient supine, place one hand under the heel and flex the knee 90 degrees with slight abduction. Apply a lateral and medial force to the knee while extending and adducting it. A palpable or audible click indicates medial meniscus injury.

Anterior cruciate ligament (ACL) tear

Ligaments may be stretched or torn if the knee is twisted or hyperextended. The ACL, located in the center of the knee, is one of the most common ligaments damaged in knee injuries. An ACL injury is often associated with an audible pop and a giving-away sensation in the knee, often with swelling from hemarthrosis. Physical examination reveals a positive Lachman's test. With the patient supine and the knee flexed 20 to 30 degrees, anchor the patient's foot to the table, then pull the tibia forward. Anterior motion is a sensitive test for ACL laxity.

Osgood-Schlatter disease

This condition, most common in adolescent males, is a painful swelling of the anterior aspect of the tibial tubercle. It is caused by strenuous activity, especially of the quadriceps muscles. The patient will often limp, and the pain will be worse with activities such as stair climbing and kneeling. Examination will reveal a warm, swollen, tender tibial tubercle, and flexion and extension will increase pain intensity. Joint examination of the knee is normal.

Baker's cyst (popliteal cyst)

A popliteal cyst occurs when fluid from the knee joint enters the connecting bursa and becomes trapped. Patients complain of a fullness or swelling of the posterior knee and calf pain aggravated by walking and alleviated by rest. Examination of the knee focuses on assessment of a change in consistency of the mass on extension (hardening) and flexion (softening), called Foucher's sign. Foucher's sign is negative with a Baker's cyst and positive with a tumor or popliteal aneurysm. The cyst can rupture and cause edema and tenderness of the lower extremity with a positive Homan's sign. Ultrasound will detect the cyst or recently ruptured cyst.

Ankle and Foot

Ankle sprain (inversion or eversion)

The most common mechanism of ankle injury is an inversion force that stresses the lateral ligamentous support of the joint. The lateral ligaments are of greater length than the medial ligaments and are more predisposed to injury. An audible pop or tear implies a rupture or tear of the ligament. Swelling of the ankle within minutes of injury indicates bleeding and soft tissue trauma. Patients with a ligamentous injury will generally be able to walk and bear weight on the injured foot, even though it may be uncomfortable. Examine the injured joint by palpating the course and attachment points of the ligaments and perform joint range of motion (ROM) to test for ligamentous integrity.

Shin splints (medial tibial stress syndrome)

Shin splints are an inflammation of the origin of muscles on the shaft of the tibia caused by overuse, often by running athletes. Patients report achy pain and tenderness over the medial tibia that increases with exercise, especially running, and improves with rest. An x-ray of the tibia will exclude fracture.

Achilles tendinitis

The gastrocnemius and soleus muscles conjoin to form the Achilles tendon. Inflammation of this tendon creates pain and swelling where the tendon inserts into the calcaneus, and a patient will report a tightness of the tendon that makes walking or running difficult. Tendinitis may be caused by overuse, especially running, or by decreased vascularity to the tendon sheath. Examination reveals tenderness over the Achilles tendon with palpation and ankle

ROM especially with dorsiflexion, crepitus over the tendon with motion, and weakness of the calf muscles.

Plantar faciitis

Plantar faciitis is caused by chronic weight-bearing stress when laxity of foot structures allows the talus to slide forward and medially, the calcaneus to drop, and plantar ligaments and fascia to stretch. Persons who are obese or who engage in excessive standing are at greatest risk. Tendons and joints become inflamed, and muscles spasm because of the misalignment of structures. Patients often complain of aching feet.

MUSCLE PAIN (MYALGIA)

Viral Infections

Viral infections can produce diffuse myalgias that are usually associated with fever, chills, upper respiratory symptoms, and malaise. A patient with influenza will have intense myalgia, high fever, and appear quite ill. Since viral illnesses are highly contagious, epidemics in both children and adults in a community may be a useful clue to diagnosis. A paraviral IgM titer is diagnostic of an acute parvovirus B19 infection.

Psychogenic

Pain that is diffuse, varies in pattern, and is unaffected by activity or rest may be psychogenic in origin. A careful history may reveal any secondary gain the patient may derive from the pain and suggest the presence of an anxiety or depression disorder. On examination, the patient may display facial expressions and descriptions of discomfort to palpation and movement that are inconsistent. This diagnosis involves excluding other causes.

Fibromyalgia

Fibromyalgia is a syndrome characterized by chronic fatigue, generalized musculoskeletal pain, and multiple trigger points of pain on physical examination. It affects primarily women between 20 to 50 years of age. Other symptoms associated with this syndrome include stage IV sleep disturbance, anxiety or depression, obsessive-compulsive behavior, and irritable bowel syndrome. Symptoms are exacerbated by stress.

SYSTEMIC DISORDERS

Acute Leukemia

Leukemia is the most common cancer in children, and bone and joint pain is the most common presenting complaint. The bone pain is diffuse, nonspecific, and may extend to adjacent joints. Laboratory findings may show the white blood count as elevated, depressed, or normal. Severe anemia is common as is a depressed platelet count. X-rays of the limb at the distal end of the femur and the proximal end of the tibia show abnormal areas of radiolucency.

Sickle Cell Disease

Sickle cell disease is a genetic disorder characterized by production of hemoglobin S, an anemia secondary to short erythrocyte survival, and sickle-shaped erythrocytes. It affects mainly African-American, Mediterranean, and Southeast Asian population groups. Sickle cell disease manifests itself after the first 6 months of life. The child presents with painful or vaso-occlusive crises characterized by symmetrical, painful swelling of the hands and feet. Older persons report pain in long bones and joints, abdominal pain, decreased appetite, fever, and malaise. The laboratory findings reveal a hemoglobin S genotype and anemia, but findings can vary depending on the hemoglobin genotype, age, gender, and presence of other organ involvement.

Systemic Lupus Erythematosus (SLE)

SLE is a systemic inflammatory condition that occurs most often in women. It is characterized by arthritis that commonly involves the small joints of the hands, wrists, ankles, and knees as well as malar rash, oral ulcers, glomerulonephritis, hematological disorders, and psychological symptoms. The pain is transient but severe. Laboratory findings show leukopenia with neutrophils predominating the peripheral count, and the ANA is positive.

Lyme Arthritis

The bite of the deer tick transmits the spirochete *Borrelia burgdorferi*. Patients may not recall a tick bite but will have been in an endemic area. The presenting complaint in Lyme disease is diffuse joint pain and swelling, a target-like skin rash (erythema migrans), fever, and chills. These symptoms may be present for weeks before the spirochete spreads via blood and lymph tissue to the myocardium and central nervous system. A chronic arthritis may appear months after the initial infection. The arthritis is asymmetrical and occurs in the large joints. The knee is a commonly affected joint. The patient has an antalgic limp with diffuse swelling and warmth of the knee joint anteriorly as well as local synovial thickening. Laboratory diagnosis reveals elevation of IgM titers and IgG antibodies against the spirochete. The ESR is elevated.

Neuroblastoma

Neuroblastoma is a malignant tumor that usually occurs in children under 5 years of age. It originates from cells in the sympathetic ganglia and adrenal medulla but can arise from any part of the sympathetic nervous system and metastasize to the bone. The presenting complaint may be varied, but bone pain, limp, pallor, and fatigue may be present. CT or MRI identify the primary location of the tumor. In the urine, 3-methoxy-4-hydroxymandelic acid and homovanillic acid levels are elevated.

Osteogenic Sarcoma

Osteogenic sarcoma is a tumor that occurs in persons 10 to 25 years old, with the most common site being the lower end of the femur or the upper end of the tibia. The patient initially complains of local intermittent pain that quickly progresses to a constant and severe pain, and an antalgic limp may develop. Palpation reveals tenderness over the area affected. Laboratory findings show an increase in serum alkaline phosphatase level; x-ray shows a "sunburst" image.

NERVE ENTRAPMENT SYNDROMES

Thoracic Outlet Syndrome (TOS)

TOS is the result of compression of nerve and vascular structures in the neck area. Arterial compression creates pallor and decreased pulses and weakness, with eventual skin and nail atrophy in the affected extremity. Nerve compression creates paresthesias, dysesthesias, and pain. History may reveal that the patient sleeps with the arm extended against the head, causing morning symptoms of pain and paresthesias. Reaching, working with the arm raised, and lifting exacerbate pain. Other risk factors include a rounded, sagging shoulder posture and shoulder muscle deformities. A common compression occurs with the cervical rib compressing the subclavian artery. A bruit may be heard over the supraclavicular fossa. EMG studies help to delineate the specific nerve involvement; however, they may not identify the vascular involvement.

Carpal Tunnel Syndrome

Carpal tunnel syndrome involves entrapment of the median nerve in the dominant hand, resulting from repeated strain that causes thickening of the flexor tendon sheath. A dull, achy pain is felt across the wrist and forearm with paraesthesia, weakness, or clumsiness of the hand; atrophy; dry skin; and skin color changes of the hand secondary to impaired nerve innervation. Symptoms are often worse at night. History reveals repetitive activity of the upper extremity. It most often occurs in women and in persons over 30 years. Examination reveals dry skin on the thumb, index, and middle finger (median nerve distribution). Thenar atrophy may be present. Tinel's sign and Phalen's test are positive (Table 9-2).

Peroneal Nerve Compression

Peroneal nerve compression can be caused by a cast, sports injury, or trauma. Pain is felt across the head of the fibula and can result in foot drop.

Tarsal Tunnel Syndrome

The posterior tibial nerve is involved, and pain is felt across the ankle and proximal foot. Tarsal tunnel syndrome is occasionally associated with motor weakness of the proximal toe flexors. Patients may not remember a specific onset but report pain and weakness of the foot muscles. Tapping

the posterior tibial nerve posterior and inferior to the medial malleolus elicits pain. Ask the patient about shoe fit and use of any orthotic devices.

Neuritis

Vascular metabolism affected by systemic disorders such as diabetes mellitus can cause a nerve to become ischemic, producing toxins that can directly damage the nerve. Inflammation can be of the nerve axon, myelin sheath, or both, Soft tissue inflammation contributing to neuropathy can be caused by collagen disorders (SLE, scleroderma).

Diabetes mellitus is commonly associated with sensory peripheral neuropathy and results in pain and sensory loss that is more intense in the lower extremities.

Alcoholism is associated with distal, demyelinating neuropathy that may resolve with cessation of alcohol ingestion.

Text continued on p. 354

Table 9-2

Selected Tests Used to Assess for Musculoskeletal Disorders

TEST	DESCRIPTION	FINDINGS
Wrist		
Finkelstein's test	Have patient flex fingers over a clenched thumb, then passively deviate the wrist ulnarly	Movement produces pain in de Quervain's syndrome (first dorsal compartment tenosynovitis)
Tinel's sign	Tap over the median nerve (palmar surface of the wrist) to assess for compression neuropathy	In a positive test, the patient reports a tingling or prickling sensation distal to the site tapped along the first three digits, wrist pain, and weak grip
Phalen's test	Ask the patient to maintain palmar flexion for 1 minute with the dorsal surfaces of each hand pressed together	Test is positive if the maneuver produces numbness and paraesthesia in fingers innervated by the median, by compressing the nerve
Knee		
Bulge sign	Apply lateral pressure to the area adjacent to the patella	Medial bulge will appear if fluid is in the knee joint

Table 9-2

Selected Tests Used to Assess for Musculoskeletal Disorders—cont'd

TEST	DESCRIPTION	FINDINGS
Knee—cont'd		
Drawer sign	With the patient supine, flex the knee 90 degrees and the hip 45 degrees with the foot on the table; apply a slow, steady, anterior pull, and in the same position gently push the tibia back	Tests for cruciate ligament stability; abnormal anterior or posterior movement of the tibia on the femur is a positive drawer sign and indicates ligamentous instability
McMurray's maneuver	With the patient supine, maximally flex the knee and hip; externally and internally rotate the tibia with one hand on the distal end of the tibia; with the other hand, palpate the joint	Pain and a palpable or audible click is a positive finding and indicates a meniscus injury
	Extend the knee with slight lateral pressure with the tibia internally rotated	Positive finding in this position indicates a lateral meniscus injury
	Extend the knee with slight internal pressure on the tibia externally rotated	Positive finding in this position indicates a medial meniscus injury
Collateral ligament test	Apply medial or lateral pressure when the knee is flexed at 30 degrees and when it is extended	Medial or lateral collateral ligament sprain will show laxity in movement and no solid end points depending on the degree of sprain
Lachman's test (cruciate ligaments)	With the knee flexed 30 degrees, pull the tibia forward with one hand while the other hand stabilizes the femur	Positive test is a mushy or soft end feel when the tibia is moved forward, indicating damage to the anterior cruciate ligament

Table 9-3

Differential Diagnosis of Common Causes of Limb Pain

Condition	History	Physical Findings	Diagnostic Studies
Musculoskeletal Inflammation			
Tenosynovitis (tendinitis)	Repetitive trauma activities; pain with movement	Swelling over tendon, crepitus	None

Continued

Table 9-3

Differential Diagnosis of Common Causes of Limb Pain—cont'd

Condition	History	Physical Findings	Diagnostic Studies
Musculoskeletal Inflammation—cont'd			
Bursitis	History of overuse; aching pain over affected bursae that radiates along the limb	Local tenderness, swelling, limited joint motion, muscle weakness	None
Fibrositis	Pain in trigger sites throughout the body, joint stiffness, disturbed sleep	Fatty, fibrous nodules in muscles, palpation of trigger points elicits pain	None
Osteomyelitis	Presentation depends on age, location of infection; history of infection, trauma, penetration, invasive procedure; refusal to bear weight (hip); constant pain	Fever, chills, vomiting, pain localized over affected area but progressively worsens; soft tissue injury or abscess	Increased WBC, ESR, C reactive protein; x-rays
Joint Inflammation			
Osteoarthritis	Older adults, asymmetrical joint pain and stiffness that improves throughout the day, history of repetitive joint trauma, obesity	DIP, PIP joints enlarged, Heberden's nodes, limited cervical spine ROM	ESR; x-ray may reveal osteophytes, loss of joint space
Rheumatoid arthritis	Morning stiffness of small joints, symmetrical involvement, anorexia, weight loss	Fever, rheumatoid nodules, ulnar deviation of wrists	Increased ESR, positive rheumatoid factor, anemia on CBC, x-ray shows bony erosion
Juvenile rheumatoid arthritis	Fatigue, weight loss, failure to thrive, refusal to walk, joint pain and stiffness	Fever, rash, guarding of joints, limited ROM; joint swelling, nodules	Elevated WBC, ESR; positive rheumatoid factor and antinuclear antibody

Table 9-3

Differential Diagnosis of Common Causes of Limb Pain—cont'd

Condition	History	Physical Findings	Diagnostic Studies
Joint Inflammation—cont'd			
Septic arthritis	History of systemic infection, malaise, diaphoresis, refusal to bear weight (hip), acute joint pain	Fever, red, swollen joint, limited range of motion	WBC, culture of joint aspirate, ESR, C-reactive protein, ultrasound of joint
Gout	Acute pain of large joint, asymmetrical, males over 30 years, history of gout	Inflamed, swollen joint, tophi, sodium urate crystals	Increased serum uric acid level, ESR, WBC
Musculoskeletal Pain Related to Trauma or Overuse			
Shoulder dislocation	History of trauma, pain	Limited rotation, arm abduction and hand supination	X-ray of shoulder
Acromioclavicular joint injury	History of trauma, pain	Limited shoulder movement; obvious deformity	X-ray of shoulder
Bicipital tendinitis	History of overuse of biceps; pain worse with movement	Positive Yergason's test; pain localized over the intertubercular groove	X-ray (Fisk view)
Rotator cuff tear	Acute: younger persons, history of trauma, severe pain; chronic: older, pain worse with overhead movement, sleep disturbance	Acute: inability to raise arm sideways, shrug shoulders; chronic: tenderness over the AC joint, crepitus, weakness in external shoulder rotation	X-ray may reveal humeral displacement or spurs
Olecranon bursitis	Repetitive motion of or pressure to the elbow, localized pain	Warmth, redness and swelling over joint, full ROM	X-ray to rule out fracture of the olecranon process
Lateral humeral epicondylitis	History of repetitive contraction of extensor and supinator muscles, pain over lateral epicondyle that progresses	Tenderness over lateral epicondyle; palpation produces pain, motion does not; supination against resistance worsens pain	None

Continued

Table 9-3

Differential Diagnosis of Common Causes of Limb Pain—cont'd

Condition	History	Physical Findings	Diagnostic Studies
Musculoskeletal Pain Related to Trauma or Overuse—cont'd			
Wrist fracture	History of fall on an outstretched hand, pain and swelling of forearm and wrist	Palpation of snuff-box increases pain; observe for joint deformity	Three-view x-rays to determine scaphoid or Colles' fracture
Finger fracture	History of trauma or fall, joint tenderness	Joint swelling, instability	Three-view x-rays (PA, lateral, and oblique)
Ganglion	Noticeable lump on dorsal surface of wrist	Gelatinous filled nodule, soft, transilluminates	None
Slipped capital femoral epiphysis	Children during rapid growth spurts, knee pain worse with activity	Limitation of medial hip rotation, limp	X-ray of epiphyseal plate
Transient synovitis of the hip	Children less than 10 years, history of upper respiratory infection, limp, pain in the anteromedial thigh and knee	Tenderness on palpation over anterior hip; hip movement increases pain and is limited; low-grade fever.	Ultrasound, ESR
Legg-Calve-Perthes disease	Boys 3-11 years, groin or medial thigh pain, limp	Decreased hip ROM	AP and frog lateral x-rays of the hip; LCPD may show increased density of the femoral head
Iliopsoas tendinitis	History of repetitive flexion of hip; pain worse with movement	With patient sitting, place the heel of affected leg on the knee of the other: test is positive if pain is elicited	None
Chondromalacia patellae	Adolescent females; history of knee trauma or misalignment, knee pain worse with activity	Tenderness to palpation over knee	Four-view x-rays of knees to rule out arthritis

Table 9-3

Differential Diagnosis of Common Causes of Limb Pain—cont'd

Condition	History	Physical Findings	Diagnostic Studies
Musculoskeletal Pain Related to Trauma or Overuse—cont'd			
Patellar tendinitis	History of overuse, especially running or jumping; dull, achy knee pain; click	Q angle greater than 10 degrees in males, 15 degrees in females, clicking or popping with knee movement	None
Medial collateral ligament sprain	History of valgus stress to knee; limp; pain	Effusion and point tenderness over knee; valgus and varus pressure to assess instability	AP and lateral x-rays may reveal a ligament avulsion of femoral origin
Medical meniscus tear	History of twisting injury to the knee, pain, difficulty flexing, bearing weight, clicking or catching of knee with movement	Positive McMurray's test, clicking or locking during joint movement	Four-view knee x-rays to rule out bony abnormality
Anterior cruciate ligament tear	History of twisting or extension knee injury; audible "pop"	Swelling; positive Lachman's test	X-ray to rule out fracture
Osgood-Schlatter disease	Adolescent males, knee pain and swelling aggravated by activity, limp	Tenderness, warmth, swelling over anterior tibial tubercle	X-ray with knee rotated inward may show soft tissue swelling
Baker's cyst	Fullness or swelling of posterior knee, aggravated by walking	Negative Foucher's sign; normal joint exam; positive Homan's sign in ruptured cyst	None
Ankle sprain	History of inversion stress with audible pop, immediate swelling	Swelling, soft tissue trauma, able to perform active ROM with ligament sprain	X-ray needed only with tenderness over the lateral malleolus to rule out fracture

Continued

Table 9-3

Differential Diagnosis of Common Causes of Limb Pain—cont'd

Condition	History	Physical Findings	Diagnostic Studies
Musculoskeletal Pain Related to Trauma or Overuse—cont'd			
Shin splints	Ache or pain over medial tibia that is worse with exercise, history of running	Tenderness over medial tibia	AP and lateral x-rays may show a stress fracture; a bone scan will be positive with increased uptake along the medial tibia
Achilles tendinitis	Pain and tightness over Achilles tendon, especially with walking or running	Tenderness over Achilles tendon; pain worse with dorsiflexion of ankle, calf weakness	Lateral ankle x-ray reveals enlarged posterosuperior tuberosity of the calcaneus
Plantar faciitis	History of chronic weight bearing, aching feet, muscle spasms, obesity	Misalignment of foot structures, especially talus, calcaneus, and plantar ligaments	None
Muscle Pain (Myalgia)			
Viral infections	History of upper respiratory infection, malaise, chills, cold symptoms, general muscle aches	Fever, ill-appearing adult or child	Viral serum titer
Psychogenic	Pain is diffuse, varies in pattern of activity, setting; history of depression or anxiety	Normal exam or patient response to exam maneuvers disproportionate to physical findings or subjective complaints	None
Fibromyalgia	Female 20-50 years, history of depression, sleep disturbance, chronic fatigue, general muscle and joint aches	Palpation of trigger points will produce pain; normal physical exam	None
Systemic Disorders			
Acute leukemia	Hip pain in children, refusal to walk	Fever, hepatosplenomegaly, bruising	CBC

Table 9-3

Differential Diagnosis of Common Causes of Limb Pain—cont'd

Condition	History	Physical Findings	Diagnostic Studies
Systemic Disorders—cont'd			
Sickle cell disease	African-American, family history; appears after 6 months of age; acute pain with swelling of hands and feet, abdominal pain, decreased appetite, malaise	Normal exam	Hemoglobin S genotype
Systemic lupus erythematosus	Female, transient arthritis of small joints, malar rash	Normal exam, may have joint tenderness on palpation	Kidney function tests, antinuclear antibody, CBC
Lyme arthritis	History of exposure to endemic areas of the deer tick, chills, diffuse joint pain and swelling, often the knee is affected	Asymmetrical swelling, warmth of joint, erythema migrans, may have myocardial involvement	Serum IgM and IgG antibodies, ESR
Neuroblastoma	Under 5 years, pain in bones	Unexplained fever	Urine for vanillylmandelic or homovanillic acid; CT scan
Osteogenic sarcoma	Persons 10 to 25 years, intermittent pain of lower femur, upper tibia, limp	Tenderness over affected area	X-ray, serum alkaline phosphatase
Nerve Entrapment Syndromes			
Thoracic outlet syndrome	History of sleeping with arm against head, morning shoulder pain, pain worse with lifting, paresthesia; rounded shoulder posture	Bruit over supraclavicular fossa; pallor, decreased pulses of upper extremity, weakness, skin and nail atrophy	EMG

Continued

Table 9-3

≣ **Differential Diagnosis of Common Causes of Limb Pain—cont'd**

Condition	History	Physical Findings	Diagnostic Studies
Nerve Entrapment Syndromes—cont'd			
Carpal tunnel syndrome	History of repetitive upper extremity motion; paresthesia, weakness, or clumsiness of hand; symptoms worse at night	Positive Phalen's and Tinel's sign, weakness of hand, dry skin over distribution of median nerve	None
Peroneal nerve compression	History of pressure to the knee from a cast, sports injury, or trauma; pain over head of fibula; clumsy gait	Unilateral foot drop	None
Tarsal tunnel syndrome	Pain in ankle and proximal foot, weakness of toe flexors, ill-fitting shoes	Tapping posterior tibial nerve elicits pain	None
Neuritis	Pain and sensory loss, usually of lower extremities; history of alcohol ingestion, diabetes	Decreased sensory and pain sensation	Liver function tests, hemoglobin A1C to rule out diabetes

≣ Acute Low Back Pain

A report of acute low back pain, although quite common, requires a thorough evaluation. The underlying pathophysiology of back pain is frequently multifactorial and includes both physiological and psychological components. About 90% of acute low back pain (ALBP) episodes in adults are related to mechanical causes that resolve within 4 weeks without serious sequelae. A smaller percentage of patients will continue to have chronic symptoms without organic pathology or will have un-derlying disease. In children, the prevalence of back pain increases with age and with involvement in sports. Anthropomorphic variations in children place them at risk for excess strain on the spine, producing back pain. These variations include reduced hip mobility, decreased lumbar extension and increased lumbar flexion, poor abdominal muscle strength, tight hamstring muscles, and lumbar hyperlordosis.

ALBP is defined as activity intolerance producing lower back or back-related leg symptoms of less than 3 months' duration. The Agency for Health Care Policy and Research (AHCPR) Guidelines provide

Nerve root	L4	L5	S1
Pain			
Numbness			
Motor weakness	Extension of quadriceps	Dorsiflexion of great toe and foot	Plantar flexion of great toe and foot
Screening exam	Squat and rise	Heel walking	Walking on toes
Reflexes	Knee jerk diminished	None reliable	Ankle jerk diminished

Figure 9-1   Testing for lumbar nerve root compromise. (From Bigos S, Bowyer O, Braen G et al: Acute low back problems in adults, *Clinical Practice Guidelines, Quick Reference Guide Number 14,* Rockville, MD, 1994, Department of Health and Human Services, Public Health Service, Agency for Health Care Policy and Research, AHCPR Pub. No. 95-0643.)

the following framework for causes of ALBP:

- Potentially serious conditions (spinal fracture, tumor or infection, or cauda equina syndrome)
- Sciatica, or leg pain and numbness of the lateral thigh, leg, and foot, suggesting nerve root compression (Figure 9-1)
- Non-specific back problems such as musculoskeletal strain, diskogenic pain, or bony deformity secondary to inflammatory disease
- Non-spinal causes secondary to abdominal involvement (gallbladder, liver, renal, pelvic inflammatory disease; prostate tumor; ovarian

cyst; uterine fibroids; aortic aneurysm; or thoracic disease)
- Psychological causes such as stress, work environment (disability, workmen's compensation, secondary gains)

When evaluating ALBP, the goals of the clinician are first to identify signs of potentially serious conditions through a careful history and physical examination. A holistic approach to the patient is needed to appreciate the extent to pain impacts the patient's daily routine or work-related activities. Because ALBP is a common occupational-related complaint and a cause of disability and lost productivity, the clinician needs to gain insight into the psychosocial and economic situation of the patient to help arrive at a correct diagnosis.

DIAGNOSTIC REASONING: FOCUSED HISTORY

What does the location of pain tell me?

Key Question
- Where does your back hurt?

Location of pain. In general, children are less specific than adults when describing location of pain. Traumatic lesions are more likely to occur in the cervical and lumbar portions of the spine where there is more motion and less protection. Generalized pain or pain over a fairly wide anatomical area is frequently seen with overuse problems and inflammatory conditions.

Back pain with neck stiffness can indicate cervical osteomyelitis. Rheumatoid arthritis produces pain in the upper back and neck. Localized pain is seen with spondylolysis and tumors. Flank pain in adults may indicate a kidney infection. Pain of gallbladder disease radiates to the subscapular areas. Compression fractures of vertebrae associated with osteoporosis may produce pain over the spinal area affected, often the midthoracic area.

Children with traumatic low back derangement will have pain and muscle spasm in the lumbar area from the pressure and shock of an impact injury collision.

Cervical spine fractures are caused by a load that exceeds the strength of the cervical spine during flexion, extension, compression, rotation, or a combination of forces.

What does the pattern of pain tell me?

Key Questions
- When did the pain start?
- How long have you had this pain?
- What does the pain feel like?

- Does it interfere with sleep?
- Have you had this pain before?

Onset. The onset of ALBP is sudden, and over half of patients with this symptom do not associate it with a specific precipitating event or injury. The vast majority of cases of ALBP resolve with conservative treatment in 4 weeks, and x-ray or further diagnostic studies are not recommended until then.

Children are frequently poor historians and parents may have a difficult time remembering when the pain started. Association with events such as birthdays, holidays, and activities is helpful in establishing the onset of the pain. Pain that is fleeting or mild and of a short duration (1 to 2 weeks) is rarely serious and can be observed for a period of time.

Back pain of greater than 4 weeks needs to be re-evaluated for further diagnostic studies.

Duration. Chronic back pain is pain of greater than 3 months' duration. In persons under 40 years of age, the cause may be postural or may indicate congenital spinal deformity (such as scoliosis) or ankylosing spondylitis. In older persons, chronic back pain is more likely to indicate degenerative disease. In children, back pain present for more than 3 weeks is often due to organic and serious causes.

Pain characteristics. In children, expression of pain depends on the child's ability to put feelings of pain into behavior; observing for these behaviors is important. Ask children to rate the pain using a pain scale from 1 to 10 or use happy to sad faces rated from 0 to 5. Ask adults to rate pain from 0 (no pain) to 10 (worst pain ever) and assess how much the pain interferes with daily activities. Intractable back pain, especially night pain with constitutional findings, is likely to indicate neoplastic disease. Painful scoliosis and stiffness are common presenting symptoms of a spinal tumor.

Night pain. Night pain is a worrisome symptom that often signals a serious problem such as tumor, infection, and inflammation. Generally, muscle pulls, overuse injuries, spondylolysis, spondylolisthesis, and Scheuermann's disease (an exaggeration of the normal posterior convex curvature of the thoracic spine) produce less pain at night. Morning stiffness that improves as the day progresses suggests ankylosing spondylitis.

Nighttime back pain is unusual and indicates the need for a complete and thorough workup.

Recurring pain. Back pain in young children who have had previous injuries or fractures may be a symptom of child abuse. In the older adult, it may be an indication of compression fractures of the spine. As with young children, it may also signal abuse by a caregiver.

What does the pain in relation to activity tell me?

Key Questions
- What makes the pain worse?
- What activities can't you do?
- What makes the pain better?
- Does the pain occur during certain movements after an activity?

Aggravating factors. Pain experienced in the lumbar area occurring after strenuous sporting activities is usually the result of macrotrauma to the muscles and tendons causing contusions and sprain. It occurs when the patient pushes the muscles and ligaments past the normal level of tolerance. Repeated injury can cause soft tissue scarring and shortening.

Stress and fatigue fractures of the pars interarticularis, the region between the superior and inferior articulating facets of the vertebra, occur when lumbar lordosis places more stress on the pars, such as in gymnastics and tennis.

Any child who has voluntarily given up a pleasurable activity because of back pain has a severe symptom.

Alleviating factors. Back pain not associated with any activity and not relieved by rest may indicate tumor. Back pain relieved with aspirin or non-steroidal antiinflammatory drugs in children may indicate osteoid osteoma, a benign tumor caused by a formation of an island of noncalcified matrix of young vascular osteoid surrounded by a margin of dense sclerotic bone.

Pain after activity. Suspect a spondylolisthesis, or forward slippage of one vertebrae over another, if the onset of pain is during hyperextension, such as with a back handspring, butterfly stroke in swimming, or a tennis serve. The defect arises from a stress fracture or stress reaction of the isthmus of the pars interarticularis in the area of L5-S1. The pain localizes to the low back and occurs during a growth spurt and after engaging in sporting events. The pain improves with rest and is worse with standing.

What does radiation of pain tell me?

Key Questions
- Does the pain travel?
- Show me where the pain travels.

Radiation of pain. Referred pain is of two types: (1) pain referred from the spine into areas lying within the lumbar and upper sacral dermatomes and (2) pain referred from the pelvic and abdominal viscera to the spine. Pain from the upper lumbar spine usually radiates to the anterior aspects of the thighs and legs and that of the lower lumbar spine radiates to the gluteal regions, posterior thighs, and calves.

Pain from visceral disease is usually felt within the abdomen or flanks. Persons with spondylolysis, a destruction of vertebral structure, or spondylolisthesis, an anterior displacement of a vertebrae, complain of hamstring tightness and buttock discomfort as well as low back pain.

Pain beginning in the back and radiating to the posterior thighs may indicate spondylolisthesis. The pain is a result of anterior displacement of the affected vertebra caused by a congenital defect in the pars interarticularis.

Is this back pain a potentially serious condition?

Key Questions

- What are your symptoms?
- Do you have control of your urine and bowels?
- Did you injure your back?
- When did this occur?

Potentially serious symptoms. Persons below 20 years and over 50 years of age are at increased risk for tumor as are those with a history of cancer. Constant LBP with saddle anesthesia, urinary retention, and fecal incontinence are symptoms of cauda equina syndrome, or compression of spinal (S1-S2) nerve roots, which is considered a surgical emergency. Children are embarrassed to talk about urinary or bowel habits and changes. Hidden spinal cord tumors might have a relationship to developmental delays in bladder and bowel control. Children under 4 years of age who have back pain should be evaluated for serious diseases, such as intraspinal tumors, dermoid cysts, and malignant astrocytomas.

History of injury. Injury to the back usually results in contusions and abrasions but can also cause spinal fracture if the force is major, such as that sustained in a motor vehicle accident or fall. In the elderly, an acute spinal fracture might result from strenuous lifting when osteoporosis is present. Injuries to the posterior structures of the spine account for most cases of low back pain in adolescents who are athletically active.

Injury to the spinal column should be suspected in anyone whose level of consciousness is impaired following an accident.

Are there signs of neurological damage?

Key Questions

- Have you been stumbling?
- Have you noticed any change in your balance or coordination?
- Does the child stumble or fall a lot?
- Do you have numbness or tingling in your extremities?

Stumbling. Spinal cord tumors such as astrocytoma or ependymoma may present as a disturbance of movement, posture, or strength in the spine or extremities. Impairment of proprioception or sensation from an upper motor neuron lesion, exhibited by foot drop or ataxia, may produce stumbling.

Numbness and tingling. Radiculopathy (nerve root pain) is sharp pain felt in a dermatomal pattern and is sometimes associated with numbness and tingling.

Is there a family history of back pain?

Key Question

- Does anyone in your family have scoliosis?

Family history. Spondylolysis and scoliosis are often seen in families, with a 40% familial occurrence in Alaskan Eskimos.

Could this pain be caused by a systemic disease?

Key Questions

- Have you been ill?
- Have you noticed any weight loss, fever, fatigue, skin rash, or joint pain?

Illness. Pharyngitis or upper respiratory infections such as pneumonia can be the precursor to diskitis in children. The intervertebral disk in children receives a blood supply from the surface of the adjacent vertebral bodies, providing the mechanism necessary for infection. Uveitis and iriditis may be associated with juvenile rheumatoid arthritis or juvenile ankylosing spondylitis.

Weight loss, fever, fatigue, skin rash, or joint pain. Infection is a likely diagnosis when there are chills and fever, weight loss, a recent history of bacterial infection, IV drug use, or in a person who is immunosuppressed. Ewing's sarcoma is a malignant tumor and can mimic spinal infection, occurring as back pain that can be accompanied by fever. Neuroblastoma is common in young children, and although it occurs in the abdomen, metastases to the spine may produce back pain. Children with diskitis will have a fever and refuse to walk because of back pain.

DIAGNOSTIC REASONING: FOCUSED PHYSICAL EXAMINATION

Observe the Patient's General Appearance

Any person appearing ill with a fever, limp, or unwillingness to walk are highly suspect for an infectious cause of back pain.

Observe for symmetry of posture and movement from a direct anterior, posterior, and lateral view of the patient. Note the amount of thoracic kyphosis (anteroposterior curve) and lumbar lordosis (anterior convexity) and the alignment of the head and neck above the center of gravity. Children with diskitis often protect their back by sitting in a hyperextended position, using the arms as support, and may lie down and cry if they are made to sit.

Observe Gait

Shifting or leaning to one side (listing) and atypical scoliosis may indicate a tumor. Listing is caused by asymmetrical sustained muscle contraction. The spinal curvature serves to relieve the discomfort and reduce pressure on a nerve root.

Severely affected gait in spondylosis is caused by hamstring tightness and results in uneven stride length with a persistently fixed knee to prevent hip flexion, which would stretch the tight hamstring muscles and increase pain.

Assess Vital Signs

Fever may indicate systemic infection as well as diskitis. Unexplained weight loss may suggest neoplasm, infection, or depression.

Examine Skin

Dermal cysts and/or a hairy patch over the spine may indicate spinal anomaly or tumor.

A doughy, fatty mass in the midline of the back (sometimes covered with hair—Faun's beard) is evidence of a lipoma, which may extend into the spinal cord and produce neurological symptoms.

Examine Eyes, Ears, Nose, and Mouth

Uveitis iriditis is seen in juvenile rheumatoid arthritis (JRA) and ankylosing spondylitis. Pharyngitis, otitis media, or infection of hematogenous origin may be the cause of diskitis in children.

Inspect the Back and Extremities

Observe for spinal alignment and symmetry of the tips of the scapula, iliac crests, and gluteal crease. If indicated, measure and compare leg lengths from the anterior-superior iliac crest to the medial malleolus. Measurements can be performed with the patient standing or supine. Legs should be of equal or less than 1 cm difference in length. Leg length differences are associated with sacroiliac, facet joint, and disk pathology.

From posterior and lateral viewpoints, observe the patient bending forward with feet together to detect scoliosis, kyphosis, or stiffness and guarding.

Percuss and Palpate Back and Spine

Painful scoliosis and stiffness is common in osteoid osteoma. Idiopathic scoliosis is usually painless without functional limitation. Point tenderness over the affected area is a finding with compression fracture of vertebrae.

Palpate and percuss the back to determine if tenderness is in the paravertebral muscular or midline spinous processes, which may indicate diskitis in children or osteomyelitis. To rule out the sacroiliac joint as the site of origin of low back pain, apply pressure over the joint with the patient's hip flexed 90 degrees and the leg adducted across the midline. This position places stress on the sacroiliac joint and will aggravate the pain if this is the site of origin.

Use fist percussion over the costovertebral angles to discriminate flank pain caused by renal disease from spinal pathology. Apply fist percussion over the costovertebral angles and over the spine to localize tenderness.

Perform Range of Motion (ROM) of the Spine

Ask the patient to flex, extend, rotate, and bend the spine laterally. Decreased mobility and back pain along the spine may indicate muscle spasm, neoplasm, or bony deformity.

Look for compensating effects of hip motion on the spine. The absence of lumbar flexion may be totally masked by a normal range of hip flexion when the patient bends forward. Lumbar flexion is tested by placing a mark over the 4th lumbar vertebra and another over the sacrum. Lumbar flexion is demonstrated by an increased distance between these two marks when the patient bends forward.

Observe for limitation of motion on forward bending caused by hip flexion contracture. Lumbar lordosis does not flatten with forward bending and is an organic cause for back pain. In children, Scheuermann's kyphosis, an exaggeration of the normal posterior convex curvature of the thoracic spine, produces pain with forward flexion, and spondylolysis produces pain with hyperextension.

Perform Straight Leg Raising (SLR)

The SLR test can assess sciatic (L5 and S1) nerve root tension. With the patient supine, place one hand above the knee, the other cupping the heel, and slowly raise the limb. Instruct the patient to say when to stop because of pain. Observe for pelvic movement and the degree of leg elevation when the patient tells you to stop. Ask the patient to tell you the most distal point of pain sensation, such as the back, hip, thigh, or knee. While holding the leg at the limit of elevation, dorsiflexing the ankle and internally rotating will add tension to the neural structures and increase the pain if nerve root tension is present.

Pain below the knee at less than 70 degrees of elevation, aggravated by dorsiflexing the ankle or hip rotation, are all signs of L5 or S1 nerve root tension suggestive of a herniated disk. This test can also be performed with the patient sitting. In a positive test, the patient will resist extension or will compensate with hyperextension of the spine.

Lift each leg in succession to detect contralateral pain in patients with nerve root compression.

A positive SLR test in children indicates disk herniation but might be unremarkable with tumor.

Check Hip Mobility

With the patient prone and supine, check active hip flexion, extension, internal and external rotation, and strength against resistance. Weakness of the gluteus maximus is associated with lumbar or referred pain from L5 nerve roots or gluteal nerve injury. In small children, check for congenital hip dysplasia with the child supine, abducting the hips. The knees should appear of equal height and should externally rotate equal degrees. Presence of a hip click, joint instability, uneven hip to knee length with hips and knees flexed, and uneven gluteal skinfolds suggest congenital hip dislocation.

Examine Feet

Perform active ROM of the ankle, feet, and toes against resistance. Weakness, pain, or limitation of dorsiflexion movement indicates an L4 nerve root injury. Similar symptoms produced by plantar flexion indicate S1, S2 involvement. Deformities of the foot, such as talipes equinovarus (clubfoot) or hallux malleus (claw toes), may aggravate misalignment of back structures because of asymmetry.

Evaluate Muscle Strength

Evaluate strength against resistance of the lower extremity muscle groups. Test the patient's ability to stand on toes and heels and to squat. A person with S1 nerve root involvement may have little motor weakness but may demonstrate difficulty in toe walking. Difficulty heel walking or squatting indicates involvement of L5 and L4 nerve roots. Leg extension at the knee against resistance tests L4 root function. In young children who are unable to cooperate for measurement of muscle strength, use measurements of like limb-girths as an estimate of the bilateral symmetry of muscle strength.

Measure Muscle Circumference

Differences in muscle circumference greater than 2 cm in two opposite limbs may signify atrophy secondary to neurological impairment.

Test Sensory Function

All neurological test results are evaluated by comparing the symmetry of responses or perceptions. Bilateral comparison is the simplest, most efficient way to determine the presence, location, and extent of any abnormality. A sensory examination is a general guide in determining the level of spinal cord involvement. Test for light touch and pain sensation in the sensory areas of L3-S1 dermatomes (see Figure 9-1). Dermatomes overlap and vary greatly in individuals, thus only gross changes can be detected by pinprick. Test 5 to 10 pinpricks in each dermatomal area if the patient reports numbness and tingling. Disk lesions rarely produce bilateral symptoms. It is sometimes difficult to distinguish numbness from cutaneous nerve versus dermatomal origin. Numbness from cutaneous nerve lesions does not occur in a dermatomal pattern. Numbness and tingling are uncommon symptoms in most children with back pain. When these symptoms are present, it suggests a serious problem.

Assess Deep Tendon Reflexes (DTRs)

Normal DTRs are symmetrical. DTRs are increased when an upper motor neuron lesion is present and decreased with a lower motor neuron lesion. A positive Babinski's sign indicates a disorder of upper motor neurons, affecting the motor area of the brain or corticospinal tracts, caused by spinal tumors or demyelinating disease. DTRs are decreased if a tumor is pressing on a peripheral nerve. Asymmetrical abdominal reflexes are seen in tumors of the spine.

An absent or decreased ankle jerk reflex suggests an S1 nerve root lesion. An L3-L4 disk herniation is the most common cause of a diminished knee jerk reflex.

Palpate the Abdomen

Palpation of the abdomen is done to detect possible visceral causes of back pain. In an elderly person, a ruptured aortic aneurysm can cause acute, severe, midthoracic back pain. If an aortic aneurysm is suspected, immediate surgical referral is critical.

Check Rectal Sphincter Tone

In cauda equina syndrome, the compression of S1-S2 nerve roots results in decreased sphincter tone and decreased sensation in the perianal area. This syndrome is a surgical emergency.

LABORATORY AND DIAGNOSTIC STUDIES

According to national practice guidelines, no diagnostic tests are warranted within the first 4 weeks for acute onset of low back pain without neurological signs.

Plain Radiographs

X-rays are useful in localizing the area of discomfort and ruling out fracture, tumor, osteophytes (bone spurs), or vertebral infection.

Standing AP and lateral views of the spine. These views of the spine accentuate any deformity, such as scoliosis, and demonstrate vertebral integrity.

Oblique and flexion views. These views increase the sensitivity for determining instability.

Spine x-ray. A flat lumbosacral spinal x-ray is done when there is a history of trauma or in persons over 50 years old who have ALBP with signs of neurological deficit. Older persons may have a history of straining or lifting.

Bone Scan

Bone scan is a radioisotope technique indicating blood flow and bone formation or destruction and can reveal inflammatory and infiltrative processes and occult fractures. The distal wrist and lumbosacral spine can be scanned to assess bone mineral density and risk of osteoporosis.

Electromyelogram (EMG)

EMG is done to assess the extent of nerve root compression and function of the peripheral nerves.

Diagnostic Imaging

Magnetic resonance imaging (MRI) is useful in evaluating soft tissue detail, such as disk herniations and spinal cord pathology, especially in vertebral osteomyelitis. Computed tomography (CT) scans are usually used for bone visualization.

Urinalysis

Urinalysis is done to assess kidney and metabolic function, including infectious processes, to rule out a visceral cause of back pain such as pain of pyelonephritis.

Erythrocyte Sedimentation Rate (ESR)

The ESR will be elevated in about 90% of patients with a serious musculoskeletal infection; however, there is no direct relationship between ESR and the severity of infection. The test is non-specific.

Complete Blood Count (CBC)

The CBC will detect anemia as well as other conditions that might manifest as back pain, such as tumor or infection. The anemia of chronic disease is usually hypochromic or normochromic with low iron indices.

DIFFERENTIAL DIAGNOSIS

POTENTIALLY SERIOUS CAUSES OF ACUTE LOW BACK PAIN

Spinal Fracture

The patient may relate a history of major trauma to the back from an impact or fall or, if elderly, a history of strenuous lifting or a minor fall. Pain is felt near the site of injury. Any suspicion of spinal fracture should be treated as an emergency. The patient is immobilized to prevent further damage and transported by emergency personnel for x-rays of the suspected area of fracture.

Tumor (Osteoblastoma, Spinal Metastasis, Osteoid Osteoma)

Primary tumors are a more common cause of back pain in children, whereas metastasis is a more common cause in adults. The lower thoracic and upper lumbar vertebrae are the most common sites of bony metastatic disease from marrow tumors. A health history and diagnostic tests may reveal other signs of general poor health such as weight loss, fatigue, weakness, and anemia.

Infection (Osteomyelitis, Diskitis)

The spine is the most common site of osteomyelitis in adults secondary to adjacent infection or following invasive instrumentation that results in bacterial seeding of the bone via the arterial blood. *Staphylococcus aureus* is the most frequently identified organism. Vertebral osteomyelitis causes stiffness and pain, usually localized over the site of infection. A tender spinous process, positive SLR test, and paravertebral muscle spasm may be seen in vertebral osteomyelitis or septic diskitis. Patients may have hip pain secondary to involvement of L2-S1.

Diskitis is usually a benign disorder in children that results in intervertebral disk inflammation. Children will be reluctant to walk, sit, or stand. Pain will be aggravated by motion and relieved by rest. History will reveal a recent bacterial infection, often secondary to pharyngitis or otitis media, IV drug use, diabetes mellitus, or immunosuppression. A small percentage of adults will report an acute onset of fever, weight loss, and general malaise; however, the majority may only have the symptom of back pain present from 2 weeks to years.

Cauda Equina Syndrome

Compression of S1 nerve root produces a constant back pain with saddle distribution anesthesia (buttock and medial and posterior thighs), fecal incontinence, bladder dysfunction, motor weakness of the lower limbs, and radiculopathy. The patient may limp and guard lumbar spine movement, will not be able to heel or toe walk, and will have abnormal or asymmetrical knee and ankle deep tendon reflexes. SLR test will be positive. This syndrome is a surgical emergency.

SCIATIC PROBLEMS

Sciatica

The most common cause of sciatica is herniated disk. History may reveal repetitive motion strain or strenuous lifting, twisting, and bending. Low back pain is associated with pain and burning that radiates along the lateral thigh, leg, and foot, sometimes associated with numbness along the dermatomal areas. SLR and sitting knee extension produces radicular pain below the knee at less than 60 degrees of limb elevation, and pain may be felt in the buttock or posterior thigh. Bowel and bladder function are normal.

NON-SPECIFIC BACK PROBLEMS

Musculoskeletal Strain (Postural, Overuse)

Back structures such as muscles and ligaments can become inflamed from overuse or strain. History often reveals no precipitating event for the onset of pain. Patients may report that pain is alleviated by rest, especially in the supine position with hips and knees flexed, and by the application of heat or cold. Pain is aggravated by sitting, walking, standing, and with certain motions. On physical examination, palpation will localize the pain, and muscle spasms may be felt. ROM of the spine will increase the pain, especially forward flexion. Neurological examination reveals no abnormalities.

Spondylolisthesis

Pain can be the result of a disruption of the vertebral spinous process, where the disruption results in subluxation of the vertebral body onto adjacent structures. This usually occurs between L5 and S1 and may be the result of a fatigue fracture that occurred years ago and failed to heal. Pain is usually chronic. Examination of the spine may reveal a palpable, prominent spinous process. Forward flexion may be limited.

Ankylosing Spondylitis

Ankylosing spondylitis is a systemic inflammatory condition of the vertebral column and sacroiliac joints. Peak incidence is in persons 20 to 30 years old; males are most often affected. Patients report chronic low back pain, worse on morning rising and lessening as the day goes on. Examination shows an excessive thoracic kyphosis and rounding of the posterior thoracic spine with forward flexion of the head, neck, and lower back. About 30% of patients will have arthritis of other joints. X-rays may reveal fusion of vertebrae, and ESR is elevated.

Spinal Stenosis

Spinal stenosis is a bony encroachment on the nerve roots of the lumbar spine. Patients report low back pain associated with lumbosacral radiculopathy, pain with walking or standing, and pain relief with sitting. Neurogenic (pseudo) claudication pain of the lower extremities is made worse with prolonged standing, walking, bending, or hyperextending the back.

Scheuermann's Disease

Adolescent males develop this disease as a result of anterior disk protrusion, causing wedging of the thoracic vertebrae and an exaggeration of the normal posterior con-vex curvature of the thoracic spine. The etiology is unknown but may come from excessive lifting or spinal flexion. The patient complains of a mild to moderate pain, worsening toward the end of the day or after physical activity but relieved by rest. Physical examination demonstrates an increase in thoracic kyphosis on lateral view, made sharper by forward bending.

Osteoporosis

Osteoporosis is a loss of mineralized bone mass that can result in a compression fracture of the vertebral body, usually occurring in the thoracic area. Back pain is often chronic and poorly localized. Multiple compression fractures may produce dorsal kyphosis and cervical lordosis. Persons at greatest risk are post-menopausal Caucasian women, especially those slight in build who have a history of inactivity. It is also common in persons over 70 years who have age-related reduction in vitamin D synthesis. Osteoporosis can also be secondary to endocrine imbalance such as hyperthyroidism, organ disease, or drugs such as corticosteroids, or excessive intake of alcohol.

NON-SPINAL CAUSES
Aortic Aneurysm (Dissecting)

Sudden onset of severe low or middle back pain in persons over 30 years might suggest a dissecting aortic aneurysm. The pain will not be alleviated by rest. The patient may exhibit pallor, diaphoresis, and confusion. Pulses and blood pressure measured on each upper extremity will be asymmetrical. Emergency surgery is indicated.

Gallstones

The presence of gallbladder problems increases with age. A gallbladder attack often follows the ingestion of a fatty meal. A crampy right upper quadrant pain (RUQ), following the ingestion of a fatty meal, is produced by spasms of the cystic duct that is obstructed with a stone. Gallbladder pain radiates around the trunk to the right scapula. Position doesn't affect the pain. Patients complain of belching, bloating, and an acidic stomach. Attacks may increase in frequency and severity and cause nighttime wakening. During an attack, palpation will show RUQ tenderness. Physical findings between attacks may be normal or there may be tenderness to palpation of the RUQ on inspiration (Murphy's sign) if the gallbladder is inflamed. RUQ mass may be felt if the gallbladder is obstructed. Obstruction is a emergency surgical situation.

Pyelonephritis

With pyelonephritis, the patient will appear ill, diaphoretic, and may complain of nausea and vomiting, headache, and back or flank pain. The patient may have a fever. Severe lumbar tenderness will be found on fist percussion for CVA tenderness. Urinalysis will reveal cloudy, malodorous urine, and microscopy will show the presence of casts and cells (i.e., RBC, WBC, epithelial).

Pleuritis

Inflammation of the pleural lining of the lungs often follows an upper respiratory infection. Pleuritic pain is sharp, worsens on inspiration or with coughing, and is lessened by lying on the affected side. Physical examination of the lungs will be normal, or crackles and bronchial breath sounds will be heard on auscultation. A chest x-ray will provide information on the condition of the lungs.

Pelvic Inflammatory Disease (PID)

The symptoms of PID depend on the extent of infection. Infection usually begins in the lower urinary tract or cervix and spreads to the endometrium, tubes, and peritoneum. The sexually active female patient may have mild to moderate dull, aching, lower abdominal, pelvic, or possibly back pain. She will report tenderness during cervical motion, uterine motion, or palpation of the adnexa. History may be positive for sexually transmitted infections (usually *N. gonorrhea* and *C. trachomatis*), vaginal symptoms, or use of an IUD for contraception.

PSYCHOGENIC CAUSES

Psychological Back Pain

A careful history is needed to gain insight into the psychosocial and economic issues surrounding report of back pain. The patient may have a history of recent life stressors, be involved in a legal injury or workmen's compensation action, or have a history of depression or alcohol abuse. The clinician should be aware of exaggerated signs of pain such as moaning, grimacing, or overreaction. A malingerer, a patient who pretends to suffer, when distracted, will show inconsistent and variable results on physical examination tests, such as straight leg raising (SLR), or will describe radiation of pain inconsistent with dermatome distribution.

Table 9-4

Differential Diagnosis of Common Causes of Acute Low Back Pain

Condition	History	Physical Findings	Diagnostic Studies
Potentially Serious Causes			
Spinal fracture	Trauma to spine or back; pain is felt near the site of injury	Palpable tenderness over site of fracture	Considered an emergency; immobilize the patient and transport for x-rays
Tumor	History of cancer; progressive pain is unremitting, occurs at night and at rest	Weight loss, fever, tenderness near tumor	ESR, bone scan
Osteoblastoma	Neck or back pain not relieved by aspirin; occurs in older adolescents and young adults	Localized tenderness, may have scoliosis with muscle spasm	Plain film shows an expansive osteolytic lesion surrounded by thin peripheral rim of bone; bone scan; CT scan
Osteoid osteoma	Occurs primarily in adolescents; rare in patients over age 40; well localized pain, which may be more severe at night and relieved by aspirin or other prostaglandin inhibitors	Painful, well-localized scoliosis may be present	Bone scan
Infection (vertebral osteomyelitis)	History of infection, invasive procedure; continuous, dull back pain; chronic back pain	Acute onset presents with fever, diaphoresis; tenderness over affected disk, positive SLR	ESR, blood culture, bone biopsy, CT scan, MRI
Diskitis	Pain aggravated by movement; more common in children	Tenderness over the affected disk	ESR
Cauda equina syndrome	Constant pain in a saddle distribution; urinary retention, fecal incontinence, radiculopathy	Positive SLR, abnormal DTRs, motor weakness	Surgical emergency

Table 9-4

Differential Diagnosis of Common Causes of Acute Low Back Pain—cont'd

Condition	History	Physical Findings	Diagnostic Studies
Sciatic Problems			
Sciatica	Acute back pain with radiculopathy; history of strain or trauma, relief with sitting	Paravertebral tenderness and spasm; positive SLR, sitting knee extension, sensory findings	EMG if chronic
Non-Specific Back Problems			
Musculoskeletal strain	Pain in back, buttocks; history of new activity or exertion; relief of pain with sitting	Paravertebral tenderness, scoliosis or loss of lumbar lordosis; no neurological signs	None
Spondylolisthesis	Young person who is in a sport that demands rapid movement between hyperflexion and hyperextension or who does excess loading in hyperextension	No neurological signs, pain localized to the low back, just below the level of the iliac crest; tight hamstrings	Lumbar spine x-rays.
Ankylosing spondylitis	Persons under 40 years, insidious onset, progressive morning back pain relieved with exercise	Painful sacroiliac joints, reduced spine mobility; may have uveitis	ESR, spinal x-rays, HLA-B27 antigen
Spinal stenosis	Pain worse throughout day, aggravated by standing, relieved by rest; pseudoclaudication	Signs of osteoarthritis of joints; may have neurological signs	Spinal x-rays
Scheuermann's disease	Affects mostly adolescent males; mild to moderately severe pain, worse at end of day, relieved by rest	Normal examination, may show an exaggerated thoracic kyphosis that is fixed in attempted hyperextension	Thoracic spine x-rays

Continued

Table 9-4

Differential Diagnosis of Common Causes of Acute Low Back Pain—cont'd

Condition	History	Physical Findings	Diagnostic Studies
Non-Specific Back Problems—cont'd			
Osteoporosis	Chronic, poorly localized back pain; post-menopausal; slight build; history of inactivity or endocrine disorder	Palpable tenderness over area of compression fracture; kyphosis or lordosis; loss of height	Bone densiometry; spinal x-ray to assess fracture
Non-Spinal Causes			
Aortic aneurysm	Severe, acute-onset pain not related to activity or movement; increased risk in persons over 30 years old; pallor, diaphoresis, anxiety, confusion	Intact aneurysm will be a visible pulsatile midline upper quadrant abdominal mass; in a dissected aneurysm, upper extremity pulse and pulse pressures are asymmetrical; posterior thoracic pain may be felt	Emergency surgical referral
Gallstones	Increased incidence with age; steady, intense pain in the RUQ with radiation to the right scapula or shoulder, belching, bloating, fatty food intolerance	Normal physical exam or positive Murphy's sign on palpation of the abdomen	Surgical referral
Pyelonephritis	Ill-appearing, sweating, nausea, back or flank pain, headache	Fever: cloudy, malodorous urine; severe lumbar tenderness on percussion	Urinalysis; urine culture
Pleuritis	History of recent URI; pleuritic pain	Normal exam or crackles and bronchial breath sounds	PPD, chest x-ray

Table 9-4

Differential Diagnosis of Common Causes of Acute Low Back Pain—cont'd

Condition	History	Physical Findings	Diagnostic Studies
Non-Spinal Causes—cont'd			
Pelvic inflammatory disease	Sexually active female, low back and abdominal pain, history of urinary or vaginal symptoms, sexually transmitted disease; IUD; multiple sex partners	Cervical and uterine motion tenderness, adnexal tenderness; cervicitis, fever	Gonorrhea, chlamydia cultures, ESR
Psychogenic Causes			
Psychological back pain	History of psychosocial stressors, depression, exaggerated expressions of pain	Exaggerated or inconsistent reactions to testing; normal exam	None

Chapter 10

Common Problems of the Neurological System

Headache

Headache is a subjective feeling of pain caused by a variety of intracranial and extracranial factors. It is one of the most common complaints in adults and children, with most headaches being self-treated with an over-the-counter analgesic. The vast majority of headaches are acute, self-limited, and do not pose imminent danger or serious sequelae. The goals for the practitioner in evaluating a headache are to (1) identify life-threatening causes of headache, (2) diagnose treatable disease associated with some headaches and (3) provide symptom relief. To accomplish these goals, the practitioner needs to conduct a careful history and focused physical examination.

Headaches can be categorized as primary or secondary. Primary headaches are characterized by the absence of structural pathology or systemic disease; they account for over 90% of all headaches. Secondary headaches are those caused by an identifiable organic pathology, one that is confined to the meninges or to the cerebral parenchyma. Pain from headache arises from stimulation of pain-sensitive structures of the head and brain caused by traction, inflammation, vascular dilatation, muscle contraction, or dysregulation of ascending brainstem serotonergic systems (Figure 10-1)

Generally, pain arising from disordered function, damage, or inflammation of structures located anterior to and above the tentorium is felt in the front of the head, whereas pain felt in the back of the head arises from structures located below the tentorium. Extracranial structures that are sensitive to pain include the skin, scalp, blood vessels, facial muscles, eyes, ears, teeth, nasal cavity, mucous membranes of the mouth and pharynx, and the temporomandibular joint (TMJ). The substance of the brain itself is not sensitive to pain, but sensitive structures include the blood vessels, sensory nerves, and ganglia. Cranial structures project pain to the surface near to the source of pain. Pain from extracranial structures is usually felt in the immediate region affected (Figure 10-2).

Headache has been divided by symptomatology into types using the diagnostic criteria proposed in 1988 by the International Headache Society

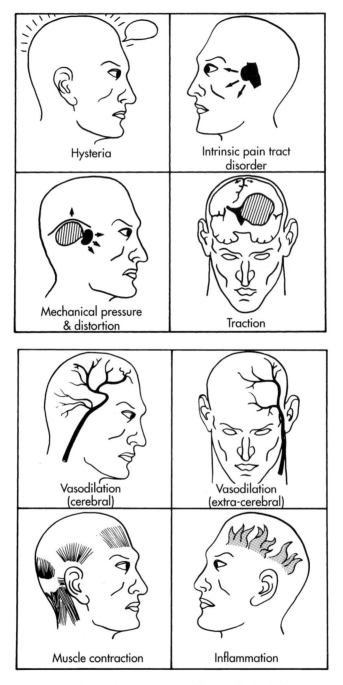

Figure 10-1 Mechanisms of cranial pain. (From Noble J et al: *Textbook of primary care medicine,* ed 2, St. Louis, 1996, Mosby.)

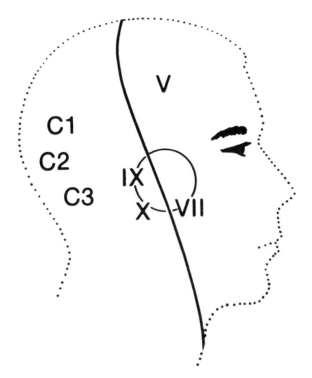

Figure 10-2 Sensory pathways for cranial pain.

(Table 10-1). Of the 13 types classified, only a few are common. Headaches can also be categorized into acute (new onset), recurrent, or chronic. Approximately 60% of new-onset headaches are migraine or tension, whereas about 90% of chronic headaches are also related to these two diagnostic categories.

DIAGNOSTIC REASONING: FOCUSED HISTORY

What clues indicate this is a potentially serious, life-threatening headache?

The clinician may first need to assess whether the patient is fully oriented before proceeding with further history. A mental status screening can be performed using the Mini-Mental Status Test (see Chapter 11, Confusion in Older Adults, pp. 408 and 409). If the patient shows a mental status deficit, transportation for immediate emergency treatment is indicated. Box 10-1 summarizes warning signs of a potentially serious cause for headache.

Key Questions
- How did the headache begin?
- On a scale from 0 (no pain) to 10 (worst pain ever) how severe is the pain?
- Is there a history of recent trauma to the head?
- Was there a loss of consciousness?
- Do you notice any other symptoms associated with the headache pain?
- Do you have any chronic health problems?

Onset, severity. Sudden onset of a severe headache without a history of chronic headache suggests an intracerebral hemor-

Table 10-1

International Headache Society Classification

CODE	HEADACHE TYPE
1	Migraine
2	Tension-type headache
3	Cluster headache and chronic paroxysmal hemicrania
4	Miscellaneous headache not associated with structural lesion
5	Headache associated with head trauma
6	Headache associated with vascular disorders
7	Headache associated with nonvascular intracranial disorders
8	Headache associated with substances or their withdrawal
9	Headache associated with noncephalic infection
10	Headache associated with metabolic disorder
11	Headache or facial pain associated with disorders of the face/cranium
12	Cranial neuralgias and nerve trunk pain; pain and sensory loss associated with interruption of peripheral nerve fibers
13	Headache not classifiable

Headache disorders: abbreviated system of classification and diagnosis, Research Triangle Park, 1992, Glaxo Pharmaceuticals.

Box 10-1

Warning Signs of Serious Causes of Headache

Stiff neck
Disturbed consciousness
Abrupt onset of severe pain
 ("worst headache ever")
Neurological deficit
Progressively worsening
Vomiting
New onset in persons 50 years or
 older

rhage (ICH) secondary to a ruptured aneurysm or vascular anomaly. Severity of headache is a very subjective measure and can sometimes be difficult to interpret. Headache of ICH without a history of trauma is rare in children and adolescents, but the incidence increases with age, especially in persons over 50 years old or in someone who is being treated with anticoagulation therapy. ICH can be catastrophic.

Onset of sudden severe headache with neurological signs is an emergency; the patient needs immediate transport to an emergency center.

Subarachnoid hemorrhage is often precipitated by physical activity and is described as the "worst headache ever." Patients also complain of a stiff neck and may have a transient loss of consciousness, nausea and vomiting, photophobia, pupillary dilatation, and seizure. Some patients who have a leaking aneurysm may complain of headache for several days but will subsequently have a worsening headache with neurological findings.

If subarachnoid hemorrhage is suspected, the patient needs transport to an emergency center for a CT scan and possible surgical intervention because early diagnosis and treatment improve prognosis.

History of trauma. Trauma to the head may cause subdural or epidural bleeding. The patient may have a brief loss of consciousness followed by a period of lucidity that can last for minutes to days, with subsequent relapse and appearance of neurological signs. Epidural hematomas are often associated with skull fracture.

Minor head trauma may result in headache because of soft tissue or extracranial injury. Pain is often localized to the site of injury and is self-limiting. Anyone who has experienced head trauma should be carefully observed for at least 24 hours for signs of neurological damage.

Associated symptoms. The entry of infectious organisms, chemical agents, and drugs into the subarachnoid space causes inflammation of meningeal structures and associated blood vessels, resulting in a headache. Headache associated with infection presents with fever and possibly meningismus (stiff neck), which can indicate meningitis or encephalitis.

ICH presents as a sudden and severe "thunderclap" headache associated with confusion, vomiting, lethargy, and focal neurological signs; it is caused by a ruptured vascular anomaly or an aneurysm. Drowsiness or confusion can be produced by increased intracranial pressure secondary to meningitis or metabolic disorders.

Brain tumors in children, especially young children, are difficult to diagnose because of the child's inability to describe headache or diplopia until about 4 years of age. Signs are vague, and the developing skull in the infant may accommodate a pathological condition for some time. However, headache as the initial manifestation of brain tumor is followed quickly by neurological signs such as vomiting, recurrent morning headaches, reflex asymmetry, and papilledema.

Presence of chronic disease. Persons with AIDS are at increased risk for cryptococcal meningitis, encephalitis, or generalized sepsis. Persons being treated with anticoagulation therapy or the elderly are at increased risk for headache from a serious cause, such as ICH or acute glaucoma. Headaches secondary to metabolic disorders can be the result of hyponatremia, uremia, hypoglycemia, and hypercapnia.

After determining the headache is not serious, how can I narrow down the causes?

Key Questions
- Where does it hurt?
- What does it feel like?
- When does it occur? What makes it worse?
- How long have you had this headache?
- Can you tell when it is coming on?

Location. Pain secondary to trauma or inflammation is perceived as near the site of insult, such as the occipital area, nape of neck, bifrontal area, or generalized to the head. Noxious stimulation from any type of disease of the eye, ear, nose, or paranasal sinuses may spread to cause pain in the head.

Adults describe tension headaches as a "hatband" distribution of pain, while children describe a generalized headache or discomfort.

Orbital pain is seen with increased intraocular pressure. Periorbital pain may be present with sinusitis, migraine, trigeminal neuralgia or it may be a sign of ocular disease. TMJ pain is located in the frontotemporal or temporal regions and may be unilateral or bilateral. Contraction of muscles of the head and neck cause headaches that are nonpulsatile, occurring in the occipital and paracervical region.

Characteristics of the pain. A moderately intense, constant throbbing headache is associated with dilatation of the cervical arteries. Severe pain indicates an expanding lesion, such as a tumor or hematoma, edema, or enlargement of the ventricles secondary to hydrocephalus.

Migraine headache pain is caused by the production of various substances on dilated arteries that sensitize those arteries to pain. The pain is steady or throbbing and is usually limited to the same side. Migraine headaches are thought to result from an initial phase of inter- or extracranial vasoconstriction, followed by a longer interval of vasodilatation. Frequently the headache takes 3 to 4 hours to reach peak pain levels.

Cluster headaches (uncommon in children) are the result of an unknown vascular change that occurs within a period of 5 minutes.

Tension (muscle contraction) headaches usually occur at school or work and often disappear on weekends and vacations or during periods of relaxation.

What does the chronicity of pain suggest?

Key Questions
- How frequently do you get a headache?
- Can you describe any pattern to the headache?
- How long does the headache last?
- Have you had this kind of headache before?
- How old were you when you first had this kind of headache?

Frequency. As a general rule, a patient who has a constant headache for more than 3 months with physical findings may demonstrate papilledema, bilateral or unilateral CN VI palsies, gait or balance disturbances, or spasticity of the lower extremities. However, in the absence of such symptoms, a recurrent headache of more than 3 months' duration is rarely related to structural or systemic findings. If a headache has been present continuously for more than 4 weeks, without accompanying neurological signs or symptoms, it is most likely psychogenic in origin, especially if coupled with prolonged school or work absences, increased stress, and depression.

Pattern and duration of headache. Headaches that occur throughout the day suggest a tension origin. Sinus headaches occur after arising and grow worse as the day goes on, especially when the person bends forward, but are less painful in the evening. Headaches associated with severe hypertension are not common and occur

only with a diastolic reading of 130 mmHg or greater. They are occipital, worse on arising, and lessen as the day goes on. Meningeal inflammation produces a pain that fluctuates throughout the day and night with no clear pattern. Migraine pain is episodic, occurring from several times a week to once a year. The pain lasts for hours and is sometimes preceded by prodromal symptoms.

Cluster headache pain demonstrates a pattern of attacks that occur daily for several weeks with long periods of remission. The pain is short, often lasting less than an hour, but is intense.

Prior history of headache. Headaches can be described as acute (new onset), recurrent, or chronic. Acute-onset headaches must be evaluated for organic causes. Recurrent and chronic headaches are usually caused by vascular inflammation or muscle tension. Chronic headaches are usually described as dull, bilateral, or bandlike. Chronic daily headaches may be mixed, produced by a combination of vascular and muscular causes.

Organic lesions may initially produce pain that is intermittent, but as the lesion progresses the duration and frequency of the attack will increase.

Psychogenic headache pain is daily, constant, diffuse, and difficult to describe.

Age of patient at first onset. The age of onset of migraines can be from 5 to 8 years old. Usually migraine headaches begin ages 10 to 30 years. New onset of migraine headaches in adults over age 50 is unusual. Tension headaches have a usual first age onset of 8 to 12 years old. Cluster headaches have a usual first onset age 20 to 40 years.

What associated symptoms does the patient have?

Key Questions
- Do you have any nausea or vomiting?
- Do you notice any vision changes?
- Does light bother you?
- Are you dizzy?

Nausea and vomiting. Nausea and abdominal pain is more common in children with migraines, whereas nausea and vomiting is more common in adults. Vomiting can be a sign of increased intracranial pressure. Headaches from tumors in the midline, cerebellar, and ventricular areas of the cranium obstruct the normal flow of the cerebrospinal fluid, producing hydrocephalus and headache and early morning vomiting that occurs usually without nausea.

Vision changes. Migraine headaches may have an aura that precedes them. A frequently reported visual aura is a scintillating scotoma or twinkling spots of brightly colored lights. In children, visual scintillation is the most common aura of migraine, often limited to one eye.

Blurred vision is seen with traction headaches.

Cluster headaches are associated with ipsilateral conjunctival injection, lacrimation, and edema of the eyelid.

Photophobia. Photophobia is often present with migraine headaches but is not present with tension headaches. Patients with meningitis often complain of photophobia.

Dizziness. Approximately one third of patients with migraine headaches experience vertigo. The vertigo may appear as an aura, occur during the headache, or occur separately.

What do the aggravating and alleviating factors suggest?

Key Questions

- Does anything make the headache better?
- Does anything make the headache worse?

Alleviating factors. Patients with meningeal irritation get partial relief from being recumbent and lying quietly. Headaches that respond to mild analgesics are more likely to be tension headaches. Children get complete relief after a brief period of rest with a migraine headache, although rest does not affect a tension headache in children. Some adults experience migraine headache relief with sleep or rest, particularly in a dark, quiet environment.

Aggravating factors. Sneezing, coughing, straining, and bending forward make a traction headache worse.

Headaches that are much worse in the early morning and improve on arising may indicate tumor. Benign exertional headaches can occur with cough or during coitus. Trigeminal neuralgia pain can be triggered by stimulation of the affected nerve, produced by rubbing the face or chewing.

What does family history indicate?

Key Question

- Does anyone else in the family have headaches?

Family history. Tension headaches have no family history. Migraines have a positive family history.

Is there anything else that would help narrow the cause or causes?

Key Questions

- Have you been ill recently?
- Have you taken any medications or vitamins?
- Could you have been exposed to carbon monoxide?

Recent health history. Any substance introduced iatrogenically into the ventricular and lumbar fluid spaces can give rise to chemical meningitis. Radiographic contrast media, antibiotics, and steroids can cause headache. Lumbar puncture can cause a severe headache in 25% of patients. The headache is eased by lying down and aggravated by sitting or standing. Chronic infection, including middle ear, mastoiditis, sinusitis, dental or pulmonary infection, cardiovascular lesions with shunting, or endocarditis, predisposes to development of a brain abscess. Half of all brain abscesses occur in children with cyanotic congenital heart disease. Penetrating skull fractures can also be a portal of entry for bacteria and contribute to the occurrence of brain abscess. Melanomas may metastasize years after excision and may first be indicated by neurological changes.

History of ingestion. Outdated tetracycline use can cause pseudotumor cerebri (increased intracranial pressure without any intracranial mass or hydrocephalus) as can excessive intake of vitamin A and substances found in some topical acne preparations.

Withdrawal from certain substances, such as caffeine or nitrates, can also produce headache.

Exposures. Exposure to carbon monoxide (CO) may cause a severe, throbbing, generalized headache. Hemoglobin values less than 10 g/dl may cause headache as a result of hypoxia.

Occupational exposure to other toxins should be assessed through an occupational history.

DIAGNOSTIC REASONING: FOCUSED PHYSICAL EXAMINATION

Observe the Patient

Assess level of alertness and orientation to person, place, and time. Any patient who complains of headache and exhibits an ataxic gait, uncoordinated movements, or reduced mental alertness should be immediately transported to an emergency center for neurological evaluation.

A patient who appears ill or toxic is a suspect for meningitis. The patient is usually lying down with the lights off (photophobia) and may complain of chills. Most toddlers cannot communicate the characteristics of a headache but instead become irritable and cranky and rub their eyes and head.

Muscle spasm may cause tilting of the head or lifting of the shoulder when there is a posterior fossa tumor, cervical spine disease, or whiplash injury. Muscle spasm from prolonged anxiety and tension may cause backward tilting of the head and half closing of the eyes.

Ptosis of the eyelid may accompany a cluster headache or brain tumor. Blinking and squinting of the eyes indicates photophobia.

Take Vital Signs

Fever may be the only indication of an infectious disease. Neonates, however, frequently have subnormal temperatures in response to infection.

In children, if the plotted height and weight chart is significantly below average, consider a hypothalamic neoplasm. Plot head circumference to assess for normal skull growth. Macrocephaly may indicate hydrocephalus or brain tumor.

Take blood pressure and pulse because bradycardia and narrowing of pulse pressure are signs of increased intracranial pressure.

Palpate and Percuss the Skull

Palpate for symmetry of contour, tenderness, and lesions on the scalp, face, and neck. Palpate the temporal arteries for quality of pulse and tenderness. Focal tenderness and induration are seen in tension headaches. Tenderness over nodular temporal arteries is a sign of temporal arteritis.

Brain abscesses cause pain by localized traction and produce tenderness on skull percussion over the area involved.

Auscultate the Cranium

Intracranial arteriovenous malformations may mimic migraine. Auscultate the orbit and skull to evaluate for cranial bruits.

Inspect the Ears, Eyes, Nose, Mouth, and TMJ

A thorough examination of the face, head, and neck structures is needed to detect organic disease. Examine the ears for signs of infection.

Unilateral ptosis, pupillary dilation, and exotropia (divergent strabismus) caused by medial rectus weakness is seen with ophthalmoplegic migraine, a functional disturbance of the oculomotor nerve.

Test extraocular movement (EOM) in all fields of gaze. If a patient cannot look completely to the right or the left (lateral gaze), suspect a CN VI palsy, possibly the result of increased intracranial pressure. If EOMs are painful, consider optic neuritis.

Observe nasal mucosa for redness and swelling that may occur with migraines. Rhinorrhea and congestion are seen with sinus headaches. Observe teeth and oral mucosa because upper molar disease and poor dentition can cause headache. Tapping on the teeth or biting down on a tongue blade can elicit pain from sinusitis.

TMJ instability can cause headache pain. See Chapter 2, Earache, for discussion of examination technique, p. 12.

Enlarged pupils seen during a headache indicate migraine; however, if they outlast a headache, then organic disease should be suspected.

Upper motor neuron facial weakness may be present in hemiplegic migraine.

Perform Ophthalmoscopy

On funduscopic examination, note contour of optic disc and clarity of margins. Note papilledema and inspect vasculature for hemorrhage or exudate, venous pulsations, and arterial spasm.

Papilledema is often caused by an expanding intracranial mass and increased intracranial pressure. Optic disc atrophy suggests a chronically increased intracranial pressure or a lesion in the optic chiasm.

Meningitis does not produce eye funduscopic changes. Retinal hemorrhage in children may indicate abuse.

Assess Cranial Nerve Function

A complete assessment of cranial nerve function may provide evidence for more serious causes of headaches secondary to inflammation, traction, or metabolic imbalance.

- *CN I—Assess for smell.* The sense of smell may be lost when the olfactory nerve is damaged by head injury or by a tumor in the vicinity of the olfactory groove.
- *CN II—Check visual acuity.* Rarely does poor vision contribute to a headache. Poor vision may contribute to eye pain, but children equate this with headache. Double vision may be the presenting ocular symptom of increased intracranial pressure caused by a unilateral 6th nerve palsy or a posterior fossa lesion.
- *CN III, IV, and VI—Check visual fields.* Unilateral or homonymous hemianopsia, a loss of the same half of the visual field of both eyes, can occur with brain tumor headaches when the tumor is in the occipital lobes or adjacent to the visual pathways. A half-field defect is seen with parietal lobe tumor. CN III palsy can cause an enlargement of the pupil from compression of the nerve by an expanding lesion. The dilated pupil is always on the side of the expanding lesion. CN VI palsy (inability to move eyes in a lateral direction) may be found with acute hydrocephalus or cerebral edema. Nystagmus suggests a brainstem or cerebellar lesion and is usually ipsilateral. Lateral gaze nystagmus is also present with an elevated blood alcohol level. Vertical and rotatory nystagmus suggests central posterior fossa abnormality.
- *CN V—Test jaw strength, pain, and touch sensation to face.* Trigeminal neuralgia pain can be triggered by stimulation of the affected nerve.
- *CN VII—Ask the patient to frown, raise eyebrows, show teeth, close

eyes against resistance, and puff out cheeks. Test taste on the anterior two thirds of the tongue for sweet and salt discrimination. Salivary and lacrimal glands are innervated by CN VII.

- *CN VIII*—Unilateral deafness should be investigated to rule out acoustic neuroma.
- *CN IX, X*—Observe swallowing; uvula rise.
- *CN XI*—Test trapezius strength and sternocleidomastoid strength against resistance.
- *CN XII—Test tongue strength.* An intracranial vascular event may cause a hemiplegia or hemiparesis that may be assessed by observing the protruded tongue drift laterally or by the inability to hold position against resistance.

Examine the Neck

Ask the patient to perform full ROM of the neck to observe for stiffness or difficulty with movement, which may indicate muscle tension or meningismus.

Test for Meningismus

Normally the chin can be flexed passively to touch the chest. If neck stiffness is present, this maneuver is not possible. With the patient supine, attempts to flex the neck cause involuntary hip flexion, and the hips rise (Brudzinski's sign). Attempts to extend the knee joint when the hip joint is flexed may cause the other limb to flex at the hip (Kernig's sign).

Assess Motor Strength and Coordination of Extremities

Unilateral upper or lower extremity weakness with loss of manual dexterity is seen in children with hemiplegic migraine. Asymmetrical increase in muscle tone on the affected side, contralateral to the hemisphere lesion, suggests a cerebral lesion.

Patients who exhibit forearm drift with arms extended and eyes closed may have a motor neuron or cerebellar disturbance with an expanding intracranial lesion.

Test Balance and Gait

Midline cerebellar abnormalities cause marked ataxia. The patient has difficulty standing on the ipsilateral leg and has a tendency to fall or stumble toward the side of the lesion. The gait is also wide-based and halting, and the patient turns with jerky movements. Minimal disturbance is observed when the patient hops on either foot or stands tandem (one foot behind the other).

Assess Deep Tendon Reflexes

Increase in or asymmetry of reflexes is seen with cerebral lesions. The plantar or Babinski response is often present with cerebral lesions.

LABORATORY AND DIAGNOSTIC STUDIES

Complete Blood Count (CBC)

CBC is done to detect for major blood dyscrasias. Hypoxia secondary to severe anemia can cause headache.

Computed Tomography (CT) Scan

CT scan is the most common non-invasive initial diagnostic tool used to detect intracranial disease and should be done with new-onset severe headache or headache associated with abnormal neurological signs.

Lumbar Puncture (LP)

Lumbar puncture can directly measure cerebrospinal fluid pressure and be analyzed for normal values of components that are altered by disease, such as lymphocytes, glucose, protein, and presence of bacteria. An LP is done when a central nervous system infection is suspected but is contraindicated if there is suspicion of increased intracranial pressure. When brain abscess is suspected, do CT before lumbar puncture.

Erythrocyte Sedimentation Rate (ESR)

ESR is a non-specific test that is elevated in the presence of inflammation. An ESR should be performed when temporal arteritis is suspected.

Skull X-Ray

An x-ray of the skull is useful in post-traumatic headache. Specific views must be obtained to better observe intracranial structures, such as the pituitary gland or paranasal sinuses.

DIFFERENTIAL DIAGNOSIS

PRIMARY HEADACHES WITHOUT STRUCTURAL OR SYSTEMATIC PATHOLOGY

Tension Headache

Tension headache is the most common type of headache in adults and occurs most often in women. The mechanism of tension headache is uncertain, but it is thought to be related to sustained muscle contraction. Tension headache produces a bilateral pain, general or localized, often described as a frontotemporal bandlike distribution. The discomfort is described as a mild to moderate, non-throbbing pain, tightness, or pressure with a gradual onset. It may last for hours or days, and recurrences may extend over weeks or months. It is associated with anxiety, depression, or stress.

Migraine Without Aura (Common)

About 20% of adults experience migraines, and episodes are not uncommon in a child as young as 5 years old. The headache is unilateral, throbbing, and accompanied by nausea, vomiting, phonophobia (noise sensitivity), photophobia, and perspiration. The headache is usually frontal or perior-

bital. Onset is rapid and crescendo is within hours. Migraines may recur daily, weekly, or less often, and are rare in persons over 50 years old and during pregnancy.

Migraine With Aura (Classic)

Classic migraine headaches are preceded by neurological signs that indicate cortical and/or brainstem involvement. Headaches may be precipitated by bright lights, noise, or tension. Auras may include visual disturbances (e.g., scintillating scotoma, a pattern of twinkling colored lights), ascending paresthesias or numbness, weakness, and aphasia. The pain may be associated with photophobia, phonophobia, nausea, and vomiting.

Mixed Headache

Mixed headaches are a combination of muscular contraction and vascular dysfunction. The headache is experienced as a throbbing, constant pain during waking hours with symptoms of tightness, pressure, and muscle contraction. Family history of migraine is not uncommon.

Cluster Headache

Cluster headaches are of vascular origin and are less common than migraines. Onset is abrupt, often during the night, and the severity increases steadily. The pain is most often unilateral and ocular or periocular. Cluster headaches occur more often in men and last 15 minutes to 2 hours. The episodic recurrences are "clustered" in cycles of days or weeks, with remission lasting months to years. Associated symptoms include ipsilateral rhinorrhea, conjunctival injections, facial sweating, ptosis, and eyelid edema. Alcohol ingestion or vasodilatation secondary to wind or heat exposure may precipitate the pain.

Benign Exertional Headache

These headaches occur suddenly and are related to coughing, sneezing, straining, running, or orgasm and are the result of stretching the pain-sensitive structures in the posterior fossa. They are more common in men. The onset is sudden and "splitting," and pain may last from seconds up to 30 minutes. They should be distinguished from headache of subarachnoid hemorrhage.

SECONDARY HEADACHES WITH STRUCTURAL OR SYSTEMIC PATHOLOGY

Infectious Origin

Sinusitis

Sinusitis is frequently associated with a sore throat irritated by post-nasal discharge, facial or tooth pain, or a headache over the affected sinus that increases in intensity with coughing or bending forward. There is also frequently a cough that worsens in a lying position, morning periorbital swelling, fever, malaise, and recent URI. The maxillary sinuses are the most frequently affected. Pain in the temporal and periorbital area suggests frontal sinusitis, while maxillary sinusitis produces pain below the eye, in the upper teeth, or both. Ethmoid sinusitis produces medial orbit pain.

Dental Disorders

Patients with dental abscess, nerve root dysfunction, or infection may have headache and facial pain located near the site of the lesion. Tenderness elicited by tapping on the maxillary teeth with a tongue blade may indicate dental root infection or maxillary sinusitis. Inspection of the mouth may reveal ulceration or infection of pain-sensitive structures in the oral mucosa and gingiva.

Pharyngitis

Bacterial infection may irritate pain sensitive structures in the oropharynx, leading to headache.

Otitis Media

Recurrent otitis media with a sequelae of mastoiditis or chronic infection may result in headache. Signs of otitis will be seen on examination of the tympanic membrane.

Meningitis

Bacterial meningitis begins as bacteria colonize in the nasopharynx and enter the CNS through the dural venous sinuses or choroid plexus into the subarachnoid space. Common causal organisms in adults are *pneumoniae* and *meningitidis*. In children, common organisms are S. *pneumoniae* and H. *influenzae*; in neonates, group B streptococcus and E. *coli*. Bacterial meningitis is usually accompanied by severe systemic toxicity and mental status changes (encephalitis). In contrast, aseptic meningitis caused by enteroviruses or mumps virus produces a mild illness sometimes without fever. Photophobia and stiff neck are present in varying degrees. The person usually appears ill with a severe headache, fever, chills, myalgias, photophobia, and stiff neck. Brudzinski and Kernig signs may be positive. A petechial skin rash may be suggestive of meningeal disease. Patients may progress to coma and have seizures.

Neurogenic Origin

Trigeminal Neuralgia

The pain associated with malfunction of CN V is characterized by a series of bursts or jabs of sharp pain lasting seconds that occur repeatedly over minutes or hours. The pain is limited to the distribution of the three branches of CN V. Headaches caused by trigeminal neuralgia are stimulated by sensory stimuli to the involved nerves, produced by rubbing or touching the face or swallowing. Trigeminal neuralgia usually occurs in persons over 55 years old and earlier onset may suggest another cause.

Optic Neuritis

Optic neuritis refers to a variety of conditions that affect the optic nerve and reduce visual function. Disorders include demyelinating disease (multiple sclerosis), inflammation, viral illness, metabolic disorders, and toxin exposure. The patient has an acute onset of blurred vision with extraocular motion pain that precedes the visual changes by several days. Funduscopic examination reveals a slightly elevated (hyperemic) disc and a blurred disc margin. Treatment is focused on the underlying disease.

Cervical Spine Disorders

The three upper cervical nerves are sensory pathways for pain sensation felt in the posterior head and ipsilateral temporal and eye areas. Disturbances in the neck may cause muscle spasms and pressure on other neck structures. Patients with neck-related headache have pain associated with motion of the neck. Downward pressure on the head makes the pain worse and may cause it to travel down the arms.

Temporal Arteritis (Giant Cell Arteritis)

Temporal arteritis is a vasculitis of the ophthalmic and posterior ciliary branches of the internal carotid artery. It almost always afflicts persons over 50 years old. It is a sharp, localized pain over a tender, nodular temporal artery. Other symptoms include fever, malaise, anorexia, weight loss, orpolymyalgia rheumatica. Ischemic jaw and face pain are rare but highly suggestive. Headaches precede the major danger of temporal arteritis, blindness, by weeks. Unilateral blindness may occur suddenly and is not reversible. Left untreated, blindness in the other eye may occur. An ESR above 50 is almost always present. Suspected temporal arteritis is an emergency, and the patient needs referral to an emergency center for immediate evaluation and treatment.

Metabolic Origin

Carbon Monoxide (CO) Poisoning

CO is a colorless, odorless gas with an affinity for binding with hemoglobin to produce carboxyhemoglobin (COHb), which impairs oxygen transport. Symptoms are non-specific and are dose related. Low COHb levels may produce mild dyspnea and tightness across the head; however, as COHb increases, the headache becomes more severe and is associated with dizziness, nausea, fatigue, and dimmed vision.

As COHb levels rise, symptoms increase in severity and lead to loss of consciousness and seizures. Blood gases and COHb blood levels are diagnostic. History may suggest recent smoke inhalation or similar symptoms in multiple family members.

Severe Hypoglycemia

Hypoglycemia is more likely to occur in persons with type I diabetes but can occur in anyone taking oral hypoglycemic agents, in younger persons who experience reactive hypoglycemia, or following excessive ingestion of alcohol. A dietary and medication history may lead to a specific causative factor. Headache is generalized and bilateral and is associated with dizziness and a sense of not feeling well. Some persons with diabetes may have nocturnal hypoglycemia and report nightmares and vivid dreams, night sweats, and a headache on awakening. Blood glucose levels can confirm the presence of hypoglycemia.

Drug Withdrawal

Withdrawal from prolonged use of steroids may cause migrainous headaches. Nitrites may precipitate headache. Other drugs causing cranial dilation and an after effect of rebound vasoconstriction include hydralazine, alcohol, histamine, nicotinic acid, and caffeine.

Dietary Ingestion

A mild to moderately severe generalized headache may occur after ingestion of tyramines (e.g., aged cheese, red wine), monosodium glutamate, and nitrites in smoked meats. A headache diary will help identify the pattern of headache related to specific foods.

Cerebrovascular Origin

Intracranial Tumor

Intracranial tumors are more common in children, and brain metastasis from primary sites in the lung, breast, or kidney are more common in adults. Pain is constant and progressive, is felt in a discrete location, changes with head position, and awakens the person from sleep.

Hydrocephalus

Hydrocephalus, or collection of cerebrospinal fluid (CSF) in the ventricles of the brain, can be caused by tumors or cysts. Headache will be progressive and may be associated with neurological findings and mental status changes similar to dementia. Radiographic techniques are diagnostic, and lumbar puncture may detect increased CSF pressure.

Subdural Hematoma

Subdural hematoma produces a sudden, severe headache that is associated with a history of head trauma, exertional physical activity, or pharmacological anticoagulation. There is transient loss of consciousness, stiff neck, nausea, vomiting, photophobia, pupillary dilation, and pain over the eye.

Pseudotumor Cerebri

Teenagers being treated with topical acne preparations, menopausal women, and persons ingesting large amounts of vitamin A are at increased risk for pain from pseudotumor cerebri. Papilledema will be present in many cases, but, without it, the-headache may be diagnosed as mixed type. A neurology referral is indicated to ensure that no local obstruction is present before a lumbar puncture is done to assess for increased intracranial pressure. Lumbar puncture can sometimes lead to herniation of the brainstem.

Brain Abscess

Pain is of gradual onset, deep, aching in nature, often worse in morning, and aggravated by coughing or straining. Other signs of increased intracranial pressure may be present, such as papilledema and widening pulse pressure. There may be a recent history of head injury, infection, or assault to the central nervous system.

Intracerebral Hemorrhage

Intracerebral hemorrhage may result in a stroke or sudden coma and is associated with neurological findings defined by the site of bleeding. A person may present with a sudden-onset, severe headache, with or without a history of trauma. The severity of symptoms from bleeding intracranial aneurysms are correlated to the rate of hemorrhage and graded from I (asymptomatic to minimal headache with nuchal rigidity) to V (deep coma, decerebrate rigidity). Elderly persons with AIDS and persons on anticoagulation therapy are at increased risk for intracerebral hemorrhage. CT scan is diagnostic.

Table 10-2

Differential Diagnosis of Common Causes of Headache

Condition	History	Physical Findings	Diagnostic Studies
Primary Headaches Without Structural or Systemic Pathology			
Tension (muscle) headache	Common in adults; bilateral pain, general or localized in bandlike distribution; history of anxiety, stress, or depression	Normal physical exam; neck muscle tightness or fasciculations may be palpated	None
Migraine without aura (common)	More common in children; unilateral, throbbing pain; nausea	Photo- and phonophobia	None

Table 10-2

Differential Diagnosis of Common Causes of Headache—cont'd

Condition	History	Physical Findings	Diagnostic Studies
Primary Headaches Without Structural or Systemic Pathology—cont'd			
Migraine with aura (classic)	Pain precipitated by environmental stimuli; visual disturbances (scintillating scotoma) precede pain	Nausea and vomiting, photo- and phonophobia	None
Mixed headache	Throbbing, constant pain during waking hours; muscle tightness; family history of migraine	Mix of findings related to tension and migraine headache pain	None
Cluster headache	Rare in children; abrupt, nighttime onset; unilateral periorbital pain that is severe	Ipsilateral rhinorrhea, nasal stuffiness, conjunctival injection, sweating, ptosis	None
Benign exertional headache	Sudden onset related to physical exertion, Valsalva, or coitus	Normal physical exam	May need to distinguish from subarachnoid hemorrhage with CT scan
Secondary Headaches With Structural or Systemic Pathology			
Infectious Origin			
Sinusitis	Frontal, upper molar, or periorbital pain; cough, rhinorrhea	Low or no fever; pain on palpation of frontal, maxillary sinuses; purulent nasal or post-nasal discharge	X-rays (Waters view)
Dental disorders	Localized pain in jaw and top of head	Malocclusion, caries, abscesses of teeth present, gum disease	Dental referral
Pharyngitis	Sore throat	Fever; injection of the posterior pharynx	Throat culture
Otitis media	Ear pain, pain with swallowing	Fever; red, bulging tympanic membrane	None
Meningitis	Severe headache, chills, myalgias, stiff neck; toxic child or adult	Positive Kernig's and Brudzinski's signs; fever, photophobia, petechial rash may be present; mental status changes	Lumbar puncture

Continued

Table 10-2

Differential Diagnosis of Common Causes of Headache—cont'd

Condition	History	Physical Findings	Diagnostic Studies
Neurogenic Origin			
Trigeminal neuralgia	Persons over 55 years; bursts of sharp pain over the face innervated by the affected nerve; triggered by stimulus to the affected nerve	Normal physical exam; stimulation of triggers may provoke pain	None
Optic neuritis	Acute onset of pain with extraocular movement (EOM), followed by blurred vision	Diminished visual acuity, decreased pupillary reflex, hyperemia of the optic disc; pain with EOM	Ophthalmology referral
Cervical spine disorders	May have a history of trauma; occipital pain, muscle stiffness	Normal physical exam or pain associated with neck motion	Cervical spine x-rays
Temporal arteritis	Age >50 years; sharp localized temporal pain; malaise, anorexia, history of polymyalgia rheumatica	Fever, weight loss; tender over a nodular temporal artery	Elevated ESR (>50); immediate referral for treatment
Metabolic Origin			
Carbon monoxide poisoning	History of exposure, throbbing headache, mild dyspnea	Nausea, vomiting, change in mental status, lethargy, loss of consciousness	Blood gases and carboxyhemoglobin level
Severe hypoglycemia	History of diabetes or medication, alcohol and food ingestion; generalized headache, dizziness, sense of not feeling well	Normal physical exam or pallor, sweating, and weakness	Blood glucose level; may need self-monitoring of blood glucose to establish pattern
Drug withdrawal	Pattern of headache associated with stopping medication or substance use	Normal physical exam	Blood chemistry
Dietary ingestion	Mild to moderately severe headache after ingestion of foods or medication	Normal physical exam	Blood chemistry

Table 10-2

Differential Diagnosis of Common Causes of Headache—cont'd

Condition	History	Physical Findings	Diagnostic Studies
Cerebrovascular Origin			
Intracranial tumor	Sudden-onset headache that is progressive, exacerbated by coughing or exercise; worse in morning; history of trauma increases risk	Papilledema, vomiting, asymmetrical reflexes, weakness, sensory deficit, or other neurological deficit	CT scan
Hydrocephalus	Progressive headache, vomiting, irritability	Rapid enlargement of head, bulging fontanels	CT scan and referral
Subdural hematoma	History of head trauma, bleeding disorders, child abuse; adult over 35 years; sudden onset of "worst ever" headache, often over the eye, transient loss of consciousness	Unequal pupils, photophobia, neurological changes, seizure	CT scan and neurosurgical referral
Pseudotumor cerebri	Teens, menopausal women, history of vitamin A or tetracycline ingestion; progressive headache	Papilledema may be present	CT scan, neurology referral to assess risk related to lumbar puncture
Brain abscess	History of chronic ear infection or cyanotic heart disease	Fever, seizures, focal neurological deficits	CT scan
Intracerebral hemorrhage	Risk factors: persons over 50 years old, with AIDS, on anticoagulation therapy, or with hypertension	If conscious, abnormal neurological findings correlated with extent of the lesion	Emergency transport for immediate evaluation (CT scan) and possible surgical treatment

Dizziness

Dizziness is a subjective symptom that patients report to account for a variety of conditions, including vertigo, lightheadedness, and loss of balance. In children the symptom is frequently a new sensation, and the complaint is usually poorly defined. The young child may not have words to explain the symptom, and family members may state that the child has trouble walking or is irritable or the child's behavior is different. Older children, like adults, tend to categorize everything from lightheadedness and unsteadiness to spinning and falling as dizziness. This section is primarily confined to the discussion of vertigo. Patients with vertigo have the sensation of either their body moving (subjective vertigo) or their environment moving around them (objective vertigo), usually described as a spinning or rotary motion.

The sensation of balance depends on interconnections among the visual, vestibular, and sensory systems. Vertigo may be thought of as a disruption of one of these three systems. Vertigo may be central, involving the brainstem or cerebellum; peripheral, involving the inner ear or vestibular apparatus; or may result from systemic causes.

Central vertigo is generally either neoplastic or vascular in origin, although any central nervous system disorder, such as multiple sclerosis, that disrupts the pathway between the vestibular apparatus and the brain may result in dizziness. Common vascular causes include recurrent intermittent vascular insufficiency, transient ischemic attack, or stroke. Migraine headache is a special vascular-related central cause of vertigo.

Peripheral vertigo is typically produced by disruption of the inner ear or vestibular apparatus. Common causes include idiopathic etiologies, vestibular nerve inflammation, inner ear inflammation or infection, or tumor. Systemic origins include psychogenic, cardiovascular, and metabolic causes. Mixed or other causes include trauma and ototoxicity.

DIAGNOSTIC REASONING: FOCUSED HISTORY

What does the patient mean by dizziness?

Key Questions
- Describe how you feel when you are dizzy without using that word.
- Do you feel as though you or the room is spinning?
- Do feel like your balance is off?
- Do feel like you are about to faint?

Sensation. Vertigo produces the sensation of either the patient spinning or the environment spinning around the patient. Some patients describe a sensation of their body moving forward or accelerating.

Patients may also complain of loss of equilibrium accompanying the vertigo. Neoplasms and progressive vestibule loss typically produce a change in vestibular function that is slow in onset and manifested as imbalance.

Loss of balance and lack of coordination in the absence of vertigo may be the result of degenerative, neoplastic, vascular, or metabolic disorders. With these symptoms, look for other nervous system abnormalities. Imbalance may also occur in adults as a result of impaired sensory input, either visual or kinetic, such as occurs with peripheral neuropathy.

Children who have a vague sense of unsteadiness may have peripheral neuropathy or a dysfunction of the vestibular or cerebellar system, whereas children who complain of a feeling of motion are more likely to have an abnormality of the vestibular system.

In contrast to dizziness and imbalance, lightheadedness is the feeling that one is about to faint (near syncope). Some patients describe it as a generalized weakness and the feeling that they are about to pass out if they do not lie down. True syncope, or a sudden transient loss of consciousness with concurrent loss of postural tone, always has a spontaneous recovery.

Orthostatic hypotension is a frequent cause of lightheadedness and is most common in elderly persons, occurring as a result of abnormal regulation of blood pressure. Neurological causes of orthostatic hypotension are less common and are usually accompanied by neurological findings.

In both children and adults, a complaint of lightheadedness may accompany anemia, hypoglycemia, or hyperventilation syndrome.

Does the vertigo result from a systemic cause?

Key Questions

- What other medical problems do you have?
- Would you describe yourself as anxious or nervous?
- Do the episodes occur in relation to any activity or movement?

Other medical problems. Cardiovascular problems are a common cause of vertigo that is systemic in origin. The mechanism of vertigo may include vasomotor instability that decreases systemic vascular resistance, venous return, or both; severe reduction of cardiac output that obstructs blood flow within the heart or pulmonary circulation; or cardiac dysrhythmia that leads to transient decline in cardiac output. Patients with hypertension may experience vertigo while taking antihypertensive or potassium-depleting medications or as a result of postural hypotension.

Anxiety. Psychogenic dizziness is one of the most common causes of vertigo. Symptoms tend to be vague and may include other symptoms such as fatigue, fullness in the head, lightheadedness, and a sense of feeling apart from the environ-

ment. Patients may describe themselves as anxious or nervous. Patients may also have other psychiatric diagnoses. Stresses and tensions affecting children, such as divorce, custody battles, and day care, can cause vertiginous-like symptoms in the older child. Anxiety with hyperventilation may cause lightheadedness in a child, who then reports the symptom as dizziness.

Relationship to activity or movement. Dizziness when turning, especially when rolling over in bed, is usually due to vertigo. However, unsteadiness while walking is often considered to be disequilibrium, which can be caused by many factors. Dizziness on standing may be the result of decreased cerebral perfusion.

In children, attacks that occur with sudden changes of posture may be the result of hypotension, vascular disease, or positional vertigo.

Is the vertigo central (brainstem or cerebellar) or peripheral (vestibular) in origin?

Key Questions

- Do you have a history of migraine headaches?
- What other symptoms do you have? (diplopia, difficulty with speech, dysphagia, paresthesia, changes in sensory and motor function)
- Do you have nausea and vomiting?
- When do the episodes occur?

Headaches. Headache is a vascular-related cause of central vertigo. Approximately one third of patients with migraine headaches experience vertigo. The vertigo may appear as an aura, occurring during the headache, or occur separately. Some of these persons will have additional symptoms that are consistent with vertebrobasilar circulation abnormalities. Migraine both with and without headache is being recognized as a source of dizziness in children.

Other symptoms. Patients with central vertigo nearly always have neurological symptoms such as double vision, facial numbness, and hemiparesis.

Cerebellar causes may produce other symptoms, such as loss of balance, that closely resemble those of a peripheral disorder, so that neurological examination findings are important in differentiating the two. Pay particular attention to complaints of motor dysfunction or lack of coordination.

Vertigo that is peripheral in origin does not produce additional neurological symptoms or signs. If the patient has nausea and vomiting, suspect a peripheral vestibular apparatus problem rather than a central cause. Nausea and vomiting are common with vestibular neuronitis and labyrinthitis and occur less often with brainstem lesions.

Timing. Vertigo that occurs on first arising in the morning is usually the result of a vestibular disorder. Vertigo that occurs while turning over in bed is characteristic of benign positional vertigo (peripheral).

What do characteristics of the episodes tell me?

Key Questions
- How long do the episodes of dizziness last?
- Is the onset sudden or gradual?
- Do you have any hearing loss?
- Do you have ringing in your ears?

Duration of episodes. Episodes that last a few seconds are typically caused by benign positional vertigo and are usually elicited by a rapid head movement. Episodes lasting minutes to hours may be caused by Meniere's disease or recurrent vestibulopathy.

Episodes that last days or weeks are commonly produced by vestibular neuronitis. Patients may feel better when they lie completely still. Stroke can also produce long-lasting episodes. The two can be differentiated based on medical history and physical examination findings.

Sudden onset of prolonged dizziness (lasting 60 minutes or more) suggests central causes such as infection, brainstem infarction, inflammation, or vestibular hemorrhage. Trauma can also produce prolonged dizziness.

The child with chronic recurrent dizziness (episodes lasting less than 30 minutes) may have central causes such as seizure problems or migraine headache. The cause may also be peripheral such as benign paroxysmal vertigo. Chronic persistent episodes may indicate brainstem lesions, anemia, diabetes, thyrotoxicosis, or a psychosomatic disorder.

Onset. A gradual onset of dizziness is typical of an acoustic neuroma or other neoplastic process that is slow growing. Benign positional vertigo (BPV) can also have a gradual onset.

Acute or sudden onset of dizziness is characteristic of labyrinthitis, Meniere's disease, stroke, or vertebral basilar causes.

Recurrent episodes are typical of BPV, vertebral basilar causes, and Meniere's disease.

Hearing loss and tinnitus. A classic triad of symptoms—vertigo, hearing loss, and tinnitus—defines Meniere's disease. Patients may also complain of a sensation of fullness in the ears. The hearing loss may be unilateral or bilateral. Patients with secondary or early tertiary syphilis may have symptoms identical to those of Meniere's disease. Tinnitus, hearing loss, and pain in the ear point to lesions in the inner ear or cranial nerve VIII.

Patients with labyrinthitis and perilymphatic fistulae may also experience hearing loss but without tinnitus, whereas an acoustic neuroma will produce unilateral hearing loss with tinnitus. Patients with recurrent vestibulopathy usually do not complain of hearing loss.

What else should I consider?

Key Questions
- What medications are you taking?
- Are you now or have you recently been ill?

- Have you had any recent injury to your head? Did you have dizziness prior to the head injury?
- Do you have ear or facial pain?
- Do you have a history of ear infections?
- Have you had any previous ear surgery?

Medications. Mediations that are salt-retaining or ototoxic may produce vertigo, lightheadedness, or unsteadiness. Salt-retaining drugs include steroids and phenylbutazone. Ototoxic medications include ethacrynic acid, streptomycin, gentamicin, aminoglycosides, aspirin, and furosemide.

Psychotropic drugs may also produce vertigo. Antihypertensive drugs may cause hypotension leading to lightheadedness. Sedatives, alcohol, and anticonvulsants may cause a sense of disequilibrium.

Current or recent illness. Vestibular neuronitis is associated with recent viral infection, often a UTI. If a patient is currently ill, consider labyrinthitis because it is frequently associated with concomitant bacterial and viral infection.

History of head trauma. Trauma to the head or ear can cause disturbance of both peripheral and central balance mechanisms. Certain traumas can cause acute destruction of the inner ear and produce vertigo. Direct trauma can occur to the labyrinth with a temporal bone fracture. A blow to the head or a whiplash injury can also produce a concussive effect on the labyrinth. Children who have a history of head trauma can present with vertigo caused by labyrinthine damage.

Vertigo often occurs as a residual symptom and usually gradually improves over the course of a year. Trauma can also produce a fistula between the middle and inner ear, causing tympanic membrane damage and ossicle disruption.

Ear/facial pain or history of ear infection. Current ear or sinus infection can produce dysfunction of the vestibular apparatus, resulting in vertigo. Recent abnormalities of middle ear ventilation and middle ear effusion are the most common cause of balance disturbance in childhood. In balance disturbance, transmission of pressure gradients through the labyrinthine windows to the inner ear fluids and the vestibular sensory receptors is altered.

Previous otology history and procedures. Patients with cholesteatoma usually have a history of chronic middle ear infection, otorrhea, and conductive hearing loss. Prior surgical procedures of the ear can produce peripheral vertigo through disruption of the vestibular apparatus or through formation of a perilymph fistula.

DIAGNOSTIC REASONING: FOCUSED PHYSICAL EXAMINATION

Take Vital Signs/Note Blood Pressure

Assess orthostatic blood pressure to rule out postural hypotension as the cause of vertigo. Assessment is done by measuring the blood pressure in both supine and standing positions. A drop in arterial blood pressure of at least 30 systolic and 20 diastolic mm Hg when the patient changes from the supine to standing position indicates orthostatic hypotension.

Note General Appearance

In a patient who is currently ill suspect labyrinthitis. In a patient who is acutely nauseated and vomiting, suspect vestibular neuronitis.

Have Patient Hyperventilate and Perform Valsalva Maneuver

Do this testing if you suspect psychogenic vertigo, as the maneuver may reproduce the vertigo in these patients. Ask the patient to perform a Valsalva maneuver and to breathe in and out or blow vigorously for 1 to 3 minutes.

Perform Vision Examination

A recent change in visual acuity or new corrective lenses may cause transient episodes of imbalance.

Perform Ear Examination

Look for the presence of effusion or infection that signals serous otitis or otitis media. Look for the presence of a cholesteatoma. It will appear as a shiny white irregular mass; foul-smelling discharge may also be present. Note the integrity of the tympanic membrane (TM) as trauma may sometimes cause its disruption. Perform pneumatic otoscopy (see Chapter 2, Earache, p. 11), which will enable you to see if changes in pressure trigger an episode of vertigo. If the patient has a fistula, changes in pressure transmitted directly to the inner ear will cause a sudden episode of vertigo.

Perform Screening Hearing Tests

Perform Rinne (AC:BC) and Weber (lateralization) tests. Expect sensorineural loss with Meniere's disease, labyrinthitis, peri-lymph fistula, and acoustic neuroma. In sensorineural loss, the sound lateralizes to the unaffected ear. With sensorineural hearing loss, bone and air conduction are both reduced in Rinne tests, but the ratio remains the same (AC>BC). Patients with a cholesteatoma, serous otitis, or otitis media may demonstrate a conductive hearing loss (Table 10-3).

Perform Positional Nystagmus Testing/Provoking Maneuvers

The presence and characteristics of nystagmus are important in determining central versus peripheral causes of vertigo. Nystagmus is defined by the axis on which it occurs (horizontal, vertical, rotary, or mixed) and by the direction in which it occurs. Nystagmus is composed of quick and slow components that can be observed. With the eye fixated, a slow drift away from the position of fixation is corrected by a quick movement back to the original position. The direction of the nystagmus is determined by the quick component because it is easier to see. The quick component depends on the interaction between

Table 10-3			
Sensorineural versus Conductive Hearing Loss			
TEST	EXPECTED FINDINGS	CONDUCTIVE HEARING LOSS	SENSORINEURAL HEARING LOSS
Weber	No lateralization, but will lateralize to ear occluded by patient	Lateralization to deaf ear unless sensorineural loss	Lateralization to better ear unless conductive loss
Rinne	Air conduction heard longer than bone conduction by 2:1 ratio *(Rinne positive)*	Bone conduction in affected ear *(Rinne negative)*	Air conduction heard longer than bone conduction in affected ear, but less than 2:1 ratio
Schwabach	Examiner hears equally as long as the patient	Patient hears longer than the examiner	Examiner hears longer than the patient

From Seidel HM et al: *Mosby's guide to physical examination*, ed 4, St. Louis, 1998, Mosby.

the vestibular system and the cerebral cortex and represents the compensatory response to vestibular stimulation. The slow component moves in the direction of the movement of the endolymph, a clear fluid within the membranous labyrinth of the inner ear.

Fixed nystagmus, which always beats in the same direction, occurs with peripheral disorders of benign positional vertigo, Meniere's disease, vestibular neuronitis, or labyrinthitis. Vestibular nystagmus typically consists of a horizontal-rotary, jerk motion of both the slow and fast component. The nystagmus associated with central causes may be horizontal, vertical, rotary, or may be inconsistent. Pronounced rotary, unidirectional upgaze or downgaze nystagmus always arises from central processes. Nystagmus that is equally rapid in both directions is characteristic of central causes. See Table 10-4 for comparison of characteristics.

Positional maneuvers (Barany or Dix Hallpike maneuvers). To determine the origin of vertigo and accompanying nystagmus, seat the patient on the table with the patient's head turned to the left or right. Quickly lower the patient to a lying position with the head lower than the table edge so that the ear faces the ground. Repeat with the head turned to the other side and then again with the head in the midline. The maneuver produces intense vertigo in patients with vestibular problems and may cause mild vertigo in patients with central causes. During this maneuver watch for nystagmus. The patient's eyes should be kept open to observe the duration and direction of the nystagmus. The nystagmus associated with peripheral causes has a 3 to 10 second delay in onset, lessens with repetition, and is in a fixed direction. In contrast, the nystagmus associated with central causes begins immediately, does not fatigue with repetition, and may be in any and changing directions. With inner ear damage, the rapid phase of nystagmus is always in the same direction regardless of the direction of gaze.

Provocation maneuvers. In patients who experience vertigo associated with position changes or rapid movement of the head, provoke nystagmus and vertigo by having the patient assume the positions that cause the vertigo. Provocation assists in the diagnosis of benign positional vertigo. If you suspect a perilymph fistula, perform pneumatic otoscopy. The pressure applied to the

Table 10-4		
Comparison of Nystagmus in Central and Peripheral Vertigo		
CHARACTERISTICS	CENTRAL	PERIPHERAL
Severity	May be disproportionate to vertigo	Proportionate to vertigo
Axis	Horizontal, vertical, rotary; unidirectional upgaze or downgaze	Horizontal, rotary
Consistency of direction	May be inconsistent	Consistent; always beats in same direction
Type	Irregular or rapid in both directions	Has both slow and quick components

middle ear may provoke nystagmus and vertigo.

Perform Neurological Examination

Look for brainstem or cerebellar dysfunction, which could cause abnormal neurological findings. Specifically test cranial nerves, looking for sensory and/or motor deficits. With the exception of hearing loss, CN function should be normal in patients with peripheral vertigo. Patients with brainstem dysfunction typically have diplopia as well as changes in sensory and motor function.

Test cerebellar function. Testing gait differences while blindfolded may be helpful. Ataxia from bilateral vestibular loss is worsened by loss of visual input, while ataxia from cerebellar disease remains about the same. The sensitivity of gait testing is increased by watching tandem gait (heel to toe). When trying to walk a straight line, the patient with a cerebellar lesion will tend to fall toward the side of the lesion. However, gait disturbances may also be present with peripheral vertigo.

Test the patient's ability to perform rapid alternating movements (RAM) either through pronation-supination or thumb to fingers, sequentially. Movements should be smooth and rhythmic, and the patient should be able to gradually increase speed. Stiff, slowed, or jerky movements indicate cerebellar dysfunction.

Do the past-pointing test. Have the patient sit with arm extended forward and index finger pointed while you sit in the same position facing the patient. The tips of your fingers should touch. Then ask the patient to close the eyes, raise the arm above the head, and bring the arm and finger back to the same position. In patients with central lesions or unilateral vestibular abnormalities, the arm will deviate toward the side of the lesion.

Test sensory and motor function. Look for focal deficits that may occur with central vertigo. Many patients with vertigo

also complain of generalized weakness, so it is important to distinguish between generalized weakness and focal motor impairment caused by brainstem disorder.

Perform Cardiovascular Evaluation

Note heart rate and rhythm and attempt to detect dysrhythmias. Auscultate carotid and temporal arteries for bruits that may alert you to a cardiovascular cause for the vertigo.

Congenital heart disease can produce episodes of syncope that might be falsely interpreted as vertiginous episodes.

LABORATORY AND DIAGNOSTIC STUDIES

Audiometry

Audiometry is used to quantify hearing loss. The patient is tested at specific frequencies (pure tones) and specific intensities. Hearing loss is measured in decibels. Audiometry is used anytime the patient presents with both vertigo and hearing loss (i.e., Meniere's disease, acoustic neuroma, labyrinthitis, perilymph fistula, or use of ototoxic medications) (see Chapter 2, Earache, p. 12).

Electronystagmography (ENG)

ENG electronically detects nystagmus that may not be detected visually. Vestibular function is evaluated using gaze testing, positional changes, and caloric stimulation. Eye movements are recorded electronically. Caloric stimulation is produced by ear irrigation with warm and then cool water.

ENG is most useful in diagnosing chronic peripheral disorders (i.e., Meniere's disease and persistent BPV) to determine the degree and progression of the vestibular deficit. It may also be useful in patients with psychogenic vertigo to provide reassurance that no organic disease is present.

Magnetic Resonance Imaging (MRI)

MRI of the brain is indicated when the history and physical examination point to acoustic neuroma or a central cause of the vertigo.

Computed Tomography (CT)

CT scan of the brain is indicated whenever there is persistent vertigo and in all cases with additional signs of neurological disturbance. In patients with medical conditions, such as renal failure, hypertension, or a hematological malignancy, who have sudden onset of vertigo, CT scan is used to look for hemorrhage into the cerebellum, brainstem, or labyrinth.

Electroencephalogram (EEG)

An EEG should be done on patients who have vertigo associated with alterations of consciousness.

Cardiac Monitoring

An electrocardiogram or Holter monitoring can provide confirmatory information on cardiovascular causes of vertigo.

Hematology and Urinalysis

Complete blood count (CBC) may reveal anemia, which can cause presyncopal lightheadedness. Urine or serum glucose will detect diabetes mellitus, which can produce vertigo. Urine testing and blood urea nitrogen (BUN) may reveal renal failure, which can also be associated with vertigo.

Serological Testing for Syphilis

Because secondary syphilis or early tertiary syphilis can produce the same symptoms that occur in Meniere's disease, screening is advocated by some to rule out syphilis as a cause.

DIFFERENTIAL DIAGNOSIS

CENTRAL CAUSES

Brainstem Dysfunction and Cerebellar Dysfunction

Central vertigo produced by disorders of the brainstem and cerebellum are usually caused by neoplastic or vascular processes, including recurrent intermittent vascular insufficiency, transient ischemic attack, or stroke. Neoplasms are usually slow growing so vestibular dysfunction is of gradual onset and usually manifests as a problem with equilibrium.

Vascular causes are more common and may produce acute-onset, long-lasting or recurrent transient episodes of vertigo. Patients usually manifest other neurological deficits. With brainstem disorders, patients may have complaints of diplopia, dysarthria, dysphagia, and paresthesia. They may demonstrate sensory and motor deficits. Cerebellar dysfunction usually results in difficulties in fine motor coordination including RAM, finger to finger testing, and gait disturbance.

Multiple Sclerosis

Multiple sclerosis can produce a wide range of neurological symptoms. Vertigo occurs in up to 50% of patients with multiple sclerosis. Disease onset is usually in the third and fourth decades of life. MRI shows characteristic demyelinating plaques.

Migraine Headache

Approximately 30% of persons with migraine headaches have vertigo. It may be present before the headache begins, during the headache, or independent of the headache. Patients may have other symptoms consistent with vertebrobasilar vascular abnormalities such as visual changes, tinnitus, decreased hearing, ataxia, or paresthesia. Diagnosis is usually made based on history.

PERIPHERAL CAUSES

Benign Positional Vertigo (BPV)

Episodes of BPV are characterized by acute onset of vertigo associated with rapid head movement or position changes. Many women complain of dizziness with position change around the time of their menses. The episodes are brief, lasting a few seconds. Nystagmus may be elicited by positional testing. Testing positional changes may provoke the vertigo. There is no hearing loss. Diagnosis is made from history and clinical findings. This is one of the most common causes of vertigo, especially in older adults.

Benign Paroxysmal Vertigo of Childhood

BPV of childhood occurs most often in preschoolers. The disorder tends to be recurrent with 1 to 4 attacks per month. The episodes occur suddenly, and the child cries out for help. Vomiting, pallor, sweating, and nystagmus are common during the episode. The neurological and audiological examinations are entirely normal. Some children may have a hypoactive or absent response to caloric testing (ear irrigation with warm and then cool water).

Meniere's Disease

Meniere's disease is characterized by a classic triad of symptoms—vertigo, hearing loss, and tinnitus. A sensation of ear fullness may also be present. The attacks are abrupt, recurrent, and last for minutes to several hours. The interval between attacks may be weeks or months. Between episodes, the patient is asymptomatic. On physical examination, sensorineural hearing loss is present in the affected ear, or it may be bilateral.

Vestibular Neuronitis

Vestibular neuronitis is frequently preceded by an acute viral infection. These patients usually present with severe vertigo, nausea, and vomiting. The vertigo lasts for days to weeks. Remaining completely motionless may help the symptoms. Auditory function is not affected. Physical examination reveals nystagmus that intensifies in amplitude when the gaze is directed away from the affected ear. Visual fixation minimizes the nystagmus.

Labyrinthitis

Frequently associated with a concurrent viral or bacterial illness, labyrinthitis produces severe vertigo that lasts for several days. Labyrinthitis may be a complication of otitis media or meningitis. This condition is distinguished from vestibular neuronitis by the accompanying hearing loss that occurs as a result of destruction of the inner ear.

Acoustic neuroma

Also called a vestibular schwannoma, acoustic neuroma is a benign tumor that originates most often in the vestibular portion of CN VIII (acoustic). It usually causes unilateral sensorineural hearing loss, tinnitus, and loss of equilibrium. The neuroma grows slowly, so loss of equilibrium is more often a symptom than is vertigo. Acoustic neuroma can also occur in CN V (trigeminal) with symptoms of paresthesia consistent with the nerve distribution. Large tumors of CN VI (abducens) may compress the brainstem.

Perilymph Fistula

Fistula formation can occur as a result of ear trauma, from a direct blow, secondary to otologic surgery, or indirectly from straining, coughing, or pressure changes. In this condition there is leakage of perilymph from either the round or oval window into the middle ear. Sensorineural hearing loss is frequently present as well as vertigo. The fistula will often heal spontaneously but sometimes may require surgery.

Sinusitis and Otitis

Serous otitis, otitis media, and sinusitis can cause disruption of the vestibular apparatus, producing vertigo. History and physical examination findings will be consistent with the specific disorder (see Chapter 2, Earache, and Nasal Symptoms and Sinus Congestion).

Cholesteatoma

Collection of squamous debris often associated with chronic middle ear infection can form a cholesteatoma, which enlarges and destroys structures in its way. On physical examination, the cholesteatoma will appear as a shiny white irregular mass. Foul-smelling discharge may be evident, and there may be visible bone destruction. A conductive hearing loss may be present.

SYSTEMIC CAUSES

Psychogenic

Psychogenic causes of vertigo are common. Patients often describe themselves as anxious or nervous and may have psychiatric diagnoses. Their symptoms are vague and imprecise. Neurological examination is normal. No nystagmus is present or elicited. The vertigo may be reproduced with hyperventilation. MRI may be useful to provide reassurance.

Cardiovascular

Orthostatic hypotension and cardiac dysrhythmias can produce vertigo. Diagnosis of postural hypotension can be made by taking orthostatic blood pressure readings. Diagnosis of cardiac conditions may involve CBC, blood chemistry, ECG, cardiac stress testing, and echocardiography.

Neurosyphilis

Secondary or early tertiary syphilis can present with symptoms similar to those of Meniere's disease. The patient demonstrates various clinical symptoms, including papilledema, aphasia, mono- or hemiplegia, CN palsies, pupillary abnormalities, or focal neurological deficits. The Argyll-Robertson pupil, which occurs almost exclusively in neurosyphilis, is a small irregular pupil that reacts normally to accommodate but not to light. Serological testing will be positive for syphilis.

OTHER CAUSES

Ototoxic Drugs and Drugs Causing Salt Retention

Medications that are ototoxic or cause salt retention may produce vertigo, lightheadedness, or unsteadiness. Drugs causing salt retention include steroids and phenylbutazone. Ototoxic medications include aspirin, ethacrynic acid, streptomycin, gentamicin, aminoglycosides, and furosemide. Psychotropic drugs may also produce vertigo. Ototoxic drugs may produce a sensorineural hearing loss. Audiometry should be performed with any noted hearing loss.

Trauma

Injury to the head or ear can produce disturbance of the vestibular apparatus and result in vertigo, resulting from labyrinthine concussion, temporal bone fracture, or perilymph fistula. Head trauma can also produce cerebral concussion involving the anterior tip of the temporal lobe. Trauma from otologic procedures can also cause vertigo.

Table 10-5

Differential Diagnosis of Common Causes of Dizziness

Condition	History	Physical Findings	Diagnostic Studies
Central Causes			
Brainstem dysfunction/ cerebellar dysfunction	Elderly; acute-onset; recurrent vertigo; tinnitus; hearing OK	Symptoms of brainstem/ vertebro- basilar vascular ab- normality: ataxia, double vision; lack of coordination; sensory/motor defi- cits; vertical, lateral, rotary nystagmus; hearing normal; cerebellar: lack of coordination; im- paired RAM, finger- to-finger testing	MRI
Multiple sclerosis	Often in 3rd-4th decade of life	May have no other findings or may have other neuro- logical symptoms	MRI
Migraine headache	Headache history; other migraine symptoms	May have symptoms of vertebrobasilar vascular abnormali- ties, as above	None
Peripheral Causes			
Benign positional vertigo	Adults: associated with positional changes; recurrent episodes; lasts seconds to minutes; some relief if motionless	Lateral or rotary nys- tagmus, *no* tinnitus or hearing loss	Provoke nystag- mus and vertigo by position that causes; ENG
Benign paroxysmal vertigo of childhood	Children: usually pre- schoolers, sudden onset with crying by child	Vomiting, pallor, sweating, and nys- tagmus common, no loss of conscious- ness; neurological and audiological exam may be normal	May have hypo- active or absent re- sponse to caloric testing
Meniere's disease	Sudden onset; lasts hours, recurrent; tinnitus and fullness in the ears	Lateral or rotary nys- tagmus; fluctuating hearing loss: low tones; sensorineural	Positional ma- neuvers, audi- ometry, ENG
Vestibular neuronitis	Sudden onset; ante- cedent viral infection	Nausea and vomiting; nystagmus; no hearing loss	Positional maneuvers

Table 10-5

Differential Diagnosis of Common Causes of Dizziness—cont'd

Condition	History	Physical Findings	Diagnostic Studies
Peripheral Causes—cont'd			
Labyrinthitis	Sudden onset, lasts hours to days	May be currently ill; lateral nystagmus; hearing loss; rarely tinnitus; nausea and vomiting may be present	Positional maneuvers, audiometry
Acoustic neuroma	Adults; gradual onset; mild vertigo; persistent tinnitus; facial numbness, weakness	Unilateral hearing loss, poor speech discrimination	MRI; audiometry
Perilymph fistula	History of trauma; hearing loss	Nystagmus and vertigo with pneumatic otoscopy; sensorineural hearing loss	Audiometry
Otitis/sinusitis	Pain in ear or face; history of ear or sinus infections; gradual onset of vertigo	Serous otitis, otitis media; tenderness over sinuses; purulent nasal discharge; no nystagmus	See Chapter 2
Cholesteatoma	History of chronic middle ear infections	Shiny white irregular mass on otoscopic exam; foul-smelling discharge may be present; bone destruction may be visible; conductive hearing loss may be present	Audiometry
Systemic Causes			
Psychogenic	Vague symptoms; recurrent; may describe self as anxious; may have other psychiatric diagnoses	Normal neurological and auditory exam	Hyperventilation to reproduce the vertigo
Cardiovascular	CV history; antihypertensive medications	Orthostatic blood pressure; dysrhythmias; carotid or temporal bruits	Depends on patient condition and symptoms

Continued

Table 10-5

Differential Diagnosis of Common Causes of Dizziness—cont'd

Condition	History	Physical Findings	Diagnostic Studies
Systemic Causes—cont'd			
Neurosyphilis	Vertigo, tinnitus, fullness in ears	Various clinical symptoms: papilledema, aphasia, mono- or hemiplegia, CN palsies, pupillary abnormalities, Argyll-Robertson pupil; focal neurological deficits	Serology for syphilis
Other Causes			
Ototoxic and salt-retaining drugs	Medication history: steroids, phenylbutazone; ethacrynic acid, aspirin, streptomycin, gentamicin, aminoglycosides, furosemide, psychotropic drugs	Sensorineural hearing loss	Audiometry
Trauma	History of trauma to the head or ear	Depends on nature and location of injury; may exhibit peripheral or central symptoms	MRI/CT

Chapter 11

Common Problems in Mental Status

Confusion in Older Adults

Confusion is characterized by disorientation and inappropriate reaction to environmental stimuli. An acute confusional state can result from hospitalization or surgery, systemic or electrolyte imbalance, organ failure, excessive medication, nutritional insufficiency, systemic infection, or cerebral insufficiency, such as stroke or transient ischemic attacks. Delirium, dementia, or depression, especially in the elderly, can also cause confusion.

Delirium, caused by alteration in brain metabolism, is characterized by abrupt onset, reduced level of acute consciousness, and sleep-wake cycle disturbance. Delirium, which is a medical emergency, can occur as a result of medications, alcohol use or alcohol withdrawal, narcotic reaction or narcotic withdrawal, Wernicke's syndrome (vitamin B_{12} deficiency), hepatic encephalopathy, acute illness, chronic illness, interacting diseases, or trauma (e.g., head injury).

Dementia, a chronic generalized impairment of brain function, affects thinking but not level of consciousness. A common early complaint in dementia is forgetfulness, with loss of concentration and loss of memory. Causes of dementia can be classified as reversible (or partially reversible), modifiable, or irreversible (Box 11-1).

Depression as a cause of confusion, especially in the elderly, is considered a reversible cause of dementia. When anxiety symptoms are also present, depression may manifest as mild delirium.

DIAGNOSTIC REASONING: FOCUSED HISTORY

Getting an appropriate history from a confused patient involves the use of another person as the historian. Preferably that person is someone who has had consistent contact with the patient and can report about usual behavioral patterns and the conditions involved with this episode.

| **Box 11-1** | | | |

Causes of Dementia

Reversible Causes of Dementia
D - Drugs/medications
E - Emotional illness/depression
M - Metabolic/endocrine disorders
E - Eye/ear involvement/
    environmental
N - Nutritional/neurological
T - Tumors/trauma
I - Infection
A - Alcoholism/anemia/
    atherosclerosis

Modifiable Causes of Dementia
Normal pressure hydrocephalus
Hepatic encephalopathy
HIV encephalopathy (AIDS dementia
    complex)

Irreversible Causes of Dementia
Alzheimer's disease
Multi-infarct dementia
Huntington's chorea

Is this a condition that requires immediate intervention?

Key Questions
- How suddenly did the confusion start?
- How long has the confusion persisted?
- Is the patient alert and aware?
- Has the patient expressed thoughts of suicide? (word or actions)
- Is there a history of substance abuse?

Confusion that is acute in onset and persistent may indicate delirium, a cerebrovascular event, cerebral infection, subdural hematoma, or neoplasm. A history of altered level of consciousness as well as the patient's current state indicates a medical condition that requires immediate intervention. Acute-onset confusion may produce paranoia and aggression. However, suicidal ideation may accompany depression and is also an indication for immediate intervention and further evaluation. If the patient has been abusing alcohol or other chemical substances, acute withdrawal may require immediate medical intervention.

If the onset is gradual and the patient is not seriously ill, consider depression or dementia. Remember that depression and dementia can co-exist. Unless the patient is suicidal or seriously ill, both depression and dementia can be handled in a more temperate manner.

What distinguishing characteristics of confusion does this patient exhibit?

Key Questions
- When did the confusion begin?
- How long has it been present?
- Is there any history of head trauma?
- Was the onset of the confusion abrupt (over a period of minutes or hours) or gradual (a few days, weeks, or months)?
- Does the confusion change within a 24-hour period (stable or fluctuating?)
- Is there a change in the sleep pattern?
- Is the patient alert and aware?
- Has the patient experienced seeing, hearing, or feeling things that are not there?

Onset and duration. Confusion that is abrupt in onset but short-lived may indicate a transient ischemic attack (TIA). Sudden onset, usually over a period of hours, is characteristic of delirium. In delirium, the condition is persistent but has been present for no longer than a month.

In an acute confusional episode, the symptoms are less severe than with delirium with a less sudden onset. The onset in depression is usually gradual, over a period of weeks, and is persistent over time. In dementia, the onset is insidious and gradual; the condition has often been present for many weeks or months.

Head trauma. Head trauma can produce confusion and disorientation. In older adults, common causes of head trauma include motor vehicle crashes, physical abuse, and falls.

Fluctuation in symptoms. With delirium, the symptoms may fluctuate over the course of a day and frequently get worse at night and with fatigue. The course is more stable with both depression and dementia, with little variation over a 24-hour period.

Disturbance in sleep-wake cycle. The sleep-wake cycle in delirium is always impaired. Either the wakefulness is abnormally increased and the patient gets little or no sleep; or the patient suffers from night insomnia and is drowsy and tired during the day. Thus the sleep-wake cycle is usually fragmented, and the patient tends to be restless, agitated, and suffers from hallucinations while awake during the night.

Level of consciousness. In both dementia and depression, the individual is likely to be both alert and aware, although the mood may be depressed. With delirium, the patient will have a decreased level of consciousness, be less alert and aware, and may be difficult to arouse. With an acute confusional state, the person will demonstrate impaired concentration and make errors in thinking.

Hallucinations. Visual, tactile, and auditory hallucinations are common with delirium, especially at night when changes in environment or activity occur. Hallucinations are uncommon in both depression and dementia, although hallucinations may occur in late-stage dementia.

Are there any associated symptoms that will point me in the right direction?

Key Questions
- Has the patient shown any tremor, especially at rest?
- Has the patient had any trouble walking?
- Has the patient complained of severe headache and/or nausea?
- Has the patient had a fever?
- Has the patient gained or lost weight?
- Does the patient engage in his/her usual activities?

Tremor, gait disturbance. Tremors are associated with parkinsonism, HIV encephalopathy, and liver disease. Gait disorder is associated with parkinsonism, medication reactions, and head trauma.

Headache, nausea, fever. Headache and nausea are associated with head trauma, stroke, and tumor. Fever is usually present with HIV infection, systemic infections, or acute alcohol withdrawal.

Vegetative symptoms. Patients with depression may exhibit vegetative symptoms (cessation of talking, eating, dressing, and toileting; insomnia; weight loss or gain; diminished interest in most activities or former pleasures) and feelings of worthlessness.

What does the pattern of cognitive losses tell me?

Key Questions
- What specific problems with mental abilities or thinking have you noticed?
- What behavioral changes or personality changes have you noticed?

Changes in mental abilities and behaviors. Patients with delirium have global cognitive losses that involve memory, thinking, perception, and judgment. These patients may become completely disoriented, irritable, and fearful. They may be difficult to arouse or conversely have insomnia. Families sometimes note visual hallucinations.

Patients in an acute confusional state may be disoriented, especially for time, less for place, and almost never for self. They show impaired concentration, experience sensory misperceptions, and make errors in thinking.

Dementia, particularly early in the disorder, presents with more selective cognitive losses. Family members complain that patients can't remember recent events, are disoriented, are irritable or depressed, have poor hygiene, show poor judgment, make financial errors, are socially withdrawn, have difficulty finding or saying the right words, are clumsy or fall, have urinary incontinence, have deteriorating interpersonal relationships, and show personality changes.

Fewer cognitive losses occur with depression. These persons may exhibit cognitive losses consistent with confusion—apathy and drowsiness, impaired concentration, and errors in thinking. The most common cognitive symptoms are severe negative thinking, guilt, and remorse.

Is the confusion caused by a concurrent medical problem?

Key Questions
- What chronic health conditions does this patient have?
- Has the patient been hospitalized recently? What for?
- Has the patient been acutely ill recently?
- Has the patient had liver, kidney, or brain disorder?
- Does this patient have hypertension, heart disease, or lung disease?
- Is there a history of mental illness or similar thought disturbance?

Current and past health status. You may need to obtain past medical records to obtain a complete medical history. Most likely you will have to use a relative or close friend to determine current and past health status. Many systemic conditions and disorders can produce alteration in mental status, particularly in older patients (Box 11-2). Chronic health problems such as alcoholism, renal failure, liver disease, severe anemia, COPD, severe cardiovascular disease, and HIV predispose individuals, especially the elderly, to the development of confusion. Patients with multiple chronic health problems are particularly at risk.

Could the confusion be caused by medication?

Key Questions
- What medications is the patient taking? (prescribed and over the counter)
- Is the patient taking the medication accurately?

Drugs that can produce altered mental status include the following:
- Alcohol
- Antibiotics (isoniazid, aminoglycosides)
- Anticholinergic agents
- Anticonvulsants
- Antidepressants
- Antihypertensive agents (reserpine, beta blockers, methyldopa, clonidine, hydralazine)
- Antiparkinsonian agents
- Cardiac drugs (digitalis, lidocaine, beta blockers, vasodilators, diuretics)
- Chemotherapeutic agents (methotrexate)
- Gastrointestinal drugs (H_2 blockers, metoclopramide)
- Illicit drugs (amphetamines, cocaine, opiates)
- Narcotics
- OTC cold/allergy preparations
- Sedatives
- Tranquilizers

Box 11-2	⎪⎪⎪⎪

Systemic Conditions Associated With Confusional States

Endocrine
Hypo/hyperthyroidism

Metabolic
Anemia (severe)
Hypo/hypercalcemia
Hypo/hypercortisolism
Hypo/hyperglycemia
Hypomagnesemia
Hypo/hypernatremia
Wilson's disease (copper disorder)
Porphyria

Infectious
AIDS
Cerebral amebiasis
Cerebral cysticercosis
Cerebral toxoplasmosis
Cerebral malaria
Fungal meningitis
Lyme disease
Neurosyphilis
TB meningitis

Cardiovascular
Congestive heart failure
Hyperviscosity

Cerebrovascular
Cerebral insufficiency (TIA, CVA)
Post-anoxic encephalopathy

Pulmonary
COPD
Hypercapnia
Hypoxemia

Renal
Renal failure
Uremia

Neurological
Hepatic encephalopathy
Hypertensive encephalopathy
Limbic encephalitis
Head trauma

Other
Alcoholism
Anemia (severe)
Leukoencephalopathy
Metastatic cancer to brain
Sarcoidosis
Sleep apnea
Vasculitis (e.g., SLE)
Vitamin deficiencies (B_{12}, folate, niacin, thiamine)
Whipple's disease

Combinations of these medications increase the probability of medication induced confusion. People who are confused may be taking medications improperly, which compounds the problem.

What risk factors do I need to consider?

Key Questions
- How old is the patient?
- How many medications is the patient taking?
- Is the patient HIV positive?
- Has the patient experienced recent life losses?

Age. Older adults are at risk for the development of confusion, delirium, dementia, and depression. Factors that place them at risk include the use of multiple medications, the existence of multiple medical conditions, and the physiological changes associated with aging. Dementia occurs in approximately 5% to 10% of people age 65 to 80 years, in 20% of people over 80 years, and in 47% of people over the age of 85 years.

Polypharmacy. Older adults who are taking multiple medications are at risk for medication interactions and resulting confusion (see also the preceding list of medications that can produce altered mental status).

HIV. Patients with HIV infection or those who are immunocompromised are at increased risk for the development of HIV encephalopathy (AIDS dementia complex) or dementia caused by central nervous system (CNS) opportunistic infections.

Recent bereavement. Recent loss and the lack of a social network place an individual at risk for depression. Both cause profound biopsychosocial stress that can easily exceed the person's resources and skills. Extreme mourning or isolation can be physically and emotionally draining.

DIAGNOSTIC REASONING: FOCUSED PHYSICAL EXAMINATION

Take Vital Signs

The presence of a fever may indicate infection or alcohol withdrawal. A diastolic blood pressure greater than 120 suggests hypertensive encephalopathy, whereas a systolic blood pressure less than 90 may indicate impaired cerebral perfusion.

Note Level of Consciousness

In both dementia and depression, the individual is likely to be alert and aware, although the mood may be depressed. With delirium, the patient will have a decreased level of consciousness, be less alert and aware, and may be difficult to arouse. With an acute confusional state, the patient will demonstrate impaired concentration and have difficulty thinking.

Perform a Mental Status Examination

A thorough mental status examination is essential. Administer the Mini-Mental State Examination (MMSE) (Figure 11-1, pp. 408-409). Patients with delirium may be unable to cooperate or answer questions. Patients with dementia are cooperative and willing to try, but make mistakes and give incorrect or "near miss" answers. Patients with depression are less cooperative and are more likely to give "don't know" answers, refuse to answer questions, or are less willing to try.

Global cognitive loss is consistent with delirium. Losses occur in the following areas: memory, thinking, perception, information acquisition, information retention, information processing, information retrieval, and information use. Thus the MMSE score will be very low with inability to perform most or all of the items.

Dementia, particularly early in the disorder, presents with selective cognitive losses that may occur in one or more of the following areas. Specific losses include:

- Apraxia: can't draw simple geometric figures
- Visuospatial problems: can't draw intersecting pentagons
- Can't perform commands
- Selective cognitive loss
- Loss of abstract reasoning
- Problems with orientation
- Problems with recent memory
- Problems with number retention

Fewer cognitive losses occur with depression than with dementia. Loss of concentration is an important symptom of depression. The individual is aware of losses and may highlight disabilities, especially memory loss. Along with loss of memory, impaired concentration and errors in judgment are common.

In older persons, also administer the Geriatric Depression scale (Figure 11-2, p. 410). The test is positive for depression if the score is above 5.

Perform a Complete Neurological Examination

Normal neurological findings are typical of early dementia and depression. Abnormal findings suggest other pathophysiological involvement.

Cranial nerves. Check vision, hearing, and sensory impairment as contributing factors in confusion. Dilated pupils suggest alcohol withdrawal; pinpoint pupils may indicate narcotic excess or eye drops. Changes in pupil size may also indicate neurological changes such as occur with stroke or neoplasm. The sense of smell is often impaired in dementia. Patients with parkinsonism may exhibit a typical facial presentation—masked facial expression, poor blink reflex, and drooling. Speech is slowed, slurred, and monotonous.

Proprioception and cerebellar function. Test coordination through rapid alternating movement (RAM), accuracy of movement, balance (Romberg), and gait. Slowed RAM is characteristic of early HIV encephalopathy. Tremor and restlessness are associated with alcohol intoxication or withdrawal. Tremor, especially resting, rigidity, and bradykinesia, indicate parkinsonism. Asterixis, sometimes referred to as liver flap or liver tremor, is an involuntary tremor of the hands, tongue, and feet that is characteristic of hepatic or metabolic encephalopathy. Postural tremor is present with HIV encephalopathy. Writhing movements (chorea) typify Huntington's disease.

Gait abnormalities are found with multi-infarct dementia, normal pressure hydrocephalus, and HIV encephalopathy.

Sensation (primary and cortical). Agnosia (failure to identify or recognize objects despite intact sensory function) is present with dementia.

Reflexes. Test deep tendon reflexes (DTRs) and the superficial plantar reflexes. Hyperreflexia and primitive reflexes are present in late dementia. Hyperreflexia is also present in multi-infarct dementia, HIV encephalopathy, and CVA.

A positive Babinski sign on testing the plantar reflex is present in multi-infarct dementia, CVA, and head injury. Cogwheeling (resistance to a passively stretched hypertonic muscle resulting in a rhythmical jerk similar to a ratchet) suggests parkinsonism.

Motor tone and function. Apraxia (impaired ability to carry out motor activities despite intact motor function) indicates dementia. Motor weakness, especially of the legs, loss of coordination, and impaired handwriting, are consistent with early HIV encephalopathy.

Language. Aphasia (language disturbance) is often present in dementia and may also occur with CVA and head injury.

Localizing and lateralizing signs in CNS. Focal neurological signs (i.e., exaggerated DTRs, positive Babinski's sign, gait abnormalities, and hemiparesis) are consistent with multi-infarct dementia. Focal deficits also occur with cerebrovascular injury.

Patients with late HIV encephalopathy demonstrate weakness greater in legs than arms, ataxia, spasticity and hyperreflexia, positive Babinski's sign, myoclonus, and bladder and bowel incontinence.

Psychomotor agitation or retardation is consistent with depression. An agitated confusional state without focal signs may occur with head trauma

Perform a Respiratory Examination

Monitor the rate and effort of respirations. Auscultate the lung fields. Tachypnea suggests hypoxia. Bibasilar crackles indicate CHF with hypoxia. Asymmetrical crackles suggest pneumonia with hypoxia. Patients with dementia or depression in the absence of concomitant lung disease will have normal findings.

Patient_____
Examiner_____
Date_____

"MINI-MENTAL STATE"

Maximum

Score   *Score*

ORIENTATION

5   ( ) What is the (year) (season) (date) (day) (month)?
5   ( ) Where are we: (state) (county) (town) (hospital) (floor).

REGISTRATION

3   ( ) Name 3 objects: 1second to say each. Then ask the patient all 3 after you
have said them.
Give 1 point for each correct answer. Then repeat them until
he learns all 3. Count trials and record.

ATTENTION AND CALCULATION

5   ( ) Serial 7s. 1 point for each correct. Stop after 5 answers. Alternatively spell
"world" backwards.

RECALL

3   ( ) Ask for the 3 objects repeated above. Give 1 point for each correct.

LANGUAGE

9   ( ) Name a pencil and watch (2 points)
Repeat the following "No ifs, ands or buts." (1 point)
Follow a 3-stage command:
        "Take a paper in your right hand, fold it in half, and put it
        on the floor" (3 points)
Read and obey the following:
        CLOSE YOUR EYES (1 point)
Write a sentence (1 point)
Copy design (1 point)
_____ Total score
ASSESS level of consciousness along a continuum

_____
Alert   Drowsy   Stupor   Coma

Figure 11-1 Mini-Mental State Test, a standardized screening tool of mental status. The maximum score is 30. Depressed patients without dementia usually score between 24 and 30. A score of 20 or less is found in patients with dementia, delirium, schizophrenia, or an affective disorder. (From Folstein MF, Folstein SE, McHugh PR: Mini-Mental State: a practical method for grading the cognitive state of patients for the clinician, *J Psychiatr Res* 12:189, 1975; Folstein M et al: The meaning of cognitive impairment in the elderly, *J Am Geriatr Soc* 33[4]:228, 1985.)

INSTRUCTIONS FOR ADMINISTRATION OF
MINI-MENTAL STATE EXAMINATION

ORIENTATION

(1) Ask for the date. Then ask specifically for parts omitted, e.g., "Can you also tell me what season it is?" One point for each correct.

(2) Ask in turn "Can you tell me the name of this hospital?" (town, county, etc.). One point for each correct.

REGISTRATION

Ask the patient if you may test his memory. Then say the name of 3 unrelated objects, clearly and slowly, about one second for each. After you have said 3, ask him to repeat them. The first repetition determines his score (0-3) but keep saying them until he can repeat all 3, up to 6 trials. If he does not eventually learn all 3, recall cannot be meaningfully tested.

ATTENTION AND CALCULATION

Ask the patient to begin with 100 and count backwards by 7. Stop after 5 subtractions (93, 86, 79, 72, 65). Score the total number of correct answers.

If the patient cannot or will not perform this task, ask him to spell the word "world" backwards. The score is the number of letters in correct order. E.g. dlrow = 5, dlorw = 3.

RECALL

Ask the patient if he can recall the 3 words you previously asked him to remember. Score 0-3.

LANGUAGE

Naming: Show the patient a wristwatch and ask him what it is. Repeat for pencil. Score 0-2.

Repetition: Ask the patient to repeat the sentence after you. Allow only one trial. Score 0 or 1.

3-Stage Command: Give the patient a piece of plain blank paper and repeat the command. Score 1 point for each part correctly executed.

Reading: On a blank piece of paper print the sentence "Close your eyes," in letters large enough for the patient to see clearly. Ask him to read it and do what it says. Score 1 point only if he actually closes his eyes.

Writing: Give the patient a blank piece of paper and ask him to write a sentence for you. Do not dictate a sentence; it is to be written spontaneously. It must contain a subject and verb to be sensible. Correct grammar and punctuation are not necessary.

Copying: On a clean piece of paper, draw intersecting pentagons, each side about 1 inch, and ask him to copy it exactly as it is. All 10 angles must be present and 2 must intersect to score 1 point. Tremor and rotation are ignored.

Estimate the patient's level of sensorium along a continuum, from alert on the left to coma on the right.

Figure 11-1, cont'd

Geriatric Depression Scale (short form)

Choose the best answer for how you felt over the past week.

1. Are you basically satisfied with your life?   yes/no

2. Have you dropped many of your activities and interests?   yes/no

3. Do you feel that your life is empty?   yes/no

4. Do you often get bored?   yes/no

5. Are you in good spirits most of the time?   yes/no

6. Are you afraid that something bad is going to happen to you?   yes/no

7. Do you feel happy most of the time?   yes/no

8. Do you often feel helpless?   yes/no

9. Do you prefer to stay at home, rather than going out and doing new things?   yes/no

10. Do you feel you have more problems with memory than most?   yes/no

11. Do you think it is wonderful to be alive now?yes/no

12. Do you feel pretty worthless the way you are now?   yes/no

13. Do you feel full of energy?   yes/no

14. Do you feel that your situation is hopeless?yes/no

15. Do you think that most people are better off than you are?   yes/no

This is the scoring for the scale. One point for each of these answers. Cut-off: normal (0-5), above 5 suggests depression.

1. no	6. yes	11. no
2. yes	7. no	12. yes
3. yes	8. yes	13. no
4. yes	9. yes	14. yes
5. no	10. yes	15. yes

Figure 11-2 Geriatric Depression Scale (short form). (From Sheikh JI, Yesavage JA: Geriatric Depression Scale: recent evidence and development of a shorter version, *Clin Gerontol* 5:165-172, 1986.)

Evaluate the Cardiovascular System

Perform a careful cardiovascular examination. Tachycardia suggests sepsis, hyperthyroidism, hypoglycemia, agitation, anxiety, or alcohol withdrawal. Be alert for indicators of cardiovascular problems that can produce hypoxia, such as congestive heart failure (CHF) or myocardial infarction (MI).

Examine the Abdomen

Examine the abdomen and percuss for costovertebral angle (CVA) tenderness. Specific findings may indicate a local or systemic cause for the confusion. For example, urinary retention suggests urinary tract infection, CVA tenderness points to pyelonephritis, and an enlarged liver may indicate hepatic encephalopathy.

LABORATORY AND DIAGNOSTIC STUDIES

Diagnostic testing is aimed at detecting or confirming a metabolic/pathophysiological cause of the confusion. If dementia seems likely, these same tests can rule in or rule out reversible or modifiable causes of the dementia. Most tests will be normal when the diagnosis is depression.

Complete Blood Count (CBC)

Leukocytosis suggests infection. Anemia as a cause of confusion in chronic illness can also be detected.

Blood Chemistry

High or low potassium or sodium, dehydration, or acidosis can all produce confusion. Elevated or depressed magnesium and calcium levels, hypoglycemia, and hyperglycemia can also cause confusion. Elevated blood urea nitrogen (BUN) and creatinine levels or an elevated BUN:creatinine ratio may indicate renal failure. Elevation in liver enzymes suggests liver dysfunction.

Thyroid Function Tests (TFTs)

Abnormal levels of thyroid-stimulating hormone (TSH) may indicate thyroid dysfunction, either thyroid toxicosis or a hypothyroid state. An elevated TSH is related to chronic symptoms of depression.

Serum B_{12}, Folate

Deficiency of B_{12} and folate are reversible causes of dementia.

Serology for Syphilis

A positive test can indicate neurosyphilis as the cause of confusion.

Arterial Blood Gases (ABGs)

ABGs are used to determine the presence or degree of hypoxia.

Toxicology Screen and Blood Alcohol Level

These tests can be used to determine alcohol or drug intoxication as a cause of confusion.

Urinalysis (U/A)

Urinalysis is used to detect infection and may point to renal indicators of systemic disease. See Chapter 6, Urinary Problems in Females and Children, p. 233 for a complete discussion of urinalysis.

Chest X-Ray

Chest x-ray is used to detect infection, congestive heart failure, chronic pulmonary disease, pneumonia, or other respiratory-associated causes of hypoxia.

Lumbar Puncture

Lumbar puncture is used to rule out bacterial, fungal, or tumor meningitis (see Chapter 10, Headache, p. 380).

Electrocardiogram (ECG)

ECG is used to rule out certain cardiovascular causes of hypoxia, such as MI or dysrhythmias.

Electroencephalogram (EEG)

EEG can identify a seizure disorder as a cause of or as a contributing factor to confusion.

Computed Tomography (CT) or Magnetic Resonance Imaging (MRI)

CT or MRI are used to diagnose cerebrovascular bleeding, injury, abscess, or tumor, or if focal neurological signs are present. These imaging tests usually do not yield useful information related to the diagnosis of dementia.

DIFFERENTIAL DIAGNOSIS

Delirium

Delirium is characterized by reduced ability to maintain attention to external stimuli, disorganized thinking, decreased level of consciousness (LOC), perceptual disturbances, disturbed sleep-wake cycle, disorientation, and memory impairment. The patient will evidence a decreased LOC and impaired arousal, increased or decreased psychomotor activity, and irritability. The onset is rapid, and the condition can last from hours to weeks. Fluctuations over the course of the day are common, with lucid intervals during the day and worse symptoms at night. The thought process is disorganized, and the patient is usually disoriented, most commonly to time. There is a tendency to mistake the unfamiliar for familiar places and patients. Hallucinations, usually visual, are common. Physical examination findings depend on the underlying cause of the delirium. The patient often exhibits asterixis or tremor. Speech is incoherent, hesitant, slow, or rapid. Box 11-3 gives DSM-IV criteria for diagnosis of delirium.

Confusion

Confusion is less abrupt and less severe than delirium, with less severe disorientation and more subtle motor signs. The diurnal variation is less severe than in delirium. The person may be apathetic and drowsy and will show disorientation, especially for time, less for place, and almost never for self. Concentration is impaired, and the person lacks direction, selectivity, and is easily distracted. Errors in thinking are common. The person may exhibit tremor and difficulty in motor relaxation.

Box 11-3

DSM-IV Criteria for Diagnosis of Delirium

- Disturbance of consciousness (i.e., reduced clarity or awareness of the environment) with reduced ability to focus, sustain, or shift attention.
- A change in cognition (i.e., memory deficit, disorientation, language disturbance) or the development of a perceptual disturbance that is not better accounted for by a preexisting, established, or evolving dementia.
- Disturbance develops over a short period of time (usually hours to days) and tends to fluctuate during the course of the day.
- History, physical examination, or laboratory evidence indicates that the disturbance is a direct physiological consequence of either a general medical condition, substance intoxication, or medication side effect.

From American Psychiatric Association: *Diagnostic and statistical manual of mental disorders,* ed 4, Washington, DC, 1994, American Psychiatric Association.

Dementia

Dementia is characterized by acquired persistent and progressive impairment of intellectual function, with compromise in at least two of the following areas:

- Language (aphasia)
- Memory
- Visuospatial skills (apraxia, agnosia)
- Emotional behavior or personality
- Cognition
- Calculation, abstraction, judgment, etc.

Boxes 11-4 and 11-5 give DSM-IV diagnostic criteria.

The onset of symptoms is insidious, with the course stable through the day and night. The condition can be present for months or years, with progressive deterioration. Recent and remote memory is impaired. The patient is alert and attention is

---

Box 11-4

DSM-IV Criteria for Diagnosis of Dementia

I. The development of multiple cognitive defects manifested by both
   A. Memory impairment (can't learn new or recall previous information)
   B. One or more of the following cognitive disturbances
      1. Aphasia (language disturbance)
      2. Apraxia (impaired ability to carry out motor activities despite intact motor function)
      3. Agnosia (failure to identify or recognize objects despite intact sensory function)
      4. Disturbance in executive functioning (planning, organizing, sequencing, abstracting)
II. The cognitive deficits in IA and IB each cause considerable impairment in social or occupational functioning and represent substantial decline from a previous level of functioning

From American Psychiatric Association: *Diagnostic and statistical manual of mental disorders,* ed 4, Washington, DC, 1994, American Psychiatric Association.

Box 11-5

DSM-IV Criteria for Diagnosis of Alzheimer-Type Dementia

Criteria as outlined in Box 11-4 for dementia plus:
III. The course is characterized by gradual onset or continuing cognitive decline
IV. The cognitive defects in criteria IA and IB are *not* the result of any of the following
   A. Other CNS conditions that cause progressive deficits in memory and cognition (CVD, parkinsonism, Huntington's chorea, brain tumor, etc.)
   B. Systemic conditions that are known to cause dementia (hypothyroid, vitamin B12 or folic acid deficiency, niacin deficiency, hypercalcemia, neurosyphilis, HIV infection)
V. The deficits do not occur exclusively during the course of a delirium
VI. The disturbance is not better accounted for by an Axis 1 disorder (major depression, schizophrenia)

From American Psychiatric Association: *Diagnostic and statistical manual of mental disorders,* ed 4, Washington, DC, 1994, American Psychiatric Association.

Box 11-6 ‖ ‖ ‖

Common Presentations of Dementia

Memory loss	Language difficulty
Depression	Social withdrawal
Irritability	Behavioral change
Poor hygiene	Urinary incontinence
Insomnia	Hallucinations (late)
Paranoia	Anxiety
Weight loss	Failure to thrive
Poor work performance	Falls, clumsiness
Financial errors	Deteriorating interpersonal relation-
Poor judgment	ships
Delirium	Personality changes

---

relatively unaffected, although orientation is usually impaired. Hallucinations are usually absent until late in the course of the disease. Speech is usually unimpaired although the person has difficulty with finding words. Sleep is often fragmented. On mental status examination, the patient tries hard and provides "near miss" answers. Physical findings are often absent. The olfactory sense may be impaired. Box 11-6 lists common presentations of dementia, and Box 11-7 lists phases of Alzheimer-type dementia.

Alzheimer-type dementia can sometimes be distinguished from multi-infarct dementia (MID) through a cardiovascular history, progression of symptoms, and the presence or absence of focal neurological signs and symptoms (Table 11-1).

Depression

Depression can produce confusion, especially in the elderly. The onset of the confusion is often abrupt, with some diurnal variation. Generally, depression is more consistent over time than delirium. The confusion is of short duration as compared to dementia. A past history of psychiatric problems, including undiagnosed depressive episodes, is common. During mental status examination, the patient tends to highlight disabilities, especially memory

---

Box 11-7 ‖ ‖ ‖

Phases of Alzheimer-Type Dementia

Limbic
2-3 years after onset
Olfactory system involved
Memory loss
Can perform tasks

Parietal
3-6 years after onset
Loss of comprehension of spoken language
Can't name common objects
Apraxia: can't perform motor skills although motor system intact
Agnosia: failure to identify or recognize objects despite intact sensory function
Misinterprets visual and auditory stimuli
Delusions

Late Frontal
6-8 years after onset
Motor disturbances: walking, swallowing, moving
Primitive reflexes
Seizures
Sensation remains intact

Table 11-1

Multi-Infarct versus Alzheimer-Type Dementia

FACTORS SUGGESTING DEMENTIA	HACHINSKI ISCHEMIA POINT SCORE*
Abrupt onset	2
Stepwise deterioration	1
Fluctuating course	2
Nocturnal confusion	1
Emotional lability	1
Relative preservation of personality	1
Depression	1
Somatic complaints	1
History of hypertension	1
History of strokes	2
Evidence of associated arteriosclerosis	1
Focal neurological symptoms†	2
Focal neurological signs†	2

*A score of 4 or more is indicative of Alzheimer-type dementia. A score of 7 or more is indicative of multi-infarct dementia.

†Focal neurological signs/symptoms: exaggerated DTRs, positive Babinski's sign, gait abnormalities, hemiparesis.

From Siu AL: Screening for dementia and investigating its causes, *Ann Inter Med* 115(92):122-132, 1991.

loss. The memory loss is equal for recent and remote events. The cognitive losses, however, are fluctuating rather than stable over time. The patient manifests a depressed or anxious mood, including sleep and appetite disturbance. Hallucinations are usually absent, although the patient may have suicidal thoughts. Depression as a cause of confusion can be easy to miss because it is often associated with anger, anxiety, and unclear thinking as well as denial.

Table 11-2

Differential Diagnosis of Common Causes of Delirium, Confusion, Dementia, and Depression

Disorder	History	Physical Findings	Diagnostic Studies
Delirium	Onset abrupt; fluctuations over course of day common with lucid intervals during day and worst symptoms at night; lasts hours to weeks; unable to maintain attention to external stimuli; disorganized thinking, perceptual disturbances, disturbed sleep-wake cycle; hallucinations, usually visual, common	Decreased LOC, impaired arousal, decreased psychomotor activity; disoriented, most commonly to time; physical exam findings depend on underlying cause of delirium; patient often exhibits asterixis, tremor, and difficulty in motor relaxation; speech incoherent, hesitant, slow, or rapid	CBC, electrolytes, glucose, BUN, creatinine, LFTs, TFTs, serum B_{12}, folate, serology for syphilis, ABGs, toxicology screen, blood alcohol level, U/A, ECG, EEG, chest x-ray, lumbar puncture, CT or MRI (when CVA or injury suspected)
Confusion	Less abrupt, less severe than delirium, diurnal variation less severe than delirium; concentration impaired, easily distracted; errors in thinking common	Apathetic, drowsy; disoriented especially for time, but less for place, almost never for self; less severe disorientation, more subtle motor signs than in delirium	CBC, electrolytes, glucose, BUN, creatinine, LFTs, TFTs, serum B_{12}, folate, serology for syphilis, ABGs, toxicology screen, blood alcohol level, U/A, ECG, EEG, chest x-ray, lumbar puncture, CT or MRI (when CVA or injury suspected)
Dementia	Onset insidious, course stable through day and night; present for months or years, with progressive deterioration; recent and remote memory impaired; hallucinations usually absent until late in course of disease; sleep often fragmented	Alert, attentive; orientation usually impaired; on mental status exam, patient tries hard, provides "near miss" answers; demonstrates one or more of following cognitive disturbances: aphasia (language disturbance); apraxia (impaired ability to carry out motor activities despite intact motor function); agnosia (failure to identify	CBC, electrolytes, glucose, BUN, creatinine, LFTs, TFTs, serum B_{12}, folate, serology for syphilis, ABGs, toxicology screen, blood alcohol level, U/A, ECG, EEG, chest x-ray, lumbar puncture, CT or MRI (when CVA or injury suspected; does not yield useful information for dementia)

Table 11-2

Differential Diagnosis of Common Causes of Delirium, Confusion, Dementia, and Depression—cont'd

Disorder	History	Physical Findings	Diagnostic Studies
		or recognize objects despite intact sensory function); disturbance in executive functioning (planning, organizing, sequencing, abstracting); physical findings often absent in Alzheimer type; olfactory sense may be impaired; speech usually unimpaired although difficulty with finding words; findings in multi-infarct dementia include focal neurological signs/symptoms: exaggerated DTRs, positive Babinski's sign, gait abnormalities, hemiparesis	
Depression	Onset of confusion often abrupt, with some diurnal variation, generally more consistent over time than delirium; confusion of short duration compared to dementia; past history of psychiatric problems common, including undiagnosed depressive episodes; cognitive losses fluctuating rather than stable over time; sleep/appetite disturbance; hallucinations usually absent although person may have suicidal thoughts	Depressed or anxious mood; tends to highlight disabilities, especially memory loss; memory loss equal for recent and remote events; PE often normal	Geriatric Depression Scale in elderly; CBC, electrolytes, glucose, BUN, creatinine, LFTs, TFTs, serum B_{12}, folate, serology for syphilis, ABGs, toxicology screen, blood alcohol level, U/A, ECG, EEG, chest x-ray, lumbar puncture, CT or MRI (when CVA or injury suspected)

Common Systemic Problems

≡ Fever

Fever is an elevation of temperature above the normal daily variation and is a symptom of an underlying process. The major common cause of fever is infection; however, noninfectious processes may present with fever. Fever of unknown origin occurs in a small percentage of cases. These fevers are usually caused by an infection that has not yet been identified. A meticulous history and physical examination supported by laboratory investigation are necessary to find the origin of the fever.

Specifically, there are three basic pathophysiological reasons for fever. The first involves the raising of the hypothalamic set point. The receptors in the area of the hypothalamus regulating body temperature are triggered to reset at a higher core body temperature. This results in an elevation of the helper T-cell production and an elevation in the effectiveness of interferon. Infection, collagen disease, vascular disease, and malignancy are commonly responsible for these fevers.

A second type of fever is a result of heat production exceeding heat loss. Here the set point is normal, and heat loss mechanisms are active. Fever occurs either because the body raises its metabolic heat production or the environmental heat load exceeds normal heat loss mechanisms. Aspirin overdose, malignant hyperthermia, hyperthyroidism, or hypernatremia may cause this type of fever.

A third type of fever is caused by a defective heat loss mechanism that cannot cope with normal heat load. Heat stroke, poisoning with anticholinergic drugs, ectodermal dysplasia, and burns are causes of this kind of fever.

For the first type of fever, antipyretics are given to lower the hypothalamic set point. They are ineffective for the second and third types of fever.

DIAGNOSTIC REASONING: FOCUSED HISTORY

Is this really a fever?

Key Questions
- How do you know you have a fever?
- Has the temperature been measured? How?

Occurrence of fever. Fever is a common presenting problem and a cardinal manifestation of disease. Patients often report a subjective fever (i.e. clinical symptoms such as flushing, chills, shaking chills, headache, malaise, or muscle aches, which are assumed by the patient to be a fever, although not validated with a thermometer). Nevertheless, the absence of fever in a single patient visit does not mean that the patient does not have a febrile illness.

Measurement of temperature. Many people use touch to determine if a fever is present. Although not a precise indication, touch can signal a high fever. During the early stages of fever, perfusion to the skin is decreased and skin temperature falls. It is only later in fever, when temperature within the muscles has risen significantly, that increased body temperature is reflected by increased skin temperature. In children, hands and feet should not be used to gauge a fever because they may be vasoconstricted and feel cold. Accurate temperature should be measured using a thermometer. Because of the diurnal variation in normal body temperature and the effect of physiological factors and body rhythms, frequent recordings throughout the day are needed to monitor fever.

Should sepsis or meningitis be of concern?

Key Questions
- Has there been any recent head trauma?
- Have you had recurrent ear infections?
- Have you had contact with anyone who has had meningococcal disease?
- Have you had any headache, lethargy, confusion, or stiff neck?
- If an infant: how old is the baby?

Head trauma, otitis media, contact. Recent head trauma, especially at the base of the skull may provide an entrance for infection. Children with recurrent or chronic otitis media may have mastoiditis spreading to the meninges. Contact with anyone with meningococcal disease and/or *Hemophilus influenzae* puts the individual at risk for contracting the disease.

Headache, vomiting, lethargy, or stiff neck. A typical history of meningitis is one of headache, fever, lethargy, confusion, vomiting, and stiff neck. However the presentation is highly variable. Any patient with even minimal neurological signs and symptoms should be evaluated for meningitis.

Infant. Fever in children less than 2 months of age is uncommon but must be viewed as serious. Generally neonates and young infants are less able to mount a febrile response, and, when they do, it is a significant finding. Fever can be viral or bacterial in nature. Fevers in the neonate may also be an indication of an underlying anatomical defect. Urinary tract infection and bacteremia are often the first indications of a structural abnormality of the urinary tract. Also, infants with galactosemia may present in the first weeks to 1 month of life with Gram-negative sepsis. Occasionally, infants present with sepsis associated with delivery (prolonged rupture of membranes) or acquired from instrumentation during delivery such as scalp electrodes or from a procedure performed in an NICU.

All infants less than 2 months of age with fever are considered to have sepsis or meningitis until proven otherwise.

What does the pattern of fever tell me?

Key Questions
- How long have you had the fever?
- What has the highest temperature been? When did this occur?

Length of fever. In adults, fevers from an acute process usually resolve in 1 to 2 weeks. Fevers that last 3 weeks or longer, that exceed temperatures of 38.4° C (101.1° F), and remain undiagnosed after a week of intensive diagnostic study are classified as fevers of unknown origin (FUO).

Fevers in children can be grouped into three categories: short-term fever, fever without localizing signs, and fever of unknown origin. Short-term fever is defined as a fever of short duration, readily diagnosed, which resolves within 1 week. Fever without localizing signs is a fever with no localizing sign and of brief duration (usually fewer than 10 days), which is not explained by findings on history or physical examination. Fever of unknown origin is a fever usually greater than 38.5° C (101.2° F) that lasts more than 2 weeks on more than four occasions.

Height of fever. Dehydration and febrile seizures are related to the height of the fever. Generally body temperatures greater than 41.1° C (106° F) are seen in heat illness, central nervous system disease, or a combination of these with infection. The higher the fever, the greater the likelihood of bacteremia.

Is the fever caused by a localized infection?

Key Questions
- Do you have any frequency, burning, or urgency with urination?
- Do you have any face or sinus pain?
- Do you have nasal discharge? What color?
- Do you have a cough? Is it productive? What color is the sputum?
- Do you have ear pain?
- Is your throat sore?
- Are you having any nausea/vomiting, diarrhea?
- Are you having any unusual vaginal discharge?
- Do you have any joint pain?

Localizing symptoms will point to the site of the infection. These diagnostic clues include headache or sinus pain, purulent nasal discharge, ear pain, toothache, sore throat, breast tenderness, chest pain, cough, dyspnea, abdominal pain, flank pain, dysuria, vaginal discharge, pelvic pain, rectal pain, testicle pain, calf pain, neck stiffness, joint stiffness, pain or heat, or focal neurological deficits (see appropriate chapters).

Urinary tract (Chapter 6). Upper urinary tract infection in adults commonly produces systemic symptoms with flank pain and fever. Fever with cystitis is uncommon in adults, but children with urinary tract infections (UTI) present with systemic rather than localized signs and symptoms. UTI is the most common infection in female children less than 2 years of age who present with a high fever and in all infants less than 90 days old with fever.

Ear, nose, throat symptoms (Chapter 2). Viral infections of the upper respiratory tract are common and usually produce fever. Otitis media is common in children. Fever may accompany both viral and bacterial pharyngitis. Pharyngitis is frequently manifested only by fever, with the infection localizing a day or two later. Acute sinusitis often produces a fever.

Respiratory and gastrointestinal (GI) symptoms (Chapters 4, 5). Most febrile illnesses are caused by viral infection of the upper respiratory tract, GI tract, or lower respiratory tract. Localized symptoms can help pinpoint the cause of the fever. Vomiting can occasionally signal pneumonia.

Joint pain. Joint pain may indicate connective tissue disorders in adults and in children over 6 years of age (see Chapter 9). Osteomyelitis or septic arthritis may also produce fever.

Can the diagnostic possibilities be narrowed or a cause be eliminated?

Key Questions
- Have you noticed a rash?
- Do you ache all over?

Skin rash (Chapter 3). The prodromal period of a rash is an important historical clue to diagnosis. The common fever and eruption periods of rashes are:
- Varicella, rubella, erythema infectiosum—1 day
- Scarlet fever—2 days
- Rocky Mountain spotted fever—3 days
- Measles—4 days
- Roseola infantum—5 days

Ache. Fevers localized to a site without general body manifestations are often bacterial in nature. Fevers accompanied by muscle aches, malaise, and/or respiratory symptoms are often viral in nature.

Does the patient have an increased risk for problems or complications?

Key Questions
- Do you have any chronic health problems?
- Have you been treated recently for any health problems?
- Have you had any recent surgery?
- Have you been diagnosed with an infectious disease recently?
- Are you sexually active? How many partners?
- Are immunizations up to date?
- Does anyone in the family have tuberculosis (TB) or hepatitis?

Chronic disease. Chronic conditions and systemic disorders, such as diabetes mellitus, HIV, malignancies, neutropenia, and sickle cell anemia, that compromise host resistance increase susceptibility to infection. Prosthetic devices, such as heart valves or joint prostheses, also increase susceptibility to infectious processes.

Health problems, surgery, recent infection. In patients with health problems, recurrent infection or incomplete treatment of infection may be the cause of fever. Also identification of any risk factors such as diabetes mellitus, neutropenia, and sickle cell anemia heightens the likelihood of bacterial disease. Patients with a past history of infectious processes such as UTI or streptococcal pharyngitis may be prone to relapse or reoccurrence. Recent surgical procedures can provide a locus for occult infection; however, a surgical procedure can also induce an inflammatory response, which causes a fever without infection. Transfusion of blood products carries a small risk of hepatitis or HIV transmission.

Sexual activity. High-risk sexual activity may raise the index of suspicion for HIV infection and additionally for pelvic inflammatory disease (PID) in women.

Immunizations. Children and adults who have not been properly immunized are more at risk for infectious diseases.

TB or hepatitis exposure. Exposure to populations with a high incidence of TB or viral hepatitis increases the risk of infection. Inquire further about constitutional symptoms such as cough or night sweats (TB) or malaise and abdominal discomfort (hepatitis).

Does the parent report a behavior change in the child?

Key Questions
- Is the child sleepier than normal?
- Is the child more irritable?
- How is the child acting?

In infants and children, behavior changes may be the only indication that the child is ill. Mildly ill infants may act alert, active, smile, and feed well. Moderately ill infants may be fussy or irritable but continue to feed, are consolable, and may smile. Severely ill infants appear listless, cannot be consoled, and feed poorly or not at all.

Could the fever be caused by something acquired while traveling?

Key Questions

- Have you been out of the country recently?
- Have you been in the woods or camping recently?

A history of travel out of the country presents the possibility of infection with amebiasis, malaria, schistosomiasis, typhoid fever, or hepatitis A and B. Camping or exposure to wooded areas may indicate exposure to ticks, Q fever, tularemia, Rocky Mountain spotted fever, *Giardia*, or Lyme disease.

Could the fever be medication-related or caused by poisoning?

Key Questions

- What medications have you taken recently?
- How much aspirin have you taken recently?
- Describe the foods you have eaten in the last 3 days.
- Could the child have eaten a poisonous plant?

Medications may hide an occult infection. Many drugs (penicillin, atropine, sulfonamides, streptomycin, and diphenylhydantoin) can induce fever in predisposed individuals. The fever starts about 7 days after the drug is taken for the first time or soon after the first dose in a patient previously sensitized. Any patient who is taking immunosuppressive agents is at a higher risk for infection. Some medications interfere with thirst recognition (sedatives, haloperidol) or sweating (anticholinergics, phenothiazines).

Aspirin overdose. Overdose of aspirin can occur with as little as 3 g per day. Toxic symptoms are also poorly correlated with serum salicylate levels. Earliest signs are vertigo and tinnitus, but fever can occur shortly thereafter and may be the only symptom patients recognize.

Food poisoning. Food poisoning fevers may occur up to 72 hours after ingestion of contaminated food.

Plants. Plants containing alkaloid atropine (deadly nightshade, jessamine, and thornapple) cause dilated pupils, flushed skin, and fever because they interfere with the normal heat loss mechanism.

Could exposure to animals explain the fever?

Key Question

- Has a cat scratched you recently?
- Have you been around any animals?

Cat scratch disease. Cat scratch disease is a bacterial infection transmitted by cats. The etiological agent is a Gram-negative bacillus. Single-node or regional adenopathy is the dominant clinical feature. A low-grade fever is also present.

Animal exposure. Also possible is brucellosis and leptospirosis from dogs, tularemia from rabbits, ornithosis, histoplasmosis or psittacosis from birds, and lymphocytic choriomeningitis from hamsters or cats. Exposure to infected animals can produce infection and fever in humans. Occupational exposure to pathogens such as brucellosis should be investigated in patients who work with animals or animal products.

Could this be a result of a recent immunization?

Key Question

- What immunizations have you had recently?

Adverse effects of immunization are rare but do occur. History of recent immunization followed by 4 hours of high temperature (39.5° C; 103° F) may indicate such an adverse reaction. Measles, mumps, rubella (MMR) immunization may cause elevation of temperature 10 to 14 days after the inoculation.

Could the fever be caused by heat exposure?

Key Questions

- Were you overdressed?
- Do you have air conditioning or windows that open?
- How warm is the room you live/sleep in?

Overdressing. Classic heatstroke occurs when the person is unable to dissipate the environmental heat burden. Mothers may inadvertently overdress children or cover them in blankets; the elderly may not be able to get out of bed when hot. Obese persons have extra adipose tissue that insulates the body, preventing loss of heat. Some cultures treat illnesses with bundling, which can cause high fevers.

Air conditioning, room temperature. During heat waves, persons may become overheated in apartments without air conditioning or with windows that will not open or are not opened because of safety concerns. The high ambient temperatures in those apartments produce elevations in core body temperature that cannot be compensated for, leading to hyperthermia.

DIAGNOSTIC REASONING: FOCUSED PHYSICAL EXAMINATION

Most fevers have an obvious cause, so look initially for localizing symptoms or clusters of symptoms that point to the cause. Remember that, in both children and adults,

---

Box 12-1

Common Causes of Fever in Children

Acute Fever

Upper respiratory tract disorders:
  Viral respiratory tract diseases
  Otitis media
  Sinusitis
Lower respiratory tract disorders:
  Bronchiolitis
  Pneumonia
Gastrointestinal disorders:
  Bacterial gastroenteritis
  Viral gastroenteritis
Musculoskeletal infections:
  Septic arthritis
Osteomyelitis
Cellulitis
Urinary tract infections
Bacteremia
Meningitis

Fever of Unknown Origin

Infectious diseases (localized and systemic)
Collagen/inflammatory diseases
Neoplastic diseases
Miscellaneous disorders:
  Drug fever
  Factitious fever
  Kawasaki syndrome
  Inflammatory bowel disease
  Immunodeficiency
  CNS dysfunction

bacterial and viral infections of the upper- and lower respiratory tracts and gastrointestinal tract are the most common causes of fevers. Look for and rule out the common causes before investigating more unlikely causes. Boxes 12-1 and 12-2 list the common causes of fever in children and adults.

Fever in a Child Less Than 2 Months Old

The younger the child, the greater the cause for concern in the presence of fever. Neonates and young infants are less able to mount a febrile response and, therefore, are more vulnerable to meningitis and other hematogenous complications. The infrequency of high fever in this age group relates to innate differences in the ability to mount a febrile response. The data suggests that fever in the first 2 to 3 months of life is relatively uncommon but that, when it does occur, it is usually significant and often ominous.

Observe the Patient

General appearance is a most important aspect of physical examination. Note how the patient looks —does he or she appear acutely ill, look dehydrated, seem lethargic, respond appropriately?

Responsiveness in children over 2 months of age has been used by pediatricians to identify febrile children with serious illness. The Yale Observation Scales for Severity of Illness in Children is commonly used to quantify observations (Table 12-1). The scale has six general areas related to the child's appearance and behavior. The results of the scale found two thirds of children with acute illness have scores of less than 10, and, of these, only 3% were found to have serious illness. Scores of greater than 10 predicted that a serious illness was likely. As the score approached 16, the likelihood that a serious illness was present was 92%.

Take Vital Signs and Note Temperature

The incidence of bacteremia, as well as specific infections, increases with the magnitude of fever. A temperature greater than 40° C (104° F) seems to be the marker for occult bacteria. However, many patients with high fever do not have major diseases.

Most infectious diseases produce tem-

Box 12-2

Common Causes of Fever in Adults

Acute Fever
Upper respiratory infections:
  Tonsillitis
  Sinusitis
  Pneumonia
Gastrointestinal:
  Bacterial gastroenteritis
  Viral gastroenteritis
  Acute abdomen
Urinary tract infection
PID
Prostatitis
Drug reactions
Alcohol withdrawal

Fever of Unknown Origin
Infectious disease
Neoplasm
Collagen/vascular; other multisystem
  disease
Drug fever
Factitious fever

Table 12-1

Yale Observation Scale Predictive Model: Six Observation Items and Their Scales

OBSERVATION ITEM	1 NORMAL	3 MODERATE IMPAIRMENT	5 SEVERE IMPAIRMENT
Quality of cry	Strong with normal tone *or* content and not crying	Whimpering *or* sobbing	Weak *or* moaning *or* high-pitched
Reaction to parent stimulation	Cries briefly then stops *or* content and not crying	Cries on and off	Continual cry *or* hardly responds
State variation	If awake, stays awake *or* if asleep and stimulated, wakes up quickly	Eyes close briefly, not awake *or* awakes with prolonged stimulation	Falls to sleep *or* will not rouse
Color	Pink	Pale extremities *or* acrocyanosis	Pale *or* cyanotic *or* mottled *or* ashen
Hydration	Skin normal, eyes normal, *and* mucous membranes moist	Skin and eyes normal *and* mouth slightly dry	Skin doughy *or* tented *and* dry mucous membranes *and/or* sunken eyes
Response (talk, smile) to social overtures	Smiles *or* alerts (<2 months)	Brief smile *or* alerts briefly (<2 months)	No smile, face anxious, dull, expressionless *or* no alerting (<2 months)

McCarthy PL, Sharpe MR, Spiesel SZ et al: Observation scales to identify serious illness in febrile children, *Pediatrics* 70(5):802, 1982.

peratures between 37.2° C and 41° C (99° F and 106° F). However, some patients with infectious diseases remain afebrile. These include neonates, immunocompromised hosts, patients with chronic renal insufficiency, and the elderly. Extreme pyrexia (i.e., temperatures exceeding 41.5° C [106.7° F]) rarely occur with an infectious disease. Conditions in which extreme pyrexia is seen include drug fevers, CNS injury, malignant hyperthermia, stroke, and HIV.

Hypothermia is always an unfavorable prognostic sign in the presence of infectious disease. This condition is seen with overwhelming sepsis (most commonly in the elderly and neonates), uremia, cold exposure, and hypothyroidism.

Observe Skin and Mucous Membranes (Chapter 3)

A macular/papular rash may indicate a viral exanthem, infectious disease, or a drug sensitivity reaction. Vesicular rashes occur with viral infection. A petechial skin rash indicates meningococcemia or Rocky Mountain spotted fever. Petechial eruptions on the hard and soft palate may indicate mononucleosis. Splinter hemorrhages found in the nail beds and petechiae of the conjunctiva indicate endocarditis.

The presence of a petechial skin rash indicates a serious infection that requires immediate referral and hospitalization.

Examine the Head and Neck (Chapter 2)

Percuss the sinuses and transilluminate for evidence of sinusitis. Examine and palpate the teeth for abscesses. Palpate the salivary glands for tenderness. Examine the throat and tonsils for signs of infection, specifically enlarged or red tonsils, lymphadenopathy, or tonsillar or pharyngeal exudate.

Inspect the ears and tympanic membrane for effusion, erythema, fluid, or purulent secretion. Inspect the optic fundi for changes associated with infectious endocarditis (i.e., Roth spots, which are small, pale retinal lesions having areas of hemorrhage with white centers, usually located near the optic disc).

In the infant, feel for a tense or bulging anterior fontanel. This is best noted if the patient is in the sitting position. The normal fontanel may feel questionably tense if the infant is supine. Tenseness may be noted in the crying child but only during expiration; this physiological bulging disappears when the patient relaxes or inspires.

Palpate the Lymph Nodes

Palpate all lymph nodes for enlargement and tenderness:
- Anterior cervical—suspect viral or bacterial pharyngitis
- Pre- or post-auricular—suspect ear infection
- Posterior cervical—suspect mononucleosis
- Supraclavicular—suspect neoplasms
- Axillary—suspect breast inflammation, local infection, neoplasm
- Localized lymphadenopathy—suspect local infectious process
- Generalized lymphadenopathy—suspect immunosuppression such as being HIV positive, neoplasm

Examine the Lungs and Chest (Chapter 4)

Percuss and auscultate the lungs. Adventitious sounds, decreased breath sounds, or areas of consolidation may indicate lower respiratory tract infection or pneumonia.

Examine the sputum for color, consistency, and presence of blood or odor:
- Yellow/green sputum—indicates bacterial infection
- Brown sputum—check smoking history
- Blood streaked—indicates upper respiratory tract infection (URI) and bronchitis
- Hemoptysis—suspect tumor, trauma, or pulmonary embolism

Palpate Breasts if Indicated (Chapter 8)

Inspect the breasts for signs of inflammation. Palpate for masses, tenderness, and discharge. Palpate axillary lymph nodes for presence and tenderness.

Examine Genitourinary System if Indicated (Chapters 6, 7)

Palpate for suprapubic tenderness, which may indicate PID or urinary tract infection (UTI), and for costovertebral angle (CVA) tenderness, which suggests pyelonephritis. Perform a pelvic examination in women without another obvious source of fever. Cervical motion tenderness, discharge, or adnexal tenderness and low abdominal tenderness may indicate PID. In men, examine for penile discharge, suggesting a sexually transmitted disease (STD), UTI, or prostatitis.

Perform a rectal examination to evaluate for tenderness and discharge, which may indicate rectal abscess or infection as well as retrocecal appendicitis.

Perform a prostate examination in men without another obvious source of fever because prostatitis may be the cause. If you suspect prostatitis, do not perform a vigorous examination or massage the prostate as this can release bacteria and produce septicemia.

Evaluate for masses and occult blood as indicators of malignancy.

Examine Musculoskeletal System if Indicated (Chapter 9)

Examination may suggest inflammation or infection of bone or joints if there is swelling, increased warmth, or tenderness. Infants may present with a picture of poor feeding, irritability, fever, or vomiting. Examination should reveal decreased mobility of affected bone or joint area, increased heat, tenderness, and swelling.

Examine the lower extremities for asymmetrical swelling, calf tenderness, or palpable vessels as an indicator of deep vein phlebitis.

Osteomyelitis may occur in young children, most commonly between 3 and 10 years of age. Septic arthritis can occur in children under the age of 3 and in young women who are sexually active.

Perform Neurological/Mental State Examination (Chapters 10, 11)

Evaluate for signs of meningeal irritation. Inflammation of the meninges from infection or blood evokes reflex spasm in the paravertebral muscles. In the cervical area, this manifests as neck stiffness. Normally the chin can be flexed passively to touch the chest. If neck stiffness is present, this maneuver is not possible. With the patient supine, attempts to flex the neck cause the knees and hips to rise from the bed (Brudzinski's sign) in order to reduce the pull on the meninges. In the lumbar region, meningeal irritation also causes spasm and can be demonstrated by passive movement of the lower limbs. Attempts to extend the knee joint when the hip joint is flexed are resisted, and the other limb may flex at the hip (Kernig's sign). Neck stiffness (nuchal rigidity) or resistance to neck flexion or rotation is a late sign and not a true sign of meningitis in infants less than 3 months old, the very old, or the severely obtunded patient. Vomiting, headache, and photophobia may also be present.

Note the presence of focal deficits, which suggests vascular occlusion or abscess formation. Assess for disturbances in mentation, irritability, lethargy, somnolence, or coma, which indicates increased intracranial pressure. Seizures occur in 20% to 30% of children with meningitis.

A seizure in a febrile infant less than 6 months old suggests meningitis rather than a simple febrile seizure. Benign febrile seizure is uncommon in very young infants.

LABORATORY AND DIAGNOSTIC STUDIES

Laboratory studies can be used selectively to confirm or negate the clinical diagnosis, especially if the history and physical findings provide strong indication of a particular infectious process. In patients with obvious viral upper respiratory tract infection, no studies are necessary. Patients with a sore throat may require a throat culture, monospot, or rapid strep test, depending on the clinical findings. In patients with urinary symptoms, a urinalysis and culture may be sufficient unless clinical findings indicate an upper urinary tract infection, which would warrant further diagnostic testing such as x-ray, ultrasound, or intravenous pyelogram.

Also see appropriate chapters for specific presenting problems and discussion of diagnostic tests.

Complete Blood Count (CBC)

Leukocytosis with a left shift suggests a bacterial infection. Atypical lymphocytes are characteristic of systemic viral infection. Immature neutrophils suggest leukemia.

Anemia may be seen in inflammatory conditions such as juvenile arthritis, malaria, and parvovirus B19 infections. Low platelet counts may be associated with Epstein-Barr virus infection, histoplasmosis, TB, spirochetal infections, or may be drug induced. Thrombocytosis is common in Kawasaki disease (an acute febrile illness in children that resembles scarlet fever) and some viral infections.

Erythrocyte Sedimentation Rate (ESR)

An elevated ESR indicates an inflammatory condition. However, the test is non-specific and does not indicate the source or cause of inflammation.

Antistreptolysin (ASO) Titer (Chapter 2)

A rise in the ASO titer is detectable by comparing two blood samples more than 2 weeks apart. An elevated titer indicates immunological response of the host following exposure to streptococcal antigen.

Urinalysis (U/A) (Chapter 6)

Use a dipstick U/A to screen for upper or lower urinary tract infection, which would reveal the presence of nitrites and leukocyte esterase. Microscopic evaluation reveals the presence of cells (WBC, RBC) and blood casts.

Urine Culture and Sensitivity (C & S) (Chapter 6)

C & S performed on a clean catch urine specimen will confirm a diagnosis of UTI and isolate the organism(s).

Stool for Leukocytes (Chapter 5)

The presence of white blood cells may suggest invasive bacterial gastroenteritis.

Stool Culture and Sensitivity (Chapter 5)

Use stool C & S to detect the presence of *Salmonella* or *Shigella*.

Stool Sample for Ova and Parasites (Chapter 5)

Have the patient collect three stool samples over a 5-day period. The first morning stool is preferred and must be delivered to the laboratory in 30 minutes or less after defecation.

Sputum for Acid-Fast Bacilli (AFB) (Chapter 4)

A sputum sample to test for AFB is used to diagnose respiratory TB. A smear is prepared from a series of three first-morning specimens collected on 3 separate days to catch the sporadic discharge of the bacilli from the tubercle.

Sputum for Gram staining

A smear is prepared from a sputum sample and stained with Gram stain. Gram-positive organisms stain purple; Gram-negative organisms stain red:

- Gram-positive cocci or diplococci indicate pneumococcal, staphylococcal, or streptococcal infections
- Gram-negative cocci indicate meningococcal, gonococcal infections
- Enteric Gram-negative bacilli indicate *E. coli, Proteus, Bacteroides, Klebsiella,* typhoid, *Salmonella, Shigella*
- Other Gram-negative bacilli indicate *Hemophilus,* pertussis, chancroid, brucellosis, tularemia, and plague

Sputum for Culture and Sensitivity (Chapter 4)

Use sputum culture to isolate a specific organism. Have the patient rinse the mouth well with water without swallowing before coughing to produce a specimen. This decreases the amount of saliva present. Do not use mouthwash because this can kill the bacteria. An early morning sample is best. The sample must contain mucoid or mucopurulent material.

Cultures of Discharge

Cultures can be prepared from any source with a discharge, e.g., vaginal, urethral, wound. Place the culture in the transport media indicated. Culture is used to isolate causative organisms.

Collect a specimen of vaginal or penile discharge on a sterile swab and place in the medium provided. For penile discharge, use a sterile urethral swab to collect a specimen from the anterior urethra by gentle insertion and scraping of the mucosa. For wound culture, use a sterile swab or aspirate with a sterile needle and syringe form the moist area. Bacteria from the center of a wound may be nonviable, so culture near the periphery.

DNA Probe (Chapters 6, 7)

DNA probes are a fast and sensitive method of detecting organisms. Probes are currently used to detect gonococcus and *Chlamydia*. Obtain a sample of vaginal or penile discharge with a sterile swab and place it in the medium provided. This test involves the construction of nucleic acid sequence (called a probe) that will match to a sequence in the DNA or RNA of the target tissue.

Blood Cultures

Two culture specimens are obtained at two different venipuncture sites. If one culture produces bacteria and the other does not, the positive culture is likely from a contaminant and not the infecting agent. Culture specimens drawn through an IV catheter are frequently contaminated. All cultures should be drawn before initiation of antibiotics if possible. Most organisms require approximately 24 hours to grow in the laboratory, and a preliminary report can be given at that time. Often 48 to 72 hours are required for growth and identification of organisms. Blood cultures may be positive in bacteremia.

Lumbar Puncture (Chapter 10)

A lumbar puncture is indicated if you suspect meningitis. Laboratory data on cerebral spinal fluid (CSF) always includes leukocytes, protein, glucose, Gram stain, cell count, and culture and sensitivity. In meningitis, expect cloudy CSF fluid with many polymorphonuclear cells containing bacteria. Glucose is decreased compared to the blood sugar, protein is increased, and the culture will be positive.

Radiographic Imaging

Chest x-rays may detect infiltrates, effusions, masses, or nodes. Kidney, ureter, and bladder (KUB) and upright abdominal films can reveal air-fluid levels in the bowel. CT scan may be used to detect abscess or tumor. X-rays are useful for detecting bone and joint involvement in osteomyelitis. Radionuclide scanning is also beneficial in detecting osteomyelitis.

DIFFERENTIAL DIAGNOSIS

Upper Respiratory Tract Infection (Chapter 6)

Viral infections can occur in any age group and are more prevalent during winter months. The fever is usually less than 38.7° C (101.5° F). Systemic symptoms are common. Known contact with others who have had similar symptoms or illness is typical but not necessary. The patient usually has a cough; any sputum is nonpurulent. Pharyngitis may be present with erythema of the oral pharynx.

Gastroenteritis (Chapter 5)

Nausea, vomiting, and diarrhea are the hallmarks of a gastrointestinal infection. Fever is usually mild. Abdominal cramping may be present.

Urinary Tract Infection (UTI) (Chapter 6)

UTIs are more common in women and female children. Localized urinary tract symptoms are common in adults; systemic symptoms are more common in children. CVA tenderness indicates upper UTI. The fever associated with an upper UTI is likely to be high, and the patient feels systemically ill. Urinalysis can support a clinical diagnosis of UTI. Urine for C & S usually confirms the diagnosis.

Pelvic Inflammatory Disease (Chapter 7)

Suspect pelvic inflammatory disease in women with a fever for which there is no other explanation. There may be vague complaints of lower abdominal pain; suprapubic tenderness may be present on abdominal examination. Pelvic examination reveals cervical motion tenderness, discharge, and/or adnexal tenderness.

Prostatitis (Chapter 6)

In men without another obvious source of fever, suspect prostatitis. The prostate will be exquisitely tender to gentle palpation. Other system examinations will be normal.

Pharyngitis (Chapter 2)

The patient complains of a sore throat. In children, fever may precede throat complaints by a day or two. The pharynx is red, and the tonsils may be enlarged or have exudate. For differential diagnosis of bacterial and viral pharyngitis, see Chapter 2. Mononucleosis occurs most often in young adults and may present with palatine petechiae, tonsillar exudate, and posterior cervical lymphadenopathy.

Sinusitis (Chapter 2)

Sinuses that are tender to percussion or do not transilluminate may indicate sinusitis, especially in the presence of purulent nasal discharge. Patients often complain of a headache, which worsens, as the patient leans forward. Patients sometimes experience a sore throat and cough from postnasal discharge, which may be apparent in the posterior pharynx.

Ear Infections (Chapter 2)

Otitis media is more common in children. The tympanic membrane will appear red and may bulge. The light reflex will be absent or diminished. TM mobility will be limited. The child may tug at the ear and act restless or irritable. The young child or infant may feed poorly. The fever may be high or low grade. Respiratory symptoms occur if the patient has concomitant respiratory infection. Ear infections are commonly associated with other upper respiratory symptoms.

Meningitis (Chapter 10)

The signs and symptoms of meningitis are related to non-specific findings associated with bacteremia or a systemic infection or to specific manifestation of meningeal irritation with CNS inflammation. Inspect skin for petechiae, cyanosis, and state of hydration and peripheral perfusion. Nuchal rigidity, back pain, Kerning's sign, Brudzinski's sign, nausea, vomiting, and bulging fontanel (in infants) may be seen. Papilledema is rarely seen. If it is present, look for other processes such as brain abscess or subdural empyema. Ataxia may be a presenting sign. Lumbar puncture confirms diagnosis.

Osteomyelitis (Chapter 9)

Bone infection is usually caused by bacteria and may arise from a clinically evident infection or from an unknown source via bacteremia. Patients complain of pain in the affected bone or joint and may exhibit soft tissue tenderness and swelling. Children demonstrate localized tenderness near the epiphysis. Diagnosis requires isolation of the responsible organism via blood cultures, pus from tissue abscesses, synovial fluid aspirate, or material from needle aspiration or bone biopsy. Radionuclide scanning, CT, or MRI may be helpful in determining the extent of infection and destruction.

Kawasaki Disease (Chapter 3)

Kawasaki disease is an acute mucocutaneous lymph node syndrome, which is classified as a vasculitic syndrome (of which fever is only one sign) affecting infants and young children under age 9. It is more common in males. It often occurs in fall and spring. The etiology is unknown. Fevers are of a high-spiking remittent pattern in the range of 38° to 40° C (100.4° to 104° F with some to 107° F) and persist despite the use of empiric antibiotics and antipyretics. Seizures may be present, and other neurological causes must be ruled out. The febrile phase lasts from 5 to 25 days with a mean of 10 days. Because of the associated rash with fever, Kawasaki disease resembles scarlet fever.

To make the initial diagnosis of Kawasaki disease, fever lasting at least 5 days with at least 4 of the following signs, in absence of known diagnosis or infection, must be present:

- Bilateral conjunctival hyperemia
- Mouth lesions—dry fissured lips and injected pharynx or strawberry tongue
- Change in peripheral extremities, edema, erythema, desquamation of skin at 10 to 14 days
- Non-vesicular erythematous rash
- Cervical lymphadenopathy

Factitious Fever

Suspect factitious fever when there is a discrepancy between oral or rectal temperature and urine temperature. The pulse rate will be inconsistent with elevated temperature. The patient has no weight loss. Repeated monitored temperature-taking does not support previous readings.

Roseola Infantum

Roseola infantum is the most common exanthem of children younger than 3 years of age. Symptoms include an irritable child who has high fever, with rapid defervescence when the rash appears on day three or four. The rash is maculopapule and lasts 1 to 2 days.

Fevers Without Localizing Signs

Often examination fails to disclose any specific signs or symptoms other than the fever itself. Most children who have a fever without localizing signs have neither an unusual nor a serious disease. In many cases, the fever will clear within a few days without a specific diagnosis. However, the longer the child has a fever without localizing signs, the less likely the fever is the result of infectious disease. Viral illness or malignancy must be considered.

Always investigate in the history and physical examination any abnormal growth suggesting any possibility of pre-existing chronic disease. Morning stiffness suggests rheumatoid arthritis, weight loss or abdominal pain suggests inflammatory bowel disease, frequent respiratory infection suggests cystic fibrosis or immunodeficiency.

Enterovirus (Chapter 4)

All enteroviruses may cause a mild, nonspecific, febrile illness lasting 2 to 5 days. Most are seasonal, occurring in late summer and early fall. Herpangina, nonexudative pharyngitis with or without lymphadenopathy, generally occurs.

Occult Bacteremia

Occult bacteremia is diagnosed in children older than 3 months who have positive blood cultures but do not have the usual clinical manifestation of sepsis or septic shock. Occult means hidden from view, and the child looks well. The majority of children who look well and are playful are at low risk for bacteremia despite fever. Those who look ill or toxic are at significant risk. The primary concern is the small but important percentage of those children who develop secondary complications from invasive bacterial disease (i.e., meningitis, bacterial sepsis, septic arthritis, or pneumonia). Peak ages for bacteremia are between 6 and 24 months, with *Streptococcus pneumoniae* as the organism most commonly responsible.

Table 12-2

Differential Diagnosis of Common Causes of Fever

Condition	History	Physical Findings	Diagnostic Studies
URI	Any age group; systemic symptoms; often known contact with ill others	Fever <38.7° C (101.5 ° F); cough; nonpurulent sputum; erythema of pharynx; viral exanthem	None
Gastroenteritis	Nausea, vomiting, diarrhea; abdominal cramping	Mild fever; abdomen may be diffusely tender	None
UTI	Female > male; burning urgency; frequency in adults; systemic symptoms/bed-wetting in children	CVA tenderness with upper UTI; fever with upper UTI	U/A; urine C & S; CBC if suspect upper UTI
PID	May have pelvic or lower abdominal pain	May have suprapubic tenderness; cervical discharge; CMT, adnexal tenderness	CBC; culture, DNA probe
Prostatitis	Perineal discomfort, frequent urination, chills and malaise	Prostate tender to palpation; fever	Segmental urine specimens; C & S of urine; C & S of prostate discharge
Pharyngitis	Sore throat; may or may not have other upper respiratory symptoms	Erythematous pharynx; may have pharyngeal or tonsillar exudate or ulcers; may have palatine petechiae in mononucleosis; lymphadenopathy	CBC; culture; rapid strep test if suspect strep; monospot if suspect mononucleosis
Sinusitis	Facial or sinus pressure or pain; headache	Purulent nasal discharge; sinuses tender to percussion; headache or pressure worsens on bending forward	X-rays or CT scan of limited value
Ear infections	Earache, pain; may have upper respiratory symptoms; child tugs at ear	High- or low-grade fever; TM red, may bulge, landmarks absent; TM mobility impaired; child irritable/restless	Pneumatic otoscopy

Continued

Table 12-2

Differential Diagnosis of Common Causes of Fever—cont'd

Condition	History	Physical Findings	Diagnostic Studies
Meningitis	Non-specific symptoms; nausea, vomiting, irritability	Petechiae, nuchal rigidity, positive Kerning's and Brudzinski's signs, petechiae; bulging fontanel in infant	Lumbar puncture
Osteomyelitis	Pain in affected bone or joint	Swelling or tenderness over affected area of joint	Culture; CBC; radionuclide scan, CT, MRI
Kawasaki disease	Under 5 years of age; males > females; fall and spring	High fever, spikes; persists despite antibiotic therapy; may have seizures; fever for 5 days with at least 4 of the following: bilateral conjunctival hyperemia, mouth lesions, edema, erythema, desquamation of skin, nonvesicular erythematous rash, cervical lymphadenopathy	WBC increased, shift to left, slight anemia, thrombocytosis, positive C-reactive protein, ESR increased, serum IgM, IgE increased
Factitious fever	Vague or no symptoms	Normal PE; no weight loss; pulse rate normal (not consistent with temperature elevation)	Discrepancy between oral/rectal temperature and urine temperature; repeated monitored temperature-taking does not support previous readings
Roseola infantum	Irritable child with fever for 4-5 days	Normal PE; when fever breaks, rash appears	None
Fevers without localizing signs	No other specific symptoms	PE usually normal initially, repeat examination in 24 hours and as needed	Urinalysis, urine C/S, chest x-ray, WBC, rule out systemic disease, malignancy
Enterovirus	Mild nonspecific febrile illness lasting 2-5 days; summer and early fall peaks	Nonexudative pharyngitis with or without lymphadenopathy frequently observed	None
Occult bacteremia	Fever in children older than 3 months	No localizing signs, child appears well	Blood culture, WBC

Altecheck A: Pediatric and adolescent gynecology, *Comp Ther* 21(5):235, 1995.

American Cancer Society: *Cancer facts and figures—1996*, Atlanta, 1996, American Cancer Society.

American Psychiatric Association: *Diagnostic and statistical manual of mental disorders*, ed 4, Washington, DC, 1994, The Association.

Armentrout D: Gastroesophageal reflux in infants, *Nurs Pract* 20(5):54, 1995.

Avner J: Occult bacteremia: how great the risk? *Contemp Pediatr* 14(6):53, 1997.

Baker R: Pitfalls in diagnosing acute otitis media, *Pediatr Ann* 20(11):591, 1991.

Barry JB, Fowler FJ Jr, O'Leary MP, Bruskewitz RC, Holtgrewe HL, Mebust WK, Cockett AT: The Measurement Committee of the American Urological Association: The American Urological Association symptom index for benign prostatic hyperplasia, *J Urol* 148:1549, 1992.

Baumann LJ, Leventhal H: I can tell if my blood pressure's up: can't I? *Health Psychol* 4:203, 1985.

Beauchamp GR, Meisler DM: Disorders of the conjunctiva. In Nelson LB, Calhoun SC, Harley RD, editors: *Pediatric ophthalmology*, Philadelphia, 1991, WB Saunders.

Berkow R, Fletcher A, editors: *The Merck manual*, ed 16, Rahway, NJ, 1992, Merck & Co.

Bigos S, Bowyer O, Braen G et al: *Acute low back problems in adults*, Clinical Practice Guideline, Pub No 95-0643, Rockville, Md, 1994, Agency for Health Care Policy and Research, US Department of Health and Human Services, Public Health Service.

Bisno AL: Acute pharyngitis: etiology and diagnosis, *Pediatrics* 97(6):949, 1996.

Bisno AL, Stevens D: Streptococcal infections of skin and soft tissues, *N Engl J Med* 334(4):240, 1996.

Boineau F, Lewy J: Evaluation of hematuria in children and adolescents, *Pediatr Rev* 11(4):101, 1989.

Brady M: The child with a limp, *J Pediatr Health Care* 7:226, 1993.

Bratton R, Agerter D: Preparticipation sports examinations, *Post Med* 98(2):123, 1995.

Bross M, Tatum N: Delirium in the elderly patient, *Am Fam Phys* 50(6):1332, 1994.

Brykcyzynski KA: An interpretive study describing clinical judgment of nurse practitioners, *Schol Inq Nurs Prac Internat J* 3:75, 1989.

Burkhart C: Guidelines for rapid assessment of abdominal pain indicative of acute surgical abdomen, *Nurs Pract* 17(6):39, 1992.

Busis S: Dizziness in children, *Pediatr Ann* 17(10):648, 1987.

Casey D, DeFazio J, Vansickle K, Lippmann S: Delirium, *Post Med* 100(1):121, 1996.

Cavataio F et al: Gastroesophageal reflux associated with cow's milk allergy in infants: which diagnostic examinations are useful? *Am J Gastroenterol* 91(6):1215, 1996.

Ceballos P, Ruiz-Maldonado R, Mihm M: Melanoma in children, *N Engl J Med* 332(10):656, 1995.

Chester A: Chronic sinusitis, *Am Fam Phys* 53(3):877, 1996.

Cibis G, Tongue A, Merrill L, editors: *Decision making in pediatric ophthalmology*, Philadelphia, 1993, BC Decker.

Cohen N: The dizzy patient: update on vestibular disorders, *Med Clin North Am Update Otolaryngol I* 75(6):1251, 1991.

Conrad E: Pitfalls in diagnosis: pediatric musculoskeletal tumors, *Pediatr Ann* 18(1):47, 1989.

Conway E, Zuckerman G: The long, hot summer, *Contemp Pediatr* 4(6):127, 1997.

Craig C, Goldberg M: Foot and leg problems, *Pediatr Rev* 14(10):395, 1993.

Dahlbeck S, Donnelly J, Theriault R: Differentiating inflammatory breast cancer from acute mastitis, *Am Fam Phys* 52(3):929, 1995.

Danilewitz M: Irritable bowel syndrome: eight questions physicians often ask, *Consultant*, p. 1310, June, 1996.

DeCherney AH, Pernoll M, editors: *Current obstetric and gynecologic diagnosis and treatment*, Norwalk, CT, 1994, Appleton & Lange.

DeGowin RL: *DeGowin & DeGowin's diagnostic examination*, ed 6, New York, 1994, McGraw-Hill.

Depression Guideline Panel: *Depression in primary care: detection and diagnosis,* Clinical Practice Guideline, Pub No 93-0550, Rockville, Md, 1993, Agency for Health Care Policy and Research, US Department of Health and Human Services, Public Health Service.

Derchewitz R: *Ambulatory pediatric care,* ed 2, Philadelphia, 1993, JB Lippincott.

Druce HM: *Sinusitis: pathophysiology and treatment,* New York, 1994, Marcel Dekker.

Dubose CD, Cutlip A, Cutlip W: Migraines and other headaches: an approach to diagnosis and classification, *Am Fam Phys* 51(6): 1498, 1995.

Dunn D: Dizziness: when is it vertigo? *Contemp Pediatr* 4(12):66, 1987.

Eddy DM: *Clinical decision making: from theory to practice,* Sudbury, 1996, Jones and Bartlett.

Edwardson BM: *Musculoskeletal disorders: common problems,* San Diego, 1995, Singular Publishing Group.

El-Mallakh R, Wright J, Breen K, Lippman S: Clues to depression in primary practice, *Post Med* 100(1):85, 1996.

Elsner P, Eichman A: Sexually transmitted diseases: advances in diagnosis and treatment. In Elsner P, Eichman A, editors: *Current problems in dermatology,* vol 24, New York, 1996, Karger.

Eviator L: Dizziness in children, *Otol Clin North Am* 24(3):557, 1994.

Facione N: Otitis media: an overview of acute and chronic disease, *Nurs Pract* 15(10):11, 1990.

Fantl JA, Newman DK, Colling J et al: *Urinary incontinence in adults: acute and chronic management,* Clinical Practice Guideline 2, 1996 update, Pub No 96-0082, Rockville, Md, 1996, Agency for Health Care Policy and Research, US Department of Health and Human Services, Public Health Service.

Farrington PF: Pediatric vulvo-vaginitis, *Clin Obstet Gynecol* 40(1):135, 1997.

Feld L, Greenfield S, Ogra P: Urinary tract infections in infants and children, *Pediatr Rev* 11(3):71, 1989.

Finelli L: Evaluation of the child with acute abdominal pain, *J Pediatr Health Care* 5(5):251, 1991.

Flynn PA, Engle MA, Ehlers KH: Cardiac issues in the pediatric emergency room, *Pediatr Clin North Am* 39(5):955, 1992.

Fox J: *Primary health care of children,* St Louis, 1997, Mosby.

Froehling D, Silverstein M, Mohr D, Beatty C: Does this patient have a serious form of vertigo? *JAMA* 271(5):385, 1994.

Garber KM: Enuresis: an update on diagnosis and management, *J Pediatr Health Care* 10(5):202, 1996.

Gerard JA, Kleinfield SL: *Orthopedic testing: a rational approach to diagnosis,* New York, 1993, Churchill-Livingstone.

Gigliotti F: Acute conjunctivitis, *Pediatr Rev* 16(6):353, 1995.

Gittes E, Irwin C: Sexually transmitted diseases in adolescents, *Pediatr Rev* 14(5):180, 1993.

Goroll AH, May LA, Mulley AG: *Primary care medicine: office evaluation and management of the adult patient,* ed 3, Philadelphia, 1995, JB Lippincott.

Gross R: Foot pain in children, *Pediatr Clin North Am* 33(6):1395, 1986.

Haberman A, Wald ER: UTI in young febrile children, *Pediatr Infec Dis J* 16(1):11, 1997.

Habif TP: *Clinical dermatology: a color guide to diagnosis and therapy,* ed 3, St Louis, 1996, Mosby.

Ham RJ, Sloane PD: *Primary care in geriatrics: a case-based approach,* ed 2, St Louis, 1992, Mosby.

Hartley A: *Practical joint assessment—lower quadrant,* ed 2, St Louis, 1995, Mosby.

Hay W, Groothuis J, Haywood A, Levin M: *Current pediatric diagnosis and treatment,* ed 13, Norwalk, CT, 1997, Appleton & Lange.

Headache disorders: abbreviated system of classification and diagnosis, Research Triangle Park, 1992, Glaxo Pharmaceuticals.

Hensinger R: Limp, *Pediatr Clin North Am* 33(6):1355, 1986.

Herr RD, Zun L, Matthews JJ: A directed approach to the dizzy patient, *Ann Emerg Med* 18(6):664, 1989.

Hickey MS, Kierman GJ, Weaver KE: Evaluation of abdominal pain, *Emerg Med Clin North Am* 7(3):437, 1989.

Hodges D: Hip pain in children: an anatomic approach, *Orthoped Rev* 17(3):251, 1988.

Hoekelman R et al: *Primary pediatric care,* ed 2, St Louis, 1996, Mosby.

Hollingworth P: Back pain in children, *Brit J Rheumatol* 35(10):1022, 1996.

Hoppenfeld S: *Physical examination of the spine and extremities,* Norwalk, CT, 1976, Appleton & Lange.

Horn JE: Urinary tract infections. In Stobo JD et al, editors: *The principles and practice of medicine,* ed 23, Stamford, CT, 1996, Appleton & Lange.

Hurst JW, editor: *Medicine for the practicing physician,* ed 4, Stamford, CT, 1996, Appleton & Lange.

Jones AK: Primary care management of acute low back pain, *Nurs Pract* 22(7):50, 1997.

Juckett G: Common intestinal helminths, *Am Fam Phys* 52(7):2039, 1995.

Kaden GG, Shenker IR, Boctman MN: Chest pain in adolescents, *J Adol Health* 12(3): 251, 1991.

Kaplan PE, Tanner ED: *Musculoskeletal pain and disability,* East Norwalk, CT, 1989, Appleton & Lange.

Kassirer JP, Kopelman RI: *Learning clinical reasoning,* Baltimore, 1991, Williams & Wilkins.

Katcher M: Cold, cough, and allergy medications: uses and abuses, *Pediatr Rev* 17(1): 12, 1996.

King KK, Cates W Jr, Lemon SM, Stamm WE, editors: *Sexually transmitted diseases,* ed 2, New York, 1990, McGraw-Hill.

Kiningham RB, Apgar BS, Schwenk TL: Evaluation of amenorrhea, *Am Fam Phys* 53(4): 1185, 1996.

Kiselica D: Group A beta-hemolytic streptococcal pharyngitis: current clinical concepts, *Am Fam Phys* 49(5):1147, 1994.

Kleiman M: Feverish children, frightened parents, *Contemp Pediatr* 6(3):161, 1989.

Kleinman A, Eisenberg L, Good B: Culture, illness, and care, *Ann Int Med* 88:251, 1978.

Kokx NP, Comstock JA, Facklam R: Streptococcal perianal disease in children, *Pediatrics* 80(5):659, 1987.

Kramer I, Kramer C: The otalgia masquerade: TMJ dysfunction, *Contemp Pediatr* 4(5):96, 1988.

Larsen R: Gastroesophageal reflux disease, *Postgrad Med* 101(2):181, 1997.

Leitman M: *Manual for eye examination and diagnosis,* ed 4, Boston, 1994, Blackwell Scientific.

Leung A, Robson W: Evaluating the child with chronic diarrhea, *Am Fam Phys* 53(2):635, 1996.

Lipsky M, Adelman, M: Chronic diarrhea: evaluation and treatment, *Am Fam Phys* 48(8):1461, 1993.

Lopez J, McMillin K, Tobias-Merrill E, Chop W: Managing fever in infants and toddlers, *Post Med* 101(2):241, 1997.

Lorin M: *The febrile child,* New York, 1982, John Wiley and Sons.

Lorin M: When fever has no localizing signs, *Contemp Pediatr* 6(2):14, 1989.

Losek JD: Diagnostic difficulties of foreign body aspiration in children, *Am J Emerg Med* 8(4):348, 1990.

Luckman J: *Saunders manual of nursing care,* Philadelphia, 1997, WB Saunders.

MacEwen GD, Dehne R: The limping child, *Pediatr Rev* 12(9):268, 1991.

Mandell GL, Rein MF, editors: *Sexually transmitted diseases,* Philadelphia, 1996, Current Medicine.

Mason J: The evaluation of acute abdominal pain in children, *Emerg Med Clin North Am* 14(3):629, 1996.

McCarthy J: Outpatient evaluation of hematuria, *Post Med* 101(2):125, 1997.

McCarthy P: *The evaluation and management of febrile children,* vol 1, no 1, Norwalk, 1985, Appleton-Century-Crofts.

McCarthy PL, Sharpe MR, Spiesel SZ et al: Observation scales to identify serious illness in febrile children, *Pediatrics* 70(5):802, 1982.

Mengel MB, Schwiebert LP: *Ambulatory medicine: the primary care of families,* ed 2, Stamford, CT, 1996, Appleton & Lange.

Micheli L, Wood R: Back pain in young athletes, *Arch Pediatr Adol Med* 149(1):15, 1995.

Middleton DB: An approach to pediatric upper respiratory infections, *Am Fam Phys* 44(5 suppl):33s, 1991.

Moffet H: *Pediatric infectious disease,* ed 3, Philadelphia, 1989, JB Lippincott.

Morrison M, Rammage L et al: *The management of voice disorders,* San Diego, 1994, Singular Publishing Groups.

Morse SA, Moreland AA, Holmes KK, editors: *Atlas of sexually transmitted diseases and AIDS,* ed 2, St Louis, 1996, Mosby-Wolfe.

Mosca V: Pitfalls in diagnosis: the hip, *Pediatr Ann* 18(1):12, 1989.

Moss AJ: Clues in diagnosing congenital heart disease, *West J Med* 156(4):392, 1992.

Murphy TP: Vestibular autorotation and electronystagmography in patients with dizziness, *Am J Otol* 4:502, 1994.

Myer C: The dizziness of children, *Emerg Med* 18(20):49, 1986.

Mygind M, Naclerio RM: *Allergic and nonallergic rhinitis: clinical aspects,* Philadelphia, 1993, WB Saunders.

Nakayama D, Rowe M: Inguinal hernia and the acute scrotum in infants and children, *Pediatr Rev* 11(3):87, 1989.

Neinstein LS: *Adolescent health care: a practical guide,* ed 3, Baltimore, 1996, Williams & Wilkins.

Newman K: Chronic cough: a step-by-step diagnostic workup, *Consultant,* p 535, October, 1995.

Newton DA: Sinusitis in children and adolescents, *Primary Care* 23(4):701, 1996.

Newton H: Common neurologic complications of HIV-1 infection and AIDS, *Am Fam Phys* 51(2):387, 1995.

Nizet V, Vinci R, Lovejoy F: Fever in children, *Pediatr Rev* 15(4):127, 1994.

Noble J: *Textbook of primary care medicine,* ed 2, St Louis, 1996, Mosby.

Norden C, Gillespie WJ, Nade S: *Infections in bones and joints,* Cambridge, MA, 1994, Blackwell Scientific.

Oberlander T, Rappaport L: Recurrent abdominal pain during childhood, *Pediatr Rev* 14(8):313, 1993.

Oski F, De Angelis C, Feign R, Warshaw J: *Principles and practice of pediatrics,* ed 2, Philadelphia, 1990, JB Lippincott.

Ott NL: Childhood sinusitis, *Mayo Clin Proc* 66(12):1238, 1991.

Paparella M, Alleva M, Bequer N: Dizziness, *Primary Care Dis Ears Nose Throat* 17(2):299, 1990.

Park Y: Evaluation of neck masses in children, *Am Fam Phys* 51(8):1904, 1995.

Parrott T: Cystitis and urethritis, *Pediatr Rev* 10(7):217, 1989.

Patter J, Burke W: When an elderly patient becomes depressed, *Fam Prac Recertif* (10):12, 1994.

Payne III WK, Ogilvie JW: Back pain in children and adolescents, *Pediatr Clin North Am* 43(4):899, 1996.

Pecina MM, Bojanic I: *Overuse injuries of the musculoskeletal system,* Boca Raton, 1993, CRC Press.

Peck D: Apophyseal injuries in the young athlete, *Am Fam Phys* 51(8):1891, 1995.

Perkins A: An approach to diagnosing the acute sore throat, *Am Fam Phys* 55(1):131, 1997.

Persaud D, Moss WJ, Munoz JL: Serious eye infections in children, *Pediatr Ann* 22(6):379, l993.

Pettel M: Chronic constipation, *Pediatr Ann* 16(10):796, 1987.

Pfenninger JL, Fowler GC: *Procedures for primary care physicians,* St Louis, 1994, Mosby.

Pichichero ME: Group A streptococcal tonsillopharyngitis: cost-effective diagnosis and treatment, *Ann Emerg Med* 25(3):390, 1995.

Presti JC, Stroller ML, Carroll PR: Urology. In Tierney LM, McPhee SJ, Papadakis MA, editors: *Current medical diagnosis and treatment,* ed 35, Stamford, CT, 1996, Appleton & Lange.

Pryor M: Noisy breathing in children, *Post Med* 101(2):103, 1997.

Putnam PE, Orenstein SR: Hoarseness in a child with gastroesophageal reflux, *Acta Pediatr* 81(8):635, 1992.

Quinn TC: Sexually transmitted diseases. In Stobo JD et al, editors: *The principles and practice of medicine,* ed 23, Stamford, CT, 1996, Appleton & Lange.

Rakel RE: *Essentials of family medicine,* Philadelphia, 1993, WB Saunders.

Rakel RE: *Saunders manual of medical practice,* Philadelphia, 1996, WB Saunders

Rakel RE: *Textbook of family practice,* ed 5, Philadelphia, 1995, WB Saunders.

Ransom SB, McNeeley SG: *Gynecology for the primary care provider,* Philadelphia, 1997, WB Saunders.

Reilly BM: *Practical strategies in outpatient medicine,* ed 2, Philadelphia, 1991, WB Saunders.

Resnick NM: Initial evaluation of the incontinent patient, *J Am Geriatr Soc* 38(3):311, 1990.

Rimell F et al: Characteristics of objects that cause choking in children, *JAMA* 274(22):1763, 1995.

Roth M: Advances in Alzheimer's disease, a review for the family physician, *J Fam Prac* 37(6):593, 1993.

Rubin RH, Voss C, Derksen DJ, Gateley A, Quenzer RW: *Medicine: a primary care approach,* Philadelphia, 1996, WB Saunders.

Ruckenstein M: A practical approach to dizziness, *Post Med* 97(30):70, 1995.

Rushton HG: Nocturnal enuresis: epidemiology, evaluation, and currently available treatment options, *J Pediatr* 114:691, 1989.

Ryan-Wenger NA, Lee JE: The clinical reasoning case study: a powerful teaching tool, *Nurs Pract* 22:66, 1997.

Sauvain KJ, Hughes RB: Back pain in children, *Orthoped Nurs* 13(6):25, 1994.

Schiffman M: Nonoperative management of blunt abdominal trauma in pediatrics, *Emerg Med Clin North Am* 7(3):519, 1989.

Schleupner CJ: Urinary tract infections: separating the genders and the ages, *Post Med* 101(6):231, 1997.

Scholer SJ, Pituch K, Orr DP, Dittus PS: Clinical outcomes of children with acute abdominal pain, *Pediatrics* 89(1):680, 1996.

Schwartz R: A practical approach to chronic otitis, *Patient Care* 21(12):91, 1987.

Seidel HM, Ball JW, Dains JE, Benedict GW: *Mosby's guide to physical examination,* ed 4, St Louis, 1998, Mosby.

Seidel JS et al: Presentation and evaluation of sexual misuse in the emergency department, *Pediatr Emerg Care* 2(3):157, 1986.

Selbst SM: Chest pain in children, *Pediatrics* 75(6):1068, 1985.

Seller RH: *Differential diagnosis of common complaints,* ed 3, Philadelphia, 1996, WB Saunders.

Settipane GA: *Rhinitis,* ed 2, Providence, RI, 1991, Oceanside Publishing.

Shilowitz M: Sudden sensorineural hearing loss, *Med Clin North Am Update Otolaryngol* 75(6):1239, 1991.

Shuttari M: Asthma: diagnosis and management, *Am Fam Phys* 52(8):2225, 1995.

Siu AL: screening for dementia and investigating its causes, *Ann Int Med* 115(92):122, 1991.

Smith J: Knee problems in children, *Pediatr Clin North Am* 33(6):1439, 1986.

Snider RK: *Essentials of musculoskeletal care,* Rosemont, IL, 1997, American Academy of Orthopedic Surgeons.

Sokic SJ, Adanja BJ, Marinkovic JP, Vlajinac HD: Risk factors for laryngeal cancer, *Euro J Epidemiol* 11(4):431, 1995.

Speroff L, Glass RH, Kase NG: *Clinical gynecologic endocrinology and infertility,* ed 3, Baltimore, 1983, Williams & Wilkins.

Spires R: Pediatric pseudotumor cerebri, *J Ophthalmol Nurs Tech* 13(4):169, 1994.

Sponseller R: Evaluating the child with back pain, *Am Fam Phys* 54(6):1933, 1996.

Stern R: Pathophysiologic basis for symptomatic treatment of fever, *Pediatrics* 59(1):92, 1977.

Stevenson R, Ziegler M: Abdominal pain unrelated to trauma, *Pediatr Rev* 14(8):302, 1993.

Stinson JT: Spondylodesis and spondylolisthesis in the athlete, *Clin Sports Med* 12(3):517, 1993.

Stool SE, Berg AO, Berman S et al: *Otitis media with effusion in young children,* Clinical Practice Guideline, Pub No 94-0622, Rockville, MD, 1994, Agency for Health Care Policy and Research, US Department of Health and Human Services, Public Health Service.

Tierney LW Jr, McPhee SJ, Papadakis MA: *Current medical diagnosis and treatment,* ed 3, Stamford, CT, 1996, Appleton & Lange.

Tietjen DN, Husmann DA: Nocturnal enuresis: a guide to evaluation and treatment, *Mayo Clin Proc* 71(9):857, 1996.

Treseler KM: *Clinical laboratory and diagnostic tests: significance and nursing implications,* ed 3, Norwalk, CT, 1995, Appleton & Lange.

Ullom-Minnich MR: Diagnosis and management of nocturnal enuresis, *Am Fam Phys* 54(7):2259, 1996.

Uphold CR, Graham MV: *Clinical guidelines in adult health,* Gainesville, 1994, Barmarrae Books.

Wagner R: The differential diagnosis of the red eye, *Contemp Pediatr* 8:26, 1991.

Wallach, J: *Interpretation of diagnostic tests,* ed 6, Boston, 1996, Little, Brown.

Weiner M: Alzheimer's disease: what we now know and what you can now do, *Consultant,* p 313, March, 1995.

Weiss AH: Chronic conjunctivitis in infants and children, *Pediatr Ann* 22(6):366, 1993.

Wiens S et al: Chest pain in otherwise healthy children and adolescents, *Pediatrics* 90(3):350, 1992.

Willett LR, Carson JL, Williams JW: Current diagnosis and management of sinusitis, *J Gen Int Med* 9:38, 1994.

Williams JW, Simel DL: Does this patient have sinusitis? Diagnosing acute sinusitis by history and physical examination, *JAMA* 270:1242, 1993.

Wilson D: Assessing and managing the febrile child, *Nurs Pract* 20(11):59, 1995.

Wisdon A: *Diagnosis in color: sexually transmitted diseases,* ed 2, London, 1996, Mosby-Wolfe.

Woll ER: Sinusitis in infants and children, *Ann Otol Rhinol Laryngol* 155(suppl 1):37, 1992.

Woods ER et al: Bacteremia in an ambulatory setting, *Am J Dis Child* 144(5):1195, 1990.

Worman SG, Ganiats T: Hirschprung's disease: a cause of chronic constipation in children, *Am Fam Phys* 51(2):487, 1995.

Wortmann D, Nelson A: Kawasaki syndrome, *Rheum Dis Clin North Am* 16(2):363, 1990.

Youngkin EQ, Davis MS: *Women's health: a primary care clinical guide,* Norwalk, CT, 1994, Appleton & Lange.

Zavaras-Angelidou KA, Weinhouse E, Nelson DB: Review of 180 episodes of chest pain in 134 children, *Pediatr Emerg Care* 8(4):189, 1992.

Index

Normal Hematology Values for Children

Age	Term babies	RBC count (10^6/mm³)	Hematocrit (packed RBC volume/dl) (%)	Mean corpuscular volume (MCV) (m³)	Mean corpuscular hemoglobin (MCH) (pg)	Mean corpuscular hemoglobin concentration (MCHC) (g/dl)
1 week	19.6	5.3	52.7	101	37	37
4 weeks	15.6	4.7	44.6	91	33	35
2 months	13.3	4.5	38.9	85	30	34
6 months	12.3	4.6	36.2	78	27	34
1 year	11.6	4.6	35.2	77	25	33
2 years	11.7	4.7	35.5	78	25	33
4 years	12.6	4.7	37.1	80	27	34
6 years	12.7	4.7	37.9	80	27	33
10-12 years	13.0	4.8	39.0	80	27	33

Modified from Lanzkowsky P et al, editors: *Primary pediatric care,* St. Louis, 1987, Mosby, p. 860.

Lumbar Cerebral Spinal Fluid (CSF) Reference Ranges

Albumin/globulin ratio   16.2-2.2
Albumin, quantitative   10-30 mg/dl
Calcium   4.2-5.4 mg/dl
Cell count   WBC/mm³

Modified from Stein JH, editor: *Internal medicine,* ed 5, 1998, Mosby.